D1570348

Handbook of Psychiatric Education and Faculty Development

Handbook of Psychiatric Education and Faculty Development

Edited by

Jerald Kay, M.D.
Edward K. Silberman, M.D.
Linda Pessar, M.D.

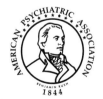

Published by the American Psychiatric Association
WASHINGTON, DC

Copyright © 1999 American Psychiatric Association
ALL RIGHTS RESERVED
Manufactured in the United States of America on acid-free paper
02 01 00 99   4 3 2 1
First Edition

American Psychiatric Press, Inc.
1400 K Street, N.W., Washington, DC 20005
www.appi.org

Library of Congress Cataloging-in-Publication Data
Handbook of psychiatric education and faculty development / edited by
   Jerald Kay, Edward K. Silberman, Linda Pessar. — 1st ed.
        p.   cm.
     Includes bibliographical references and index.
     ISBN 0-88048-780-1
     1. Psychiatry—Study and teaching—Handbooks, manuals, etc.
   2. Medical colleges—Faculty—Handbooks, manuals, etc.   3. Mental
   health personnel—Training of—Handbooks, manuals, etc.   I. Kay,
   Jerald.   II. Silberman, Edward K., 1944– .   III. Pessar, Linda,
   1944– .
     [DNLM: 1. Psychiatry—education.   2. Faculty, Medical.   WM 18
   H2363   1999]
   RC459.H357   1999
   616.89'0071'1—dc21
   DNLM/DLC
   for Library of Congress   98-32453
                                                                          CIP

British Library Cataloguing in Publication Data
A CIP record is available from the British Library.

Contents

Section III. Psychiatric Education

Section IV. Psychiatric Administration

Contributors

Linda Andrews, M.D.
Director of Residency Education, Department of Psychiatry and Behavioral Science; Assistant Dean of Student Affairs, Baylor College of Medicine, Houston, Texas

George W. Arana, M.D.
Professor and Associate Dean for Graduate Medical Education, Medical University of South Carolina; and Chief of Psychiatry, VA Medical Center, Charleston, South Carolina

James C. Ballenger, M.D.
Professor and Chairman, Department of Psychiatry and Behavioral Sciences, Medical University of South Carolina, Charleston, South Carolina

Gwyn Barley, Ph.D.
Assistant Professor; Course Director, Primary Care, The University of Colorado School of Medicine, Denver, Colorado

Nancy L. Bennett, Ph.D.
Director of Educational Development and Evaluation, Department of Continuing Education, Harvard Medical School, Boston, Massachusetts

Carol A. Bernstein, M.D.
Director of Residency Training in Psychiatry and Associate Professor of Clinical Psychiatry, New York University Medical Center, New York, New York

David Bienenfeld, M.D.
Professor, Vice Chair, and Director of Residency Training, Wright State University, Dayton, Ohio

Soo Borson, M.D.
Associate Professor, Department of Psychiatry and Behavioral Sciences, University of Washington, Seattle, Washington

Jonathan F. Borus, M.D.
Professor of Psychiatry, Harvard Medical School; Psychiatrist in Chief, Brigham and Women's Hospital; and Former Editor, *Academic Psychiatry*

Amy C. Brodkey, M.D.
Clinical Associate Professor of Psychiatry, University of Pennsylvania School of Medicine; Attending Psychiatrist, Friends Hospital, Philadelphia, Pennsylvania

Vivien K. Burt, M.D., Ph.D.
Associate Professor of Clinical Psychiatry, UCLA School of Medicine, UCLA Neuropsychiatric Institute and Department of Psychiatry, West Los Angeles VA Medical Center, Los Angeles, California

Mantosh Dewan, M.D.
Professor and Interim Chair, Department of Psychiatry, SUNY Health Science Center at Syracuse, Syracuse, New York

Dorcas Dobie, M.D.
Assistant Professor, Department of Psychiatry and Behavioral Sciences, University of Washington, Seattle, Washington

Larry R. Faulkner, M.D.
Vice President for Medical Affairs and Dean of the School of Medicine, University of South Carolina, Columbia, South Carolina

Theodore B. Feldmann, M.D.
Director of Medical Student Education in Psychiatry, Department of Psychiatry and Behavioral Sciences, University of Louisville School of Medicine, Louisville, Kentucky

Paul E. Garfinkel, M.D.
Professor and Chair, Department of Psychiatry, University of Toronto and President and CEO, Centre for Addiction and Mental Health, Toronto, Ontario, Canada

Carl Greiner, M.D.
Vice Chair for Education, Department of Psychiatry, Creighton/Nebraska University Medical Center, Omaha, Nebraska

John B. Herman, M.D.
Director of Continuing Medical Education and Adult Psychiatry Residency, Department of Psychiatry, Massachusetts General Hospital, Boston, Massachusetts

Allan S. Kaplan, M.Sc., M.D., F.R.C.P.C.
Head, Program for Eating Disorders, The Toronto Hospital, Director, Postgraduate Education, Associate Professor of Psychiatry, University of Toronto Faculty of Medicine, Toronto, Ontario, Canada

Jerald Kay, M.D.
Professor and Chair, Department of Psychiatry, Wright State University School of Medicine, Dayton, Ohio

Steven Kick, M.D.
Assistant Professor, Department of Medicine, The University of Colorado School of Medicine, Denver, Colorado

William M. Klykylo, M.D.
Associate Professor and Director, Division of Child and Adolescent Psychiatry, Department of Psychiatry, Wright State University School of Medicine, Dayton, Ohio

Kewchang Lee, M.D.
Clinical Instructor of Psychiatry, University of California, San Francisco

Ellen Leibenluft, M.D.
Chief, Unit on Rapid Cycling Bipolar Disorder, Clinical Psychobiology Branch, National Institute of Mental Health, Bethesda, Maryland; and Clinical Associate Professor of Psychiatry, Georgetown University School of Medicine, Washington, D.C.

James W. Lomax, M.D.
Associate Chairman and Director of Educational Programs, Baylor College of Medicine, Houston, Texas

Francis G. Lu, M.D.
Clinical Professor of Psychiatry, Co-Director, Cultural Competence and Diversity Program, University of California, San Francisco

Myrl R. S. Manley, M.D.
Director of Medical Student Education in Psychiatry and Associate Professor of Clinical Psychiatry, New York University Medical Center, New York, New York

Emily Borus McCort, M.D.
Assistant Clinical Professor, Department of Psychiatry, The University of Colorado School of Medicine, Denver, Colorado

Paul C. Mohl, M.D.
Professor and Residency Training Director, Department of Psychiatry, University of Texas Southwestern Medical Center at Dallas, Dallas, Texas

Nancy Morrison, M.D.
Assistant Professor of Psychiatry and Director of Residency Training, University of New Mexico School of Medicine, Albuquerque, New Mexico

Carol C. Nadelson, M.D.
Professor of Psychiatry, Cambridge Hospital, Cambridge, Massachusetts

Michele T. Pato, M.D.
Associate Professor, Department of Psychiatry, State University of New York at Buffalo and Buffalo General Hospital, Community Mental Health Center, Buffalo, New York

Harold Alan Pincus, M.D.
Deputy Medical Director, Office of Research, American Psychiatric Association, Washington, D.C.

Sudha Prathikanti, M.D.
Clinical Instructor of Psychiatry, University of California, San Francisco

Nyapati R. Rao, M.D.
Director of Psychiatry for Education and General Residency Training, Clinical Associate Professor of Psychiatry, State University of New York Health Science at Brooklyn, Brooklyn, New York

Donald R. Ross, M.D.
Director, Division of Education and Residency Training, Sheppard Pratt Health System; and Clinical Associate Professor of Psychiatry, University of Maryland School of Medicine, Baltimore, Maryland

Alberto B. Santos, M.D.
Professor and Director of Residency Training, Department of Psychiatry and Behavioral Sciences, Medical University of South Carolina, Charleston, South Carolina

Stephen C. Scheiber, M.D.
Executive Vice President, American Board of Psychiatry and Neurology, Inc., Deerfield, Illinois; Adjunct Professor, Department of Psychiatry, Northwestern University Medical School, Chicago, Illinois; Adjunct Professor, Department of Psychiatry, Medical College of Wisconsin, Milwaukee, Wisconsin; and Senior Attending Physician, Evanston Hospital, Evanston, Illinois

Steven S. Sharfstein, M.D.
Clinical Professor of Psychiatry, University of Maryland; and President, Medical Director, and Chief Executive Officer, Sheppard Pratt Health System, Baltimore, Maryland

Frederick S. Sierles, M.D.
Professor and Chairman, Department of Psychiatry, Finch University of Health Sciences/The Chicago Medical School, North Chicago, Illinois

Edward K. Silberman, M.D.
Clinical Professor of Psychiatry and Director of Residency Education, Jefferson Medical College, Philadelphia, Pennsylvania

Deborah A. Snyderman, M.D.
Instructor in Psychiatry and Human Behavior, Jefferson Medical College, Philadelphia, Pennsylvania

John J. Spollen, M.D.
Resident in Psychiatry, Medical University of South Carolina, Charleston, South Carolina; and American Psychiatric Association/Mead Johnson Fellow in Public Psychiatry

Stefan Stein, M.D.
Professor of Clinical Psychiatry, Cornell University Medical College; and Director of Residency Education, New York Hospital–Cornell Medical Center, Payne Whitney Clinic, New York, New York

Terri Tanielian, M.A.
Research Manager, American Psychiatric Association, Washington, D.C.

Bryce Templeton, M.D., M.Ed.
Professor of Psychiatry, Chief of Psychiatric Education, Eastern Pennsylvania Psychiatric Institute, Philadelphia, Pennsylvania

Troy L. Thompson II, M.D.
Professor, Department of Psychiatry and Human Behavior, Jefferson Medical College, Philadelphia, Pennsylvania

David Trachtenberg, M.D.
Clinical Teaching Assistant, New York University Medical Center, New York, New York

Gary J. Tucker, M.D.
Professor and Chairman, Department of Psychiatry and Behavioral Sciences, University of Washington, Seattle, Washington

Natalie Walders, M.A.
Graduate Student, Clinical Psychology, Case Western University, Cleveland, Ohio

Michael Weissberg, M.D.
Department of Psychiatry, The University of Colorado School of Medicine, Denver, Colorado

Sidney H. Weissman, M.D.
Professor of Psychiatry, Loyola Medical Center, Maywood, Illinois

Joel Yager, M.D.
Professor of Psychiatry and Vice Chair for Education, University of New Mexico School of Medicine, Albuquerque, New Mexico

Introduction

These are challenging times for academic psychiatrists. Pressures to contain costs have begun to halt, or even reverse, the general expansion of medical school psychiatry departments under way since World War II. Over the next decade departments can expect decreasing clinical revenues from third-party payors, traditionally the major source of faculty salaries, decreasing federal government contributions to graduate medical education, and decreasing proportions of federal research grant applications approved for funding. Thus, support for the core academic activities of teaching, research, and scholarship is less secure than at any time in the careers of currently practicing psychiatrists.

Present economic pressures, and possibly the societal values underlying them, are affecting academic health centers and their teaching programs in a variety of ways. Under pressure from managed care companies, whose mission is to contain costs and/or enhance profits and not to support academic activities, both paid and volunteer faculty are devoting more time to generating clinical revenues and less to teaching medical students and residents. Second, medical schools have fewer resources to dedicate to new educational programs, and in some cases, even to the continuing support of medical student teaching programs. Third, residency programs are being advised to recruit smaller training classes, with the potential effect of requiring faculty to spend yet more time providing clinical services, and less in teaching, research, and scholarship. Fourth, the essential role of the psychiatrist is being reconsidered, and with it, estimates of the number of psychiatrists needed in the coming decades. Psychiatry is being viewed increasingly as a supporting service for primary care medicine, bringing new emphasis on accessibility of psychiatric concepts in medical student education and collaboration with primary care physicians in residency training. Fifth, the explosion in psychiatric knowledge has challenged educators continually to update and integrate new knowledge into curricula and also has contributed to tensions within some programs regarding what to include and what to delete. Sixth, with more researchers competing for a limited pool of extramural research funding, faculty have needed to develop new strategies for pursuing scholarship. Seventh, as faculty are more pressed to produce clinical revenues and have increasing difficulty obtaining research grants, academic promotion by traditional criteria becomes increasingly problematic. Medical schools have been required to diversify criteria for promotion to reflect the realities of academic life, and psychiatry departments have had to find ways to facilitate progress of faculty along the new lines of professional development.

This volume provides a comprehensive guide to psychiatric education and scholarship in the context of current dilemmas and challenges. The *Handbook of Psychiatry Residency Training,* which appeared in 1991, was directed exclusively to directors or associate directors of residency training programs. The new *Handbook* aims to reach a wider audience including faculty involved with undergraduate, graduate, and continuing medical education, as well as those with interests in research and administration. In this spirit, the new *Handbook* is edited by a chair, a residency training director, and a medical student education director.

The *Handbook of Psychiatric Education and Faculty Development* represents the collective wisdom of outstanding psychiatric educators, researchers, and administrators addressing the themes of program administration and career development. We have included appendices in many chapters aimed at providing specific, up-to-date information on topics ranging from honorary resident fellowships to sources of research funding. It is our hope that this guide will be a resource for those newly entering academic careers, a source of information (and, we hope, inspiration) for residents contemplating such a career, and a useful reference volume for more experienced faculty. We welcome comments from our colleagues about the usefulness of these chapters, as well as their ideas about what might be included in future editions of the *Handbook.*

Jerald Kay, M.D.
Edward K. Silberman, M.D.
Linda Pessar, M.D.

Career Pathways in Academic Psychiatry

1

The Development of Academic Psychiatrists

**Joel Yager, M.D., Nancy Morrison, M.D.,
and Vivien K. Burt, M.D., Ph.D.**

Many psychiatrists aspire to academic careers, but considerable variation exists in exactly what an academic career signifies. According to some surveys, about a third of medical students entering psychiatry indicate interest in academic careers, about 15% wish to take research fellowships, and about an additional 25% are interested but still undecided about such fellowships (Association of American Medical Colleges 1986; Bashook and Weissman 1987; Haviland et al. 1987; Yager et al. 1990). Most students want careers that mix teaching, patient care, clinical or applied research, and administration in academic medical centers; only 1% to 2% envision careers that focus on basic research. At the "output" end, for residents graduating in 1986 to 1988, program directors reported that 9.7% of graduating residents took a half-time or greater academic position as an initial postresidency job (El-Mallakh and Riba 1990).

As with most choices, whether or not an individual prefers an academic career depends in part on the person's other options. With massive, largely unwelcome changes rapidly occurring in private practice, academic careers may look better than ever to young graduates. Nevertheless, since academic lives are also changing rapidly, new faculty are well advised to have realistic expectations as to what awaits. Academic medicine's future is far more uncertain now than in the past (Alpert and Coles 1988; Freedman 1991; Romano 1991).

Because few people entering academic careers know much about the different career options available, the requirements for each one, and the rules for successful career building, this chapter puts these options into perspective. We consider the early professional life cycles of academic psychiatrists, factors determining success, the impact of academic careers upon personal life, the financing of academic positions, considerations regarding entering one's first position, and strategies that promote junior faculty development. We conclude with the observation that the most critical element for fashioning a successful academic career, in addition to luck and determination, is considerable self-awareness regarding personal needs, values, motives, and capacities. After all, one's assessment of success depends not only on achievement but also on what one really wants.

Interests, Personality, and Cognitive Style in Relation to Academic Career Path

Individual aptitudes, motivations, competing needs, and current opportunities all contribute to the evolution of careers. For the beginning academic, "know thyself" is an excellent place to begin. To start, those contemplating academic careers should identify which aspects of academic life they find most attractive, what personal needs would be served by such a career (and at what cost), and how their professional and personal life are to be balanced. If one adds the increasingly demanding leg of academic administration to the classic "three-legged stool" on which academics perch (service, teaching, and research) (Freedman 1991), and allows time and space for family and other personal interests, the result is a very complex piece of furniture on which to balance. Attaining academic tenure, a rapidly disappearing element of academic life anyway, may not be all it's imagined to be, and getting there may be too much of an ordeal relative to an individual's other needs.

We find in our experience that each academic path favors certain types of people. Some personality-related "demand characteristics" of prototypical paths, admittedly overdrawn and stereotyped, are shown in Table 1–1. These qualities reside along a continuum. Primary researchers veer toward the left column, and individuals favoring the roles of teaching/clinician/administration tend to move toward the right.

Another way to decide on the most appropriate academic career path is via the following, somewhat whimsical, academic motivation self-assessment test (to be answered with a minimum of self-deception). Con-

Table 1–1. Personality and task-related demand characteristics for academic pathways

Professor/Research series	Professor/Clinician educator
Inner directed	Outer directed
Quantitative	Qualitative
Idea oriented	Person oriented
Competitive (with self or others)	Group oriented
Goal oriented	Process oriented
Single-minded	Multitrack
Driven by academic reward systems	Driven by other rewards
Enjoy research > teaching	Enjoy teaching > research
Original research	Original or applied research
Laboratory research	Clinical research
Analytic research	Descriptive research
Analytic scholarship	Synthetic scholarship
Research team leader	Research collaborator
Long hours	Long hours
Self-sacrificing	Self-sacrificing
Persistent	Persistent

sider the extent to which you are drawn to an academic life by answering the following questions:

1. Do you truly aspire to gain new scientific knowledge and enjoy *doing* research; that is, are you willing to spend tedious hours writing elaborate grant proposals that have about a 10% to 20% chance of getting funded, gathering detailed data, meticulously going over results, arduously writing up results for publication, and subjecting yourself to the critical review of hawklike peers whose job it is to nitpick and find fault with what you've produced? Furthermore, can you accept that much of the work you publish is unlikely to ever be cited by anyone else (Hamilton 1990)? Will presenting your findings at national meetings, seeing your results accepted into the corpus of scientific knowledge, and obtaining a modicum of renown for your accomplishments provide you with adequate satisfaction for your efforts?

2. Are you drawn to the apparent collegiality of the academic life, and although you don't fancy yourself as a genius researcher in your own right, will you be gratified to contribute in some small way to ongoing research efforts?

3. Do you crave the excitement of juggling multiple activities: clinical work, administration, research, and teaching?

4. Do you hope that an academic life will protect you to some degree from potentially contaminating motivations that might afflict you in a fee-for-service private practice setting?

5. Are you drawn to the idea of being in a "stimulating" environment where your colleagues and students keep up with the latest developments, and you can feel that you're up-to-date on new developments in research, teaching, and clinical care?

6. Do you enjoy creative speculation and original ideas? Even though you don't have the patience to test the validity of your ideas in formal research projects, would you like to have a serious audience for your ideas?

7. Does your motivation for an academic career derive largely from the high status accorded to "Professors" in your family, a status that may even be higher than that accorded to physicians? That is, do you see entering an academic life as one way to compensate and reduce your need to apologize for having selected psychiatry instead of another field of medicine, believing that, for psychiatry, "academics" is not having to say you're sorry?

Responses to such questions will permit those aspiring to academic careers to assess how their particular interests and aptitudes correspond to various academic paths. Affirmative responses to question 1 suggest tendencies toward the research scientist, professorial, traditional "triple-threat" track. Affirmative responses to questions 2 through 6 suggest tendencies toward the compensated and voluntary clinical faculty. Affirmative responses to question 7 suggest the need for some sort of academic role, regardless of series.

The Evolution of Contemporary Academia

The large academic medical complex as we know it today evolved primarily over the past 50 years, starting with the massive infusion of federal money into medical centers via the National Institutes of Health (NIH) and the National Institute of Mental Health (NIMH) (Freedman 1991). During that time, university medical schools, expanding their clinical bases for medical students and house staff, became affiliated with a wide variety of county, city, Veterans Administration (VA), state, nonprofit community and private hospitals. Thus, many departments grew extremely large and bestowed a wide variety of academic and semiacademic titles upon their many affiliated physicians, so that psychiatry departments with up to hundreds of academic, paid clinical, and voluntary appointments became commonplace (Freedman 1991; Romano 1991).

However, over the past 25 years, resources have been shrinking. The NIMH clinical training grants for psychiatric education, once a major source of financial support, are now virtually nonexistent (Freedman 1976). For years the amount of federal money available to fund actual psychiatric research has also not kept constant with inflation (Freedman 1985; Pardes and Pincus 1983), and the odds that an approved grant proposal will actually be funded have fallen to roughly 1 in 10. Furthermore, recent policy decisions at the NIMH favoring basic research over clinical research means that support for the clinical research conducted by many psychiatry departments has been further compromised. As a result, academic psychiatrists have been forced to generate more of their salaries through clinical activities.

Concurrently, cuts in Medicare and Medicaid and reduced reimbursement for physicians by managed care systems also threaten the clinical revenues upon which academic departments rely. Faculty now increasingly work in environments dominated by managed care, leading to increased clinical work, less compensation, and, looming on the horizon, fewer psychiatric residents. The very existence of many academic centers is threatened. Within this setting, today's academic lives are fashioned.

Academic Path Options

Medical schools currently use a confusing array of university academic titles and series: examples include professor, professor of clinical psychiatry, clinical professor of psychiatry, compensated clinical professor, adjunct professor, professor-in-residence, and research professor, among others. There are no universal conventions as to what these terms signify, and universities are currently experimenting with ways to condense the number of titles. For example, at many schools, individuals promoted to associate or full professor may use those titles without additional modifying terms—regardless of tenure, clinician versus researcher status, or salary source. This shift reflects a growing awareness that researchers, clinicians, administrators, and teachers are all valued in the work of the contemporary medical school.

Differences among the various academic titles are meaningful only to academic insiders. Although at some universities real differences exist among the series with regard to eligibility as principal investigator on a research grant, academic senate membership, and eligibility for usually poorly paid sabbatical leave, many of the differences are purely symbolic. Academic series usually differ with respect to the types of activities expected of the faculty member, the predominant value systems, and funding. The professor of psychiatry/research series refers to those full-time faculty appointments that at the assistant professor level are associated with the notion of "publish or perish." Review for promotion is based on original scientific or scholarly contributions, publications, and grants, but teaching and clinical and/or administrative service are also considered: hence, the notion of the "quadruple threat" faculty member. Requirements for academic review from assistant to associate professor resulting in "up or out" after seven years are usually reserved for this series. At least part of the salary is usually paid by the university once tenure is awarded. Characteristics of some common types of appointments are outlined in Table 1–2. These arrangements, typical for the University of California and some others, may vary considerably elsewhere.

Departments differ considerably with regard to the attitudes and atmosphere that exist among faculty about these various series. Inequities regarding how faculty in the different series perceive they are to be dealt with may generate feelings of envy, shame, competition, superiority, inferiority, haughtiness, and resentment. Depending on local circumstances, members of some academic series may feel that the grass is always greener in the other series. In departments where such splits in value truly occur, two or three class systems may arise. The manner, values, and quality of department leadership determine how well faculty members feel esteemed for what they contribute to the department's overall missions.

Funding Sources

Academic salaries are funded through a variety of sources. These commonly include: academic full-time equivalent (FTE) positions funded directly by the university; academic funding from the university to be used flexibly by departments without formal allocation of official FTE positions; hospital or medical center funds and positions (from university, private,

Table 1–2. Characteristics of academic series

Professor of psychiatry, research series	Professor clinician-teacher academic series	Professor part-time or volunteer
Full-time vs. part-time		
▪ Usually full-time. —Strict full-time (all income in department's practice plan). —Geographic (i.e., permitted an outside private practice).	▪ Usually full-time. —Strict full-time (all income in department's practice plan). —Geographic (i.e., permitted an outside private practice).	▪ Most part-time. —May have full-time appointments in university-affiliated hospitals. ▪ Voluntary appointments may be a few hours per week, or specified number of hours per month or year.
Salary sources		
▪ Usually includes university "base" or part of base or supplement. ▪ May be entirely from nonuniversity sources such as hospitals.	▪ Sometimes includes university "base" or part of base or supplement. ▪ Often entirely from nonuniversity sources such as hospitals.	▪ Usually hospital staff or practice income. ▪ Volunteer faculty derive no income per se from the university.

(continued)

Table 1–2. Continued

Professor of psychiatry, research series	Professor clinician-teacher academic series	Professor part-time or volunteer
Promotion		
■ Based on research/scholarly productivity, grants >> teaching. ■ Promotion to Associate Professor may require 15–50 peer-reviewed publications, most as first author. —In research medical schools, case reports, reviews, chapters, textbooks, and drug company protocols generally count little.	■ Often based primarily on outstanding teaching and administration, and to some extent on research/scholarly productivity and grants. —Some use this series for clinical investigators rather than laboratory investigators.	■ Based on —Documented outstanding teaching. —Local, regional, national recognition for leadership. —Contributions to university, professional community. —Excellence in practice. —Scholarship.
Tenure		
■ May be tenured. —Many universities have nontenured series as well. —Tenure may be linked to salary source (e.g., VA position).	■ May be tenured. —Tenure may be linked to salary source (e.g. coterminus with VA, state hospital position). ■ Many universities have nontenured series as well. ■ Some universities use "term appointments" (e.g., 5 years). ■ Some universities limit the percentage of positions assigned in this series.	■ None ■ Appointment usually contingent on ongoing contributions. —May be on an annual basis. —Many departments review voluntary appointments less frequently.

10

Teaching expectations

■ Usually several hours per week. —Often in laboratories (with fellows, postdocs) and clinical settings as much as courses or seminars.	■ Strong expectations for outstanding teaching and teaching administration. ■ Promotion often requires innovative teaching, local, regional, and national recognition as an outstanding teacher, major contributions to teaching administration (e.g., running a training program, acquiring training grants).	■ Strong. Usually specified re hours per week, month, or year. ■ Some appointments related to hospital staff, university, or community service activities rather than to teaching per se.

Clinical practice expectations

■ May be none. Depends on salary.	■ Depends on salary sources.	■ High expectations for excellence as clinical practitioner.

Administrative expectations

■ Ordinarily requires participation in academic departmental committees. —Hospital committee obligations depend on other salary sources.	■ Depends on salary sources. —Often large administrative responsibility for educational and training programs.	■ Depends on salary source. ■ Some departments permit contributions of administrative time in lieu of direct teaching or clinical work to satisfy requirements.

(continued)

11

Table 1–2. Continued

Professor of psychiatry, research series	Professor clinician-teacher academic series	Professor part-time or volunteer
	Research/scholarly expectations	
▪ Strong research and scholarly expectations. —Creation of new knowledge (original rather than derivative). —Increasingly reserved for quantitative laboratory sciences, especially in the 25 or so "research medical schools." —Conceptual originality counts as much as data production. —Work judged primarily by peer-reviewed grants and quality and quantity of peer-reviewed publications.	▪ Often considerable, although usually not necessarily in quantitative laboratory research. —Clinical research is acceptable. —Producing original teaching material (reviews, textbooks) matters.	▪ Ordinarily few. ▪ Reviews, chapters, textbooks, case reports help with promotion. ▪ Presentations at national, regional conferences encouraged.

12

community, VA, state, county, or city sources); grants and contracts (federal, state, foundation, private donors, industry); and, increasingly, clinical practice (often funneled through a university physicians' group practice plan). Most universities give very little money to their medical school departments. Consequently, the large majority of psychiatric faculty are funded by medical facilities, and salaries are often linked to specific patient care, administration, and teaching assignments. Paradoxically, junior faculty whose salaries are paid by *non*university sources are often at less risk of losing their jobs due to inadequate research productivity and/or grant writing than their university-funded colleagues, because they can often transfer to clinical jobs at their home institutions if necessary. Junior faculty hired into full-time federal, state, or county-based university-affiliated positions often become "tenured" into these civil service positions after only 6 months to 2 years of probationary employment.

Tenure

The meaning of "academic tenure" varies widely among universities, and rules concerning tenure are changing rapidly. A 1989 survey of U.S. medical schools revealed that among responding schools, 78% were actively changing and redefining requirements for tenure track promotion, 65% were changing criteria for nontenure track promotions, and 50% were developing nontenured tracks in 50% (Bickel 1991). According to this survey the use of tenure in medical schools is decreasing: Full-time faculty with tenure dropped from 41% in 1985 to 38% in 1989 (Higgins 1986; Whiting et al. 1990). Five schools awarded tenure to basic sciences faculty only, and seven had no tenure system. Many schools were freezing or severely limiting tenure awards compared with previous years (Bickel 1991).

The percentage of academic psychiatrists who actually get university tenure anywhere is small. Enormous differences exist with regard to what tenure means and what salary guarantees it brings. According to the 1989 survey, in 12% of schools tenure guaranteed "total salary," and in 42% tenure guaranteed "continued appointment at designated rank without salary guarantee" (Bickel 1991). In other schools, tenure generally means that some portion of salary is guaranteed, usually a specified university contribution, but not including practice plan, grants, or other contributions. Many school bylaws are silent on the matter of guarantees.

How tenure is awarded varies from university to university. In most instances, full-time faculty in the "regular" or "ladder" series (professor of psychiatry series) who meet the university's expectations for original research and/or original scholarship and/or grant productivity are awarded tenure at the time of promotion from assistant professor to associate professor. However, some universities grant tenure only upon promotion from associate professor to full professor, and in other universities the decision to award tenure is made entirely independent of decisions regarding promotion.

Problems with the current tenure system are considerable. First, the abolition of mandatory retirement for tenured faculty (American Association of University Professors Committee on Retirement 1990) may further plug the tenure system, requiring some process to clear a path for younger faculty on the way up. Second, physicians entering academic careers are usually faced with having to prove themselves as "quadruple threats" (as researchers, teachers, clinicians, and administrators), whereas nonphysician academics are usually required only to produce research or scholarly work and teach. Finally, most medical school–affiliated positions do not equate security of employment with academic tenure. Even full professors whose salaries depend entirely on grant-derived funds may become unemployed if their grants aren't funded.

Factors Fostering Academic Careers

The following environmental factors are prominent in stimulating and shaping academic careers:

1. Academic psychiatrists are well served by taking postresidency fellowships. In selecting a fellowship, trainees should make sure that they will gain experience in the research, teaching, and administrative as well as clinical methods that will be a focus for later work. It is also important that fellowships provide skilled mentors who truly desire to help trainees develop their independence, for example, by guiding them to write independent grants, conduct independent research, write and publish first-authored as well as coauthored articles and chapters, and undertake independent but supervised teaching and/or administrative responsibilities.
2. In negotiating for a first academic job, junior faculty should discuss specific resources available to help develop academic careers: What will the entry-level position require with regard to direct clinical work, teach

ing, administration, and research? How much time and energy is the assigned job likely to take? What are the arrangements for office and other necessary space? Does the position come with a personal computer with time on the system, secretarial support, protected time for academic work, seed money for research, access to students, consultants for design and data analysis, travel funds and time to go to professional meetings, and faculty mentors?

3. During early faculty years, individuals should be open to discovering their own academic and clinical affinities, facilitated by frequent feedback from mentors, collaborators, division chiefs, and department chairs on individuals' research, teaching, clinical work, and administration. This is when the faculty member's aptitudes will emerge as a serious researcher, dedicated clinician-teacher, and/or skillful administrator.

4. All along, young faculty must factor in shifting and competing demands from other aspects of their lives. What are an individual's priorities and trade-offs with respect to time and energy to be devoted to family, income, and other pursuits? What mechanisms exist to encourage the career development of women who will likely begin families, or who have young families?

5. Mentors: Good mentoring is often cited as the single most important factor in fostering successful academic careers. The availability and selection of mentors are crucial aspects of academic career development, during residency, fellowship, or early faculty positions. The mentor-mentee relationship is part good luck, part interpersonal chemistry, and part thoughtful selection. Good mentors have concrete outcomes: national or local reputations as mentors, and the careers and independent assessments of those whom they've mentored.

Choosing a mentor simply on the basis of scientific, administrative, or clinical renown may prove to be a mistake if that person turns out to be self-absorbed, have little time or interest in really caring for trainees, have an obnoxious personality, or simply not be a good fit with a particular trainee for any other reason. At the same time, some mentors who are reputed to be tough to work with may, nevertheless, bring out the best in trainees by stimulating creative thinking and hard work through their demands and challenges. Those assessing mentors should strive to speak directly with all current and recent mentees to help with this assessment.

Having a variety of mentors is also useful. Some may narrowly focus on specific types of research techniques or areas of academic involvement, whereas others may serve in broader spheres—providing insightful, wise perspectives about career strategies in relation to the mentee's specific goals and interests; providing resources, networking, and direction; and often helping with "whole life planning," assisting the mentee to think about deeper values and needs in the integration of professional and personal concerns at critical choice points.

Early Academic Career Life Cycles

Most departments provide a variety of initial positions for entry-level faculty. Four common entry positions and typical associated early career paths are outlined in Table 1–3.

Laboratory scientist entry-level appointments in research-oriented departments are usually based on prior research fellowships, increasingly M.D. and Ph.D. training, and demonstrated research productivity. Sometimes entry-level research grants such as the NIMH's "First Award," a career development award, or National Alliance for Research on Schizophrenia and Depression (NARSAD) awards for young investigators have been applied for or obtained.

For **clinical service-based positions,** for example, inpatient ward/emergency room/outpatient/consultation-liaison psychiatrists, prior research or subspecialty fellowships are increasingly helpful, but less necessary. In the case of consultation psychiatry, double residency training in internal medicine or family medicine is increasingly attractive. Those starting out in service-based positions usually begin their research or scholarly work by identifying a specific clinical question followed by conducting intensive case studies and/or case series to develop pilot data, developing fruitful research collaborations, conducting pharmaceutical company supported studies to gain familiarity with measurement techniques and for discretionary research funds, writing grants, mastering necessary research techniques (which may require protected time or special leave to learn), and freeing up clinical time to do research. Running services that provide patients with a particular clinical problem may be especially helpful for clinical researchers; conversely, it's often best to focus research on the patients at hand.

Although innovative and grant-funded clinical research may result in promotion in tenure track series, most faculty in these positions are pro

Table 1–3. Common entry-level academic positions and their usual course

---

Laboratory scientist

■ Entry-level appointment based on prior research background.
—May already have entry-level grant.
■ Seed money often provided for 1–3 years, pending grants.
■ Lack of demonstrated grant-getting and/or research productivity within 3–5 years generally leads to shift in series or departure.

Clinical service-based position (e.g., inpatient ward/emergency room/ outpatient/consultation-liaison psychiatrist)

■ *Emerging researcher:* Identifies interest; Learns/knows necessary research technique; Writes/gets grant; Frees up clinical time.
—Without substantial research, usually promoted in clinician-teacher or clinician-administrator/professor of clinical psychiatry series. (Hint: running clinical services that provide sources of patients with particular problems usually facilitates research.)
■ *Emerging teacher/administrator:* Enjoys and develops career based on teaching and/or clinical work and/or administration more than research → May or may not remain with university full-time.
—Usually promoted in clinician-teacher/clinician-administrator or professor of clinical psychiatry or clinical professor series.

Training director (or assistant/associate training director)

■ Often attached to another service as well.
—Most work time in service, teaching, and administration.
■ May develop independent laboratory/clinical research program if previously trained in research.
■ Commonly promoted in clinician-teacher or professor of clinical psychiatry series.

Paid part-time clinician/instructor/lecturer

■ Rare for pure teaching activities due to funding cutbacks.
■ Most remain part-time positions, tied to specific departmental courses or clinical tasks.
■ Usually untenured, sometimes of relatively short duration.
■ Appointments usually in "clinical professor" series.

---

moted in the clinician-teacher series. Most clinician-teachers focus on teaching, clinical work, and administration rather than research and are promoted in this series.

Educator-administrators (e.g., training directors, assistant/associate training directors, and medical student directors) often have positions linked to additional administrative or clinical service roles. Scholarly work often takes the form of research collaboration, chapters, "thought pieces," or survey research. Individuals with prior research backgrounds may be able to develop and maintain independent research programs while devoting substantial time and energy to administration. Generally, promotion is in the clinician-teacher series.

As academic educational funds have dried up, **paid part-time clinician/instructor or lecturer** positions that pay faculty exclusively for teaching have become much more difficult to sustain. Such positions are not tenured, are renewed based on immediate past performance on a year-to-year basis, and are at great risk during times of departmental upheaval. Appointments are generally in the clinical series.

New and Emerging Faculty Roles

Changes in medicine are creating opportunities for faculty with new skills (Yager 1995). Those now embarking on academic careers should consider contributing to academic departments as follows:

1. **Total Quality Management (TQM) officer:** Will conduct strategic planning and ongoing management using concepts based on the works of Deming (Walton 1986) and Drucker (1973) for continuous quality and productivity improvement. Departments will constantly ask themselves "What is our business?," and "How can we do it better, cheaper, faster, and more satisfyingly?" These faculty will serve as both efficiency and effectiveness experts, scrutinizing not only clinical services, but rituals governing research, administration, and education as well.
2. **Clinical computerologist:** Faculty capable of initiating and maintaining clinical information systems, instructing others in their use, and innovating applications in clinical care, education, and both basic and applied research.
3. **Public education/marketing:** To survive, departments will be required to constantly attract patients and money. Faculty will be needed who can convincingly "sell" their departments to various public and private "customers," "stakeholders," and charitable donors.
4. **Program developer-entrepreneur:** In today's business-like academic departments, creative, risk-taking entrepreneurial faculty who initiate successful new programs will be highly valued. Academic en-

trepreneurs will exploit opportunities affecting market share, costs, outcomes, and patient satisfaction.

5. **Primary care psychiatrist:** In lieu of old-style consultation-liaison psychiatrists, the new faculty member works on-site in primary care settings, in a collaborative, shoulder-to-shoulder relationship with primary care physicians. This type of involvement helps develop primary care physicians and trainees who are knowledgeable about psychiatric management and may result in closer interdepartmental linkages and more referrals.

6. **Stand-up supervisor:** In contrast to "sit-down" psychotherapy and case supervisors typical of past eras of training, contemporary supervisors are needed to provide direct, hands-on supervision, seeing patients together with residents during the initial assessment and follow-ups. The "stand-up supervisor" is present immediately, "on-line," to staff the residents' work, as in traditional primary care teaching clinics. Such supervision tends to be extremely pragmatic, directly addressing pressing concerns as well as longer-term issues.

7. **Mobile faculty:** Faculty will need to get comfortable out of their offices, serving in multiple settings. They might follow patients and trainees from setting to setting in the British model of "firms"; serve as attendings for psychiatric "swat teams" in emergency centers, community settings, and general hospitals; serve as rotating unit chiefs on inpatient services; or work as "circuit riders," covering sites in communities that may be linked to the academic medical center's extended services.

Junior Faculty Development Strategies

New faculty may benefit from the following strategies to enhance research skills and productivity, teaching abilities, and/or administrative skills, based in part on the recommendations of Wyatt (1982):

1. Learn the histories of successful and unsuccessful faculty. How have others with similar interests, series, and track records fared? How important are research, publications, grants, teaching administration, clinical practice, and university, community, and professional service? Spend your time proportionally doing what matters most, but make sure that these efforts match to a large extent what you most enjoy and do best.

2. Prepare well for your career. Those developing research careers should take enough time to learn the required research methodologies, biostatistics, and protocol preparation. Most entry-level faculty are too busy to permit adequate "on-the-job" learning of research and grant-writing skills. Serious research usually requires an initial fellowship period of several years. Those primarily interested in teaching should learn about modern educational methods, and evaluation theory and techniques.

Meetings of the Association for Academic Psychiatry (AAP), American Association of Directors of Psychiatric Residency Training (AADPRT), and/or Association of Directors of Medical Student Education in Psychiatry (ADMSEP) can be helpful sources for cutting-edge educational ideas, skill building, and networking. Many medical schools now offer additional faculty development in instructional technique. Those interested in administrative careers may benefit from supplemental MBA and/or MPH courses, or from one of the available national programs for executive physician development. All faculty can benefit by reading the literature of academic career development (McGaghie and Frey 1986; Pincus 1995; Whitman et al. 1989).

3. If interested in doing research, join an ongoing, funded research group where both senior- and intermediate-level mentors are available in order to experience first hand day-to-day research, learn how to develop and organize ideas for grants, and then learn how to write those grants.

4. If aiming toward a traditional tenure track research-oriented career, guard your calendar to ensure sufficient time to prepare grants, conduct research, and write. Teaching will count, but quality will often be preferable to quantity. Teach as much as possible in conjunction with your research and scholarly activities. Although it is essential to contribute as a "team player" to department activities, it is also essential to use time carefully to pursue academically focused tasks (Davison 1995).

5. If aiming toward a traditional tenure track or clinician-educator career, make every effort to obtain peer-reviewed grant funds for research and/or special programs. Although these funds are increasingly difficult to obtain, they carry considerable weight in promotion and tenure decisions.

6. For traditional tenure track careers, strive to publish as first author in respected, peer-reviewed journals. The prestige of the journals and your authorship position within a group matter. Many promotions committees are focusing more on quality than quantity (e.g., faculty may have

to submit their 10 best papers rather than their entire bibliography to committees).

For clinician-educator careers, keep open for opportunities to write about what interests you. Many successful clinician-educators have set themselves minimum quotas of two to three publications per year as a writing discipline, for example, case reports, reviews, chapters, and collaborative research publications.

7. Find a mentor, usually a successful full (or at least associate) professor in your series of choice who shares interests and life issues, and set up regular meetings regarding work and career plans. This mentor should be asked to review your curriculum vita and provide feedback at regular intervals.

8. Pick areas of focus that are both timely and important. Such areas are more likely to be funded, published, and cited.

9. Explore all sources of funding (grants, contracts, fellowships, departmental seed funds) and discretionary time (sabbaticals, other leaves) that can promote academic activities. If necessary and feasible, schedule some time out of the office to write. Some faculty take writing time in lieu of conference time; some use personal leave if no other options are available, and if this practice doesn't clash with family needs.

10. If possible, serve on the promotions committee or other departmental and/or medical school committees likely to provide views from the top as well as helpful networking.

11. Make yourself useful. Take on an important task and role in the department so that others know that you are working for the common good and "pulling your oar."

12. Become active in regional, and especially national and international, professional organizations. Through presentations, holding offices, chairing committees, and serving on peer review committees, you will be able to establish a network of colleagues who may be called on to write to promotions committees.

13. Maintain a list of colleagues and students and keep adequate track of their whereabouts, so that promotions committees can easily request letters of reference.

14. Maintain file copies of teaching evaluations, references to or reviews of published or presented work, funding agency's reviews of grants, clinical and administrative reviews, and any other documented external evaluation of your work.

15. Keep colleagues notified of your work by sending them preprints and reprints of publications, announcements of presentations and awards, and other relevant information.
16. Take advantage of established support systems for junior faculty, for example, systematic linkages with senior faculty advisers and peer-group support mechanisms. Where such arrangements don't exist, try to foster their development.
17. Realize that getting promoted is not the most important thing in the world, nor is it the only measure of success. Achieving satisfaction, fulfillment, balance, and a sense of having contributed comes in different ways for different people.

Having an important sense of personal priorities and knowing how to carefully allocate time between career, family, and other activities are essential for success in life, and in that much smaller piece of it called academics (Pincus 1995).

References

Alpert JS, Coles R: Careers in academic medicine: triple threat or double fake. Arch Intern Med 148:1906–1907, 1988

American Association of University Professors Committee on Retirement: Ending mandatory retirement in higher education. Academe 76:52–54, 1990

Association of American Medical Colleges: Medical Student Graduation Questionnaire, 1986: Subset Report: Psychiatry and Child Psychiatry. Washington, DC, Association of American Medical Colleges, 1986

Bashook PG, Weissman SH: Career plans of new psychiatrists. Paper presented at the annual meeting of the American Psychiatric Association, May 9–14, 1987. CME Syllabus and Proceedings Summary. Washington, DC, American Psychiatric Association, 1987

Bickel J: The changing faces of promotion and tenure at U.S. medical school. Acad Med 66:249–256, 1991

Davidson J: The Complete Idiot's Guide to Managing Your Time. New York, Alpha Books, 1995

Drucker PF: Management: Tasks, Responsibilities, Practices. New York, Harper & Row, 1973.

El-Mallakh RS, Riba M: Post-psychiatry residency career choice: current trends. Acad Psychiatry 14:86–91, 1990

Freedman DX: Research funds are down—take heart! Arch Gen Psychiatry 42:518–522, 1985

Freedman DX: The alma mater is sinking—this is dangerous to your health. Arch Gen Psychiatry 33:407–410, 1976

Freedman, DX: Of chairs and stools—or, what's academic about academic medicine? Perspect Biol Med 35:87–96, 1991

Hamilton D: Publishing by—and for?—the numbers (News and Comment). Science 251:1331–1332, 1990

Haviland MG, Pincus HA, Dial TH: Career, research involvement, and research fellowship plans of potential psychiatrists. Arch Gen Psychiatry 44:493–496, 1987

Higgins EJ: Women and Minorities on U.S. Medical School Faculties, 1985. Washington DC, Association of American Medical Colleges, 1986

McGaghie WC, Frey JJ: Handbook for the Academic Physician. New York, Springer-Verlag, 1986

Pardes H, Pincus H: Challenges to academic psychiatry, Am J Psychiatry 140:1117–1126. 1983

Pincus HA (ed): Research Funding and Resource Manual: Mental Health and Addictive Disorders. Washington, DC, American Psychiatric Press, 1995

Romano J: The battered chairman syndrome. Arch Gen Psychiatry 48:371–374, 1991

Walton M: The Deming Management Method. New York, Prigree Books, 1986

Whiting B, Godley C, Sherman E: Women and Minorities on U.S. Medical School Faculties, 1989. Washington DC, Association of American Medical Colleges, 1990

Whitman N, Weiss E, Bishop FM: Executive Skills for Medical Faculty, Salt Lake City, UT, Department of Family and Preventive Medicine, 1989

Wyatt GE: Ethnic minorities and tenure. Am Psychol 37:1283–1284, 1982

Yager J, Yager AR, Siegel D, Strauss GD: Professional interests among residency applicants in psychiatry: A pilot study of autobiographical statement. Acad Psychiatry 14:80–85, 1990

Yager, J: New roles for psychiatric faculty. Paper presented at meeting on Educational Issues in Managed Care, American Association of Chairmen of Departments of Psychiatry-American Association of Directors of Psychiatric Residency Training combined meeting. Baltimore, MD, August 1995

2

Development as an Educator

Jerald Kay, M.D.

As many authors in this *Handbook* have noted, medical school faculty rarely have just one responsibility or role. Nearly all medical schools have professorial tracks for their voluntary (nonpaid) faculty who provide limited but significant teaching as well as tracks that emphasize research, education and clinical/administrative service, and, more recently, clinical service alone. This last track has been created in some medical schools as a response to managed care, which, by and large, has refused to support training and education. Faculty on this new track deliver patient care and teach for very small amounts of time, to generate resources to support basic academic missions previously funded through more readily available grants and higher rates of reimbursement for teaching and clinical service. Regardless if an individual is a researcher, an administrator, a clinician-educator, or a clinician with a faculty appointment, he or she is likely to be devoting professional time to teaching.

The rightful importance of research within academic health centers is reflected in the number of chapters in this book that address the development of research skills. Although significant departmental efforts are made usually to promote a junior faculty member's acquisition of research attitudes and skills, the same degree of attention is not often paid to the young professor's development as an educator. It may be trite, but the old adage of "see one, do one, and teach one" remains the guiding principle of learning how to teach in many institutions. Teaching is indeed its own virtue, but it does not follow that teaching skills are automatically acquired. Advancement and promotion as an educator requires thoughtful career planning; in this sense, it is no different from advancement in research, administration, or clinical service. This chapter argues for a broader definition of medical school scholarship, summarizes the traditional teaching opportunities within an academic psychiatry department, discusses how to acquire and strengthen teaching skills, and proposes techniques and methods to maximize one's opportunity for promotion as an educator.

Scholarship Reconsidered: Beyond "Teaching Versus Research"

The late Ernest Boyer, president of the Carnegie Foundation for the Advancement of Teaching, noted that American university scholarship has become more narrowly defined over the last 90 years. Basic research within the medical school has become the quintessential form of scholarly activity. Boyer (1990) proposed four types of scholarship:

1. The scholarship of discovery—what we usually think of as "research"
2. The scholarship of integration—"serious disciplined work that seeks to interpret, draw together, and bring new insight to bear on original research"
3. The scholarship of application—"scholarly service that applies and contributes to human knowledge"
4. The scholarship of teaching—"a dynamic endeavor ... not only transmitting knowledge but *transforming* and *extending* it as well" (pp. 17–24)

The scholarship of discovery needs no further elaboration and is at the very heart of academic life. The scholarship of integration is the pursuit of making connections among disciplines, of explicating the meaningfulness of apparent isolated facts. It has become even more important as medical school departmental boundaries are broken down and new interdisciplinary bridges are built. The scholarship of integration requires interpretation. The consolidation of neurobiological findings into a framework for understanding how psychotherapy might work is one example of the scholarship of integration.

The scholarship of application struggles with questions of how new knowledge can be of assistance to both individuals and institutions. It raises the evocative question of whether social problems can be approached through rigorous scholarly activities. The scholarship of application should not be confused with academic service activities such as membership on medical school or departmental committees. The scholarship of application is often characterized by reciprocity. Faculty members, for example, learn much from their patients when new treatment approaches are applied and evaluated.

The focus of this chapter is on the scholarship of teaching. Unfortunately, as external economic forces drive academic health centers, less attention seems to be paid to the scholarship of teaching, and teaching is experienced by many faculty as one more obligation in a busy and demanding work week. The scholarship of teaching aims at educating students and attracting future scholars. It requires that the teacher be widely read, be up-to-date, and have a firm grasp of his or her field. The effective teacher strives to stimulate the student through active, not passive, learning and transmits the importance of lifelong learning. The latter is critical to the professional growth of the physician because much of what is taught in medical schools becomes rapidly outdated. It is often said that most successful academicians can trace their inspiration to an exciting teacher or mentor. In this sense, teaching is at the very heart of scholarly pursuit, since outstanding teaching pushes students into new and creative directions. It is probably also true that most effective physicians have acquired certain values and approaches to their work from highly engaging teachers.

Although scholarly activity is required in all medical schools, many medical schools do not constrain the content of faculty scholarship. Accomplishments that represent excellence in any of the four scholarship styles, if appropriately documented (most often through publications in peer-reviewed journals and other formal evaluation methods to be discussed), are considered in the promotional process. Thus, articles describing curricular innovations or pedagogical approaches are considered as examples of the scholarship of teaching just as published case reports may be considered as examples of the scholarship of application.

Teaching Opportunities

The teaching opportunities in medical student education, residency training, and continuing medical education that are available to faculty within a traditional academic department of psychiatry are described in detail in

Section I of the *Handbook*. Table 2–1 summarizes some of the challenges and rewards of these major educational activities.

Educational Career Paths

For many educators, a natural career path or trajectory is implied in Table 2–1. Learning how to teach invariably begins in medical school where every student is impressed with one or two especially effective teachers. In residency, one is responsible for teaching and supervising medical students on the clerkship. Many programs also offer residents the opportunity to lead or colead small-group discussions as part of the preclinical psychiatry/ behavioral sciences courses. These experiences provide the trainee with the opportunity to observe seasoned teachers who deliver lectures and facilitate groups. Psychiatry departments that are committed to undergraduate and graduate medical education invariably conduct specific resident teaching sessions on how to become an effective teacher in multiple teaching formats. They also provide residents with some instruction on how to give useful feedback and instruction in the principles of evaluation. As part of their didactic and treatment experiences, residents are exposed to a host of teachers, many of whom become instrumental in the resident's professionalization experience. If these activities are gratifying, then some residents will consider a career path in psychiatric education.

Although a new faculty member can become a residency training director or director of education immediately after graduation, it does not happen frequently for several important reasons. First, experience in teaching medical students and/or directing a medical student course is an invaluable opportunity to develop and refine teaching, evaluation, and administrative skills. The challenges of directing a training program are considerable and require a fair amount of administrative sophistication, which is quite difficult to learn on the job. Second, a close proximity in age between a residency director and his or her residents, or a very large difference between the training director's age and that of the faculty and chair, may be a disadvantage in commanding the necessary respect usually accorded to a faculty member in that position. Third, just as few people would seek the help of a teenage psychotherapist, a young and inexperienced faculty member is likely also to have had relatively limited life experiences and clinical experiences as a psychiatrist, experiences that often are essential in counseling and evaluating trainees.

Table 2–1. Some challenges and rewards of teaching positions

Position	Challenges	Rewards
	Medical Student Education—Preclinical	
Preclinical lecturer	Neutralizing antipsychiatry stereotypes	Demonstrating usefulness of psychiatry
	Developing effective lecture styles	Elucidating psychiatric treatment efficacy
	Framing material to future nonpsychiatrists	Teaching many idealistic students
	Developing fair tests and evaluation procedures	Identifying and nurturing potential interest in psychiatry
	Teaching to a broad range of student sophistication	
	Integrating new teaching technology	
Discussion leader	Integrating lecture material, reading, and personal responses to material	Promoting student-centered learning
	Building a safe and productive small-group milieu	Teaching critical-thinking and problem-solving skills
	Integrating relevance of psychiatry to primary care	Development of meaningful teacher-student relationships that often persist throughout four years
	Engaging nonproductive or reticent students	Helping students begin to achieve tolerance for ambiguity
	Encouraging problem solving	
	Helping students listen critically	
	Fostering individual and group development simultaneously	

(*continued*)

Table 2–1. Continued

Position	Challenges	Rewards
	Medical Student Education—Preclinical *(continued)*	
Discussion leader	Becoming comfortable with multiple roles of group leader, moderator, formal authority figure, facilitator, transference object	
Interdisciplinary course teacher	Achieving balance between espousing psychiatry's importance as referral speciality versus teaching psychiatric skills useful to all M.D.s	Demonstrating the relevance of psychiatry to all of medicine
	Dealing with antipsychiatry bias from other teachers and their overestimation of their psychiatric skills	Espousing the biopsychosocial model of illness and health
		Maintaining psychiatry's identity as medicine specialty
Course director	Developing a working relationship with large groups of students	Opportunities to work with schoolwide curriculum committees
	Constructing fair and valid examinations and evaluation process	Collaboration with basic scientists and clinicians from other departments
	Meeting the needs of subgroups of student minority, women, gays and lesbians, etc. and their criticisms	Identifying and assisting those students with psychological problems
	Fighting for equity for your course versus other basic science courses	Successful integration of behavioral sciences as legitimate basic science of medicine
	Recruiting sufficient faculty for small groups	Above-average scores on USMLE Part I
	Integrating USMLE Part I objectives	

Medical Student Education—Clinical

Clinical supervisor/seminar leader	Demonstrating the power of the doctor–patient relationship in students who underrate their clinical skills	Gratifying personal student-teacher relationships
	Teaching effective interview and assessment skills	Establishing positive attitudes about psychiatry that may influence future referral practice to psychiatry
	Providing meaningful but sensitive performance feedback	Instilling correct practices regarding diagnosis, treatment, psychopharmacology
	Developing new technological approaches to teaching and learning	
Clerkship director	Demonstrating to students that psychiatric patients get well	Teaching residents to become effective teachers
	Organizing clinical experiences that provide maximum clinical responsibility but are phase appropriate to the learning level	Recognition from other clerkship directors regarding student knowledge of psychiatry and sensitivity to psychosocial needs of patients
	Designing an evaluation process that is fair	Appreciation from the training director, chair, and department regarding students enthusiastic about entering psychiatry
	Assisting students with major resistance to psychiatric patients	Above-average scores on standardized tests (USMLE Part II, NBME shelf exams)
	Identifying students with interfering characterological problems	
	Integrating USMLE Part II objectives	
	Rewarding faculty for teaching similar content throughout entire academic year	

(continued)

Table 2–1. Continued

Position	Challenges	Rewards
Medical Student Education—Clinical (continued)		
Director of medical student education	Planning a three-year curriculum that integrates behavioral science and clinical psychiatry in a rigorous and interesting fashion Fostering appreciation and respect for psychiatry in a generation of physicians Protecting psychiatry curricular time in medical school education Ensuring that psychiatric skills and knowledge are included in primary care and other interdisciplinary curricula	Mentoring medical students Nurturing student interest in psychiatry Collaborating with colleagues in creating medical school policies through work in curriculum, student affairs and year committees Collaborating with educators in other specialties locally and nationally to protect and advance medical education Gaining local, regional, and national recognition for directing a high-quality program Having the pleasure of one's students become one's residents and one's colleagues
Graduate Medical Education (GME)		
Supervisor	Teaching residents the power of doctor–patient relationship Helping residents to accept patient's emotional pain and conflict without judging them Teaching residents to engage patients by listening to patient communication beyond manifest content level	Observing, firsthand, professional growth and development in residents Staying up-to-date on literature and practice Developing mentoring relationships Improving supervisory skills through experience

	Supporting residents to integrate psychotherapy skills into their medical role	Assisting residents to receive appropriate psychological help when needed
	Integrating the neurobiological with the psychological	Being an advocate for resident issues
	Teaching sophisticated diagnostic and treatment techniques	Direct input into curriculum process
	Identifying learning inhibitions and providing meaningful interventions	
	Providing useful feedback	
	Sharing your own experiences in an appropriate fashion	
Service chief (inpatient, outpatient, C/L, etc.)	Coping with residents who drop out of rotations unexpectedly	To maximize educationally what your service can contribute to residency education within a limited amount of time
	Developing innovative ways to address growing problem of increasing patient acuity, decreasing length of stay, and increasing paperwork	Solving teacher–resident disputes
		Advocating for your institution in a balanced fashion
Seminar/course leader	To organize concise and effective courses with limited curricular time	Intellectual gratification from give-and-take of seminars
	To evaluate strengths and weakness of seminar and provide corrections	Being challenged to learn more yourself
	To integrate your subject matter with other seminars	Demonstrating that residents have indeed mastered course material

33

(continued)

Table 2–1. Continued

Position	Challenges	Rewards
	Graduate Medical Education (GME) (continued)	
Seminar/course leader	To understand the role your seminar plays in the entire educational process for the resident	Identifying those residents with exceptional talent and guiding them into increasingly challenging activities
Residency training director	Developing/refining a professional curriculum in a field that is rapidly changing and at a time of decreased support for GME	Achieving the status of a role model who can synthesize many aspects of psychiatry
	Bridging ideological schisms among the faculty	Assisting residents to begin scholarly activities
	Maintaining high morale in the residency training program	Gaining local, regional, national recognition for directing a high-quality program
	Successfully recruiting talented new trainees	Working with residents on a close basis and providing counseling for professional career development
	Establishing fair and equitable evaluation processes	Assisting residents in receiving national fellowships
	Dealing with the "problem" resident and uncooperative faculty	Increasing respect for psychiatry in academic center by training quality psychiatrists
	Establishing a productive and rewarding relationship simultaneously with residents, faculty, hospital administration, and the chair of psychiatry	Developing new and successful educational technologies
		High PRITE scores

34

	Creating reputable educational scholarship for him/herself	High ABPN pass rates
	Establishing an effective and harmonious residency training committee	
	Passing the accreditation process	
Continuing Medical Education (CME) Course Director	Assessing correctly CME needs	Meeting psychiatrists and other health professionals
	Constructing effective, balanced and credited programs	Developing new professional relationships
	Establishing hospitable program	Gaining knowledge of community practice standards and challenges
	Ensuring profitable programs	Helping practitioners become more effective clinicians
	Developing a reliable evaluation process	
Director of Education	Remaining on top of numerous education programs	Creating a cohesive educational philosophy across all stages of professional development
	Fighting for sufficient resources for education/ training programs	Capacity to instill significant values in all education programs
	Mentoring young teachers who may not appreciate the importance of teaching activities	
	Acquiring new educational/technological methods	
	Establishing a scholarly approach to teaching and sustaining educational research programs	

One academic career path of the psychiatric educator, therefore, begins with extensive experience in medical student education, then onto residency education as a teacher, supervisor, and ultimately administrator, followed by responsibility in some departments for both programs. Along the way, such a person would be wise to develop a circumscribed research or clinical interest that complements these educational responsibilities. For some, a chair of psychiatry is then a reasonable next step, since it requires considerable knowledge of education, research, and administration. For others, becoming the very best medical student or residency director is an admirable professional goal, and, in fact, the career paths for directors of medical student education and residency training are quite similar with regard to age, job longevity, and academic rank. And yet for another group deeply committed to undergraduate and graduate medical education, there are opportunities in the medical school as either deans of student affairs, deans of curriculum, or deans of house staff affairs. Regardless of the position, the successful academic advancement of a psychiatric educator follows a prescribed process, which will be addressed later in this chapter.

Some Basic Principles of Learning and Teaching

A thorough discussion of pedagogy is beyond the scope of this chapter, but it is helpful to remember that there are fundamental tenets of effective medical education. Psychiatric educators should not have to learn them exclusively through experience. Appendix 2–A includes some general texts on teaching as well as specific resources on psychiatric education. George Miller (1962), the grandfather of American medical education, enumerated more than 35 years ago 10 succinct basic principles of successful learning:

1. Learning involves a change in behavior of the learner.
2. Different people learn different things by different means and at different rates.
3. Learning is more efficient if the intermediate course goals are seen to be related to the final objectives.
4. Success tends to raise a student's level of aspiration and failure lowers it, with the degree of movement roughly related to the degree of success or failure.
5. Emotion is involved nearly as much as intellect in the learning process.
6. Retention of information, of skills, of understanding, or of attitudes is

significantly increased if the learning is accomplished in a context that has meaning for the student.

7. The rapidity and the degree of forgetting can also be reduced by over-learning facts beyond simple recall, overlearning skills beyond minimal proficiency.

8. If efficiency and effectiveness of learning is an important goal, then there is sound experimental basis for the efforts directed toward integration and correlation of subject matter.

9. Learning how to be a doctor and being one are obviously different things.

10. More generalized training may also be transferred when there is similarity between the new situation and the one in which that behavior was learned as appropriate. (pp. 50–64)

Miller also postulated five principles of teaching that, in conjunction with his principles of learning, comprise a pithy summary of the pedagogical principles that make for effective educational experiences for students, residents, and practitioners. These include:

- Learning is personal.
- Learning must be meaningful.
- Learning must be aimed at realistic goals.
- Learning should be accompanied by feedback.
- Learning should be based on good interpersonal relationships. (Miller 1962, pp. 69–72)

Although space does not permit a complete exposition of all of Miller's principles, and many are self-evident, some comments on his ideas about motivational and emotional factors in learning, the centrality of the teacher-student relationship, and the retention and transfer of knowledge are in order. Motivation to learn about psychiatry obviously resides within the student. The effective teacher, however, is skilled in enhancing this motivation, which is accomplished through the establishment of a positive, reinforcing, and empathic relationship. Mutual trust, shared goals, and shared evaluation methods and criteria characterize the instructional relationship. This is accomplished also through appreciating the many learning styles of students. Think about, for example, the approaches of recently graduated psychiatrists who are sitting for the Part I (written) American Board of Psychiatry and Neurology (ABPN) examination. Some psychiatrists review by reading comprehensive textbooks from cover to cover to ensure that every topic is revisited. Others can read comfortably with synopses of text-books. Some prefer to rely heavily on review books of questions and an-swers as a method of identifying the limits of their knowledge base. Many candidates prefer lectures and practice sessions and therefore enroll in board review courses. Still others opt for audiocassettes because they have found learning through listening to be especially effective.

Miller's principles are useful in conceptualizing another common and enduring educational challenge for many psychiatric educators. Providing medical students and nonpsychiatric residents with phase-appropriate and successful ambulatory experiences with psychiatric patients that relate directly to the practice of primary care medicine builds enthusiasm for learning and promotes the transfer and integration of knowledge, skills, and attitudes into an ambulatory practice. If the relevance of psychiatry to primary care medicine is demonstrated consistently by the educator, then these learners will have an easier time appreciating the importance of the goals of the psychiatry rotation as it applies to their eventual career interest. This in turn is likely to promote greater retention of psychiatric principles, better ability to tolerate ambiguity in psychiatric patient encoun-ters, and, it is hoped, greater problem-solving abilities and continuing pro-fessional interest and development in the behavioral aspects of primary care medicine.

What Constitutes Ideal Teaching?

In a meta-analysis of 31 educational studies (Feldman 1988), the following knowledge, attitudes, and skills of the teacher were found by students and educators to be critical:

- Awareness and concern with students' abilities and their progress —The teacher communicates at an appropriate level for the students, uses reading materials that are neither overwhelming nor boring, and realizes when one student's learning problem is shared by others.
- Preparation and organization of teaching sessions—The teacher is well prepared for class, organizes the course in a logical fashion, and builds on previously mastered material.
- Knowledge of subject—The teacher conveys a comprehensive and up-to-date mastery of his or her field.
- Enthusiasm—The teacher conveys enthusiasm and interest in the subject, students, and the course.
- Clarity and understandableness—The teacher explains clearly and

uses well-chosen examples; students can follow and understand lectures or presentations; the teacher answers students' questions and summarizes important points.

- Helpfulness and availability—The teacher is clearly willing to provide personal assistance, keeps appointments and is timely with students, provides special "group help" sessions when needed, is available to students outside of regular teaching times, and makes a readily apparent effort to develop rapport with students.
- Fairness of evaluation—Concepts emphasized in class are tested in exams; the teacher explains the evaluation process; exams cover material on which students expect to be tested, are fair, and require synthesis of course material and not merely recall of facts; the teacher uses multiple evaluation techniques and assigns appropriate weight to each of them.

Principles of Effective Feedback

The provision of feedback to the learner is the one principle that warrants further discussion, because it remains one of most poorly understood and practiced instructional activities at virtually all levels of medical education. Giving feedback has actually become more problematic within the last 10 years or so because of the increasing tendency toward litigation in our society. However, medical educators should know that the courts have upheld the right of the faculty to assess and dismiss students and residents based on institutional standards of performance and conduct. That is not to say that some teachers may treat their students in an abusive manner and that the student is correct to complain. As well, there are times when due process is not followed in medical student and residency education programs and important advancement decisions are made on arbitrary and capricious bases. All of these issues notwithstanding, the most central problem in providing feedback is that very few teachers are comfortable making critical comments about students. All directors of medical student education and residency training struggle with overly positive evaluations of students and residents. It is not uncommon for some students to progress through a number of years of medical school only to be discovered as having significant educational, characterological, or ethical deficiencies in their final year of school. Residents too are passed on from year to year in some programs without adequate remediation plans. Although teachers may wish not to hurt students' feelings, ultimately they do a terrible disservice to the student by withholding appropriate feedback.

No therapeutic contract exists between a student and teacher, but providing helpful feedback shares many features of an effective psychotherapeutic interpretation. Feedback, like an interpretation, is effective when the teacher pays close attention to timing, dosage, specificity, and delivery. The following are characteristics of growth-promoting feedback:

- Comments about improving performance or knowledge base should not address the student's personality.
- To avoid humiliating a student, feedback should be given in a private and safe setting.
- Effective feedback is highly specific in characterizing weaknesses.
- Feedback should not be limited to describing areas needing improvement but should also be complementary in assessing strengths.
- Feedback should be directed toward skills, attitudes, or knowledge that can be improved; it should not focus on those things that the student cannot change.
- It is important to be empathic with the student's or resident's plight in providing feedback—there is no place for embarrassing and demeaning the learner.

With respect to the administrative skills needed to oversee courses, programs, and curricula, and to negotiate effectively within an academic health center, Dr. Faulkner's chapter in this book, Chapter 28, has much to offer the individual wishing to advance as a career educator.

How Are Teaching Skills Acquired?

Excellent teachers are made, not born. Yet, at the same time, there are some personal qualities that often distinguish the effective teacher from the ineffective one. First and foremost, the effective teacher has an innate ability to empathize with students. It has been noted as well that unbridled enthusiasm for teaching is critical. Strong personal commitment to what you teach is also appreciated by students. For some teaching, like in large lectures, it helps to be more extroverted, to enjoy performing before others, and to have a reasonable amount of showmanship.

Many aspects of showmanship can be broken down into its effective components and therefore can be taught to novice instructors. For example, knowing all of your medical students by their first names sends a powerful message that a teacher truly cares about students. Each medical school produces a photographic composite of its students by year, which allows a teacher to identify those who ask questions in the clerkship didactics program and, with extra effort, those in the preclinical behavior sciences courses. A teacher's ability to make eye contact with students, especially in large groups, is critical for understanding the effectiveness of your delivery as well as assessing the students' level of understanding. Drama in the classroom can be achieved in a host of ways. For example, lecturers who can walk among the students as they are teaching often create an intimate teaching environment regardless of the size of the audience. Selecting evocative affective-laden clinical material can provide an engaging experience. Achieving comfort in utilizing your own clinical and personal life experiences in your teaching is yet another stimulating technique. The use of humor can be very captivating, providing the teacher never disparages students and avoids topics that are likely to offend and polarize students in the class.

It is a very intimidating, but often highly rewarding experience to tape a lecture and then review it alone and subsequently with a senior educator. The camera does not lie and provides the educator with a very accurate view of his or her teaching techniques. This can be done in individual supervision as well as in larger teaching venues. Taping a teaching session permits examination of the rate of information and dynamics of delivery, its appropriateness to an audience, and even how body language is utilized.

Substantial enjoyment from being in the role of the expert and mentor is vital, as is deriving personal satisfaction from associating with students and fostering their professional development. For other teaching opportunities, such as in individual supervision of psychotherapy, it is often helpful to be more reflective and to establish a clear learning milieu that is safe for the discussion of highly personal feelings about a patient and about oneself. Above all, individuals who either resent having to teach or have little tolerance or patience for novices probably should spend their professional time in other than educational activities.

There is a body of knowledge about teaching effectiveness, some of which has been described, with which all psychiatric educators should be familiar. Like any other aspect of medicine, educational techniques are introduced and evolve constantly. The psychiatric educator has an obligation to keep up with medical and psychiatric education literature (see Appendix 2–A for a bibliography of helpful readings). This requires reading, at a minimum and in addition to general psychiatry and subspecialty journals, the following publications:

Academic Medicine

Academic Psychiatry

Medical Education

Journal of the American Medical Association

These journals help the educator to keep abreast of nationwide trends about course content, pedagogical approaches, evaluation techniques, student characteristics, educational research, and innovative teaching technologies such as computer-assisted instruction and distance learning. The first three journals are, by the way, the most likely forums for the publication of your own manuscripts (see Chapter 3 for more in-depth information on writing).

The role of an educator mentor cannot be overestimated. Just as mentors play a role in psychiatric research or administration, a knowledgeable senior mentor can play a pivotal role in advancing the educational career of a protégé. Although it is possible to succeed in psychiatric education on your own, it is much easier to do so with the help of a skilled psychiatric teacher. A mentor is helpful in three broad areas: getting to know the academic institution, career development, and professional development. First, a mentor teaches the novice about the culture of their institution and their department, which is often helpful in preventing conflict. The ability to identify resources to support teaching and research is invaluable. An appreciation of the social and political dynamics of a department allows a smoother integration into the academic world. Second, the mentor advises on the advancement and promotion process and provides general support and encouragement. Third, with respect to professional development, suggestions for building effective teaching strategies and selecting long-term research and writing plans can be exceptionally helpful. Young teachers can learn from their mentors how to develop and deliver effective lectures, run engaging small groups, use educational technology, collaborate with educators from other medical school departments, develop and monitor a curriculum, evaluate students and their teachers, and provide feedback to students and teachers. A helpful mentor facilitates appointments to key medical school committees that are vital for professional advancement as well as assists, for example, with the first appointment to a component of the

American Psychiatric Association Council on Medical Education. Successful mentors also introduce their mentees to accomplished educators at national meetings as well as inform mentees about how to join committees in national educational organizations.

In addition to mentorship, joining psychiatric educational organizations is enormously helpful to the young teacher. Psychiatry is fortunate in having effective organizations that advocate for medical student and resident education. For the young professor whose primary responsibility is with medical students, the Association of Directors of Medical Student Education in Psychiatry (ADMSEP) and the Association for Academic Psychiatry (AAP) are exciting groups in which to participate. For training directors, membership in the American Association of Directors of Psychiatric Residency Training (AADPRT) is a must. All these organizations provide the opportunity to network with other educators around the country, begin collaborative multicenter educational research, compare curricula from other institutions, have access to model curricula and teaching resources developed by experienced educators, and to learn from the most exciting teachers in the country through workshops, lectures, and informal meetings. These organizations provide camaraderie and the opportunity for skill development and knowledge acquisition that is vital for professional growth. They make it unnecessary for each new educator to redevelop the wheel at his or her own institution. In addition, promotion in the academic ranks is very much dependent on extrainstitutional recognition of teaching skills and accomplishments. The psychiatric educational organizations provide opportunities for developing national reputations.

All medical student educators should seek appointment to a United States Medical Licensing Examination (USMLE) test committee of the National Board of Medical Examiners. Similarly all educators involved heavily with graduate medical education should volunteer to perform site visits on behalf of the Psychiatry Residency Review Committee, our specialty's accreditation arm of the Accrediting Council for Graduate Medical Education. All psychiatric educators should volunteer to examine for the American Board of Psychiatry and Neurology (ABPN), which provides a glimpse into the state of knowledge of many recent residency graduates and is yet another vehicle for meeting educators and establishing new networks.

One additional valuable resource exists in many, but not all, academic health centers—an office of medical education. The responsibilities of those faculty and or deans assigned to an office of education include scientifically evaluating curriculum and teachers, assisting in the construction of reliable and valid examinations, supporting research in medical education, coordinating curriculum revision, and developing new teaching technologies. A large portion of the efforts of such organizations are devoted to assisting faculty to become more effective teachers. Not only will members of an office of education observe your lectures and discussion groups but most will tape your teaching activities and help you improve your delivery, style, and organization. In addition, an office of education typically sponsors regularly scheduled workshops for faculty and often will bring to the medical school nationally recognized experts in medical education. The office of medical education can assist the young educator in developing a methodology for studying research questions in undergraduate and graduate medical education.

How to Get Promoted as an Educator

How teaching is defined has much to do with how teaching is evaluated. Serious educators conceptualize teaching activities much in the same way that psychiatrists conceptualize their clinical approach to patients. The seven areas listed in Table 2–2 represent a framework for teaching (Cashin 1989). Some areas are more appropriate to the behavioral science course director or residency educator responsible for seminars. Other areas are relevant to all psychiatric teachers regardless of their teaching responsibilities.

The Teaching Portfolio

It comes as no surprise that most faculty are evaluated and rewarded for research publications. However, it may come as a surprise that substantial evidence indicates that research productivity and teaching effectiveness are unrelated (Feldman 1987; Webster 1996). A recent meta-analysis of 58 studies once again demonstrated that research activities do not enhance teaching (Hattie and Marsh 1996). Teaching performance, be it outstanding or mediocre, is largely ignored in many medical schools. The undervaluation of teaching accomplishments in tenure and advancement decisions is due in large part, to the lack of evidence and precision about the quality of teaching performance. One solution to this problem is the development of the teaching portfolio that is composed of samples of an educator's most

Table 2–2. An expanded definition of teaching

    I.   Subject matter mastery
        A.   Content areas
        B.   Comprehensiveness of content
        C.   Currency and relevance of content
        D.   Objectivity of coverage
   II.   Curriculum development
        A.   Course fit with other courses
        B.   Course revisions
  III.   Course design
        A.   Instructional goals and objectives
        B.   Appropriateness of teaching methods
        C.   Appropriateness of assessment methods
  IV.   Delivery of instruction
        A.   Methods: lecture, small-group discussion, supervision
        B.   Skills: speaking, explaining
        C.   Aids: handouts, audiovisual tools, CAI, supplementary readings
   V.   Assessment of instruction
        A.   Tests: multiple choice, essays, case discussion, AV clinical presentation, patient interviews
        B.   Papers, projects
        C.   Grading/evaluating practices
        D.   Ongoing vs. episodic
  VI.   Availability to students
        A.   Office hours
        B.   Informal meetings
        C.   Telephone (especially with clinical supervision)
 VII.   Administrative requirements (completed and on time)
        A.   Book orders
        B.   Library reserve
        C.   Course or seminar syllabi
        D.   Reporting of grades or evaluations

---

outstanding teaching as well as reflective statements about that work (Figure 2–1).

Teaching portfolios are not only useful for professional advancement but also can be of great help in faculty development and even in the annual faculty review process and merit determination conducted by all university-based departments. Additionally, the teaching portfolio is a testimony of intellectual and scholarly discussion about teaching—it makes teaching a more serious endeavor. It also places the responsibility for evaluating in-

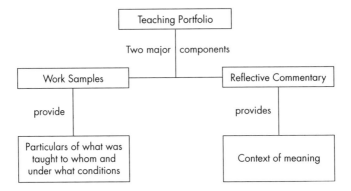

Figure 2-1. The composition of the teaching portfolio.
Source: Wright State University, Teaching and Learning Center Newsletter, February, 1994.

struction, and not relying simply on student evaluations, in the hands of the psychiatric educator. Teaching portfolios also hold the promise for evaluating one another's teaching. In the process of collecting documentation that illustrates teaching effectiveness, the educator is drawn into thinking about his or her teaching activities and achievements, rearranging priorities, rethinking teaching strategies, and planning for the future (Seldin 1991).

What belongs in a teaching portfolio? Appendix 2–B lists the possible items that might be included in an effective teaching portfolio. Appendix 2–C is an outline for another model that appraises faculty performance. I have found the following items to be especially central to compiling the portfolio:

- Student course and teaching evaluations, particularly those that produce overall ratings of satisfaction and effectiveness and describe needs for correcting deficiencies
- Listing of all course titles, enrollments, and brief course descriptions
- Description of course material prepared for students
- Participation (and presentations) in national educational meetings, seminars, workshops focused on instructional improvement
- Unstructured and, if available, unsolicited written evaluations by students after course completion
- Statements about your teaching from colleagues in your department or other departments (e.g., in interdisciplinary courses) who have attended your lectures or conferences
- The formal evaluation of educational innovations you have introduced

- Written comments from students, residents, and colleagues about your availability to discuss educational issues
- Listing of participation in curriculum development
- Publication of a textbook or other educational materials
- Research and publications based on your teaching or course development
- Student scores on standardized tests (USMLE for medical students, PRITE and ABPN for residents, and recertification rates for practitioners)
- Honors and awards received for educational accomplishments and talents

One of the benefits in compiling a teaching portfolio is that it can be incorporated directly into the "Teaching" section of a curriculum vitae. This provides a powerful statement about the role of education in your professional work.

Some Concluding Thoughts on the Promotion of an Educator

Schools of medicine sustain faculties that support their unique mission. Some of these schools are strongly identified with a particular type of research productivity. Others have a more broad-based approach to their mission. All medical school faculty have the responsibility to achieve academic growth and development in the areas of teaching scholarly activity and of service. Usually any one of these areas can be the primary area of achievement, *if* the faculty member accomplishes this in a unique way that fits the mission of his or her psychiatry department. Since each department of psychiatry is responsible for a balance of teaching, scholarly activity, and professional service, the distribution of the departmental mission to departmental faculty members and the professional development of individuals are the responsibility of the chair.

This view has several implications for the development and advancement of a psychiatric educator. First, to be an effective teacher one must be an effective collaborator and colleague. Second, an effective teacher must demonstrate achievement in a rigorous manner that is consistent with departmental goals. Third, advancement as a teacher requires the absolute support of your chair and educational administrators (residency and medical student directors or directors of education). In competitive medical schools in recent years, probably no faculty member focusing exclusively in education (i.e., has no other area of productive research) received promotion without the strong support of his or her chair to school and university promotion committees and deans. Excellence in teaching can be recognized, but it requires dedication and vigilance; in this respect, advancement as a psychiatric educator is no different from advancement as a basic and clinical researcher or a medical administrator.

To conclude on a positive note, the majority of schools have established promotion criteria for clinician-educators regardless of whether the school has an explicit clinician-educator track (Beasley et al. 1997). Teaching and clinical skills, mentoring, academic administration, developing educational programs, nonresearch scholarship, clinical research, and service coordination are important considerations in the advancement of the clinician-educator. Moreover, schools have determined that, compared with investigators, fewer peer-reviewed publications are required for advancement of educators. Perhaps now more than ever, recognition for outstanding educational contributions is uniformly possible.

References

Beasley BW, Wright SM, Cofrancesco J, et al: Promotion criteria for clinician-educators in the United States and Canada. JAMA 278:723–728, 1997

Boyer EL: Scholarship reconsidered: priorities of the professoriate. Princeton, NJ, Carnegie Foundation for the Advancement of Learning, 1990, pp 13–25

Cashin WE: Defining and evaluating college teaching (IDEA Paper No 21). Manhattan, KS, Kansas State University Center for Faculty Evaluation and Development, September 1989

Feldman KA: Research productivity and scholarly accomplishment of college teachers as related to their instructional effectiveness: a review and exploration. Research in Higher Education 26:227–298, 1987

Feldman KA: Effective college teaching from the students' and faculty's view: matched or mismatched priorities? Research in Higher Education 28:291–344, 1988

Hattie J, Marsh HW: The relationship between research and teaching: a meta-analysis. Review of Educational Research 66:507–542, 1996

Miller GE: Teaching and Learning in Medical School. Cambridge, MA, Harvard University Press, 1961, pp 50–64, 69–72

Seldin P: The teaching portfolio: a practical guide to improved performance and promotion/tenure decisions. Bolton, MA, Anker, 1991

Seldin P: Successful Faculty Evaluation Programs: Multi-Source Information for Appraising Faculty Performance. Crugers, NY, Coventry Press, 1986

Webster D: Research productivity and classroom teaching effectiveness. Instructional Evaluation 9:14–20, 1996

Wright State University: The teaching portfolio. Center for Teaching and Learning Newsletter (February): pp 1–4, 1994

Educational Bibliography

Continuing Medical Education

Strauss G: Continued professional development, in Psychiatry, Vol 2. Edited by Tasman A, Kay J, Lieberman JA. Philadelphia, PA, WB Saunders, 1997, pp 1892–1900

Faculty Development

Brown GR: The inpatient database as a technique to prevent junior faculty burnout. Academic Psychiatry 14:224–229, 1990

Jarvis D: Junior Faculty Development: A Handbook. New York, Modern Language Association of America, 1991

Rittelmeyer LF: Leadership in an academic department of psychiatry. Academic Psychiatry 14:57–64, 1990

Sparr LF, Bloom JD, Marcel LJ, et al: The organization and regulation of voluntary faculty. Academic Psychiatry 15:61–68, 1991

General Education

Boice R: The New Faculty Member: Supporting and Fostering Professional Development. San Francisco, CA, Jossey-Bass, 1992

Boyer EL: Scholarship Reconsidered: Priorities of the Professoriate. Princeton, NJ, Carnegie Foundation for the Advancement of Learning, 1990, pp 13–25

Janes J, Hauer D: Now What?: Readings on surviving (and even enjoying) your first experience at college teaching. Littleton, CO, Copley, 1987

Katz J, Henry M: Turning Professors into Teachers. New York, ACE and Macmillan, 1988

McKeachie WJ: Teaching Tips: A Guidebook for the Beginning College Teacher, 8th edition. Lexington, MA, D. C. Heath, 1986

Schwenk T, Whitman N: The Physician as Teacher. Baltimore, MD, Williams & Wilkins, 1987

Weimer M, Neff RA: Teaching College, Collected Readings for the New Instructor. Madison, WI, Magna Publications, 1990

Medical Student Education

American Psychiatric Association: Teaching Psychiatry in Medical School: The Working Papers of the Conference on Psychiatry and Medical Education, 1967. Washington, DC, American Psychiatric Association, 1969

American Psychiatric Association: A Guideline for a Medical Student Curriculum in Psychiatry and Behavioral Science. Washington, DC, American Psychiatric Association, 1994

Kay J: The psychiatry club: enhancing the career choice of psychiatry. J Psychother Pract Res 50:62–63, 1984

Kay J: Child psychiatry recruitment and medical student education. Academic Psychiatry 13:208–212, 1989

Kris K: Distress precipitated by psychiatric training among medical students. Am J Psychiatry 143:1432–1435, 1986

Langsley DG, McDermott JF, Enelow AJ (eds): Mental Health Education in the New Medical Schools. San Francisco, CA, Jossey-Bass, 1973

Miller GE (ed): Teaching and Learning in Medical School. Cambridge, MA, Harvard University Press, 1961

Reiser LW, Sledge WH, Edelson M: Four-year evaluation of a psychiatric clerkship 1982–1986. Am J Psychiatry 145:1122–1126, 1988

Ross RH, Fineberg HV: Innovators in Physician Education: The Process and Pattern of Reform in North American Medical Schools, New York, Springer, 1996

Residency Training

Alpert MC: Videotaping psychotherapy. J Psychother Pract Res 5:93–105, 1996

American Psychiatric Association: Psychiatric Residents as Teachers. Washington, DC, American Psychiatric Association, 1989

Arif A, Westermeyer J: Guidelines for teaching in medical and health institutions, in Manual of Drug and Alcohol Abuse. Edited by Awni Arif and Joseph Westermeyer. New York, Plenum, 1988, pp 9–33

Borus JF, Groves JE: Training supervision as a separate faculty role. Am J Psychiatry 139:1339–1342, 1982

Bowden CL, Sledge WH, Humphrey FJ, et al: Educational objectives in psychiatric residency training: a survey of training directors and residents. Am J Psychiatry 140:1352–1355, 1983

Caligor E: Annotated psychodynamic bibliography for residents in psychiatry. J Psychother Pract Res 5:319–340, 1996

Katzelnick DJ, Gonzales JJ, Conley MC, et al: Teaching psychiatric residents to teach. Academic Psychiatry 15:153–159, 1991

Kay J: Handbook of Psychiatry Residency Training. Washington, DC, American Psychiatric Press, 1991

Kay J, Bienenfeld D: The role of the residency training director in psychiatric recruitment. Academic Psychiatry 16:127–133, 1992

Lewis JM: To Be a Therapist: The Teaching and Learning. New York, Brunner/Mazel, 1978

Lewis JM: Swimming Upstream. New York, Brunner/Mazel, 1991

Mohl PC, Lomax J, Tasman A, et al: Psychotherapy training for the psychiatrist of the future. Am J Psychiatry 147:7–13, 1990

Rao NR, Meinzer AE, Berman SS: Countertransference: its continued importance in psychiatric education. J Psychother Pract Res 6:1–11, 1997

Reiser MF: Are psychiatric educators "losing the mind"? Am J Psychiatry 145:148–153, 1988

Sacks MH, Sledge WH, Warren C: Core Readings in Psychiatry: An Annotated Guide to the Literature. Washington, DC, American Psychiatric Press, 1995

Yager J, Borus JF: A survival guide for psychiatric residency training directors. Academic Psychiatry 14:180–187, 1990

Yager J, Linn LS, Winstead DK, et al: Characteristics of journal clubs in psychiatric training. Academic Psychiatry 15:18–32, 1991

Supervision

Altshuler KZ: Common mistakes made by beginning therapists. Academic Psychiatry 13:73–80, 1989

Greben SE, Ruskin R (eds): Clinical Perspectives on Psychotherapy Supervision. Washington, DC, American Psychiatric Press, 1994

Kline F, Goin MK, Zimmerman W: You can be a better supervisor! Journal of Psychiatric Education 1:174–179, 1977

Rodenhauser P: Toward a multidimensional model for psychotherapy supervision. J Psychother Pract Res 3:1–15, 1994

Shanfield SB, Mohl PC, Matthews KL, et al: Quantitative assessment of the behavior of psychotherapy supervisors. Am J Psychiatry 149:352–357, 1992

Watkins CE: Psychotherapy supervisor development: on musings, models, and metaphor. J Psychother Pract Res 4:150–158, 1995

Teaching Portfolio Table of Contents

DEPARTMENT NAME
UNIVERSITY NAME

Source: Wright State University 1994.

Multisource Information for Appraising Faculty Performance

From Students
- an assessment of teaching skills, content and structure of the course
- workload
- teacher-student interactions
- organization of course material and clarity of its presentation
- student advising

From Faculty Peers
- a review of teaching materials (assignments, handouts, tests, papers)
- mastery and currency of subject matter
- original research
- professional recognition
- participation in the academic community
- interest in and concern for teaching
- service of the nonacademic community

From Administrators
- an appraisal of the workload and other responsibilities
- student course enrollment
- teaching improvement
- service to the institution

From the Professor
- self-appraisal as a teacher
- self-appraisal as a faculty member with added academic responsibilities
- illustrative course material
- evidence of professional accomplishment
- student advising
- committee memberships
- service to the academic community other than committees
- service to the nonacademic community
- professional recognition

Source: Seldin 1986.

3

Writing for Publication

Jonathan F. Borus, M.D.

Writing for publication has traditionally been an essential component of a successful career in academic medicine, and the infamous dictum "publish or perish" bespeaks the fact that in academic systems, promotion and tenure decisions are heavily influenced by a faculty member's publication record (Batshaw et al. 1988). In many universities and medical schools there is a hierarchy of "academic credit" given to different types of publications, with first-authored publication of original research reports in widely read, peer-reviewed journals usually having the highest valence, followed by significant non-first-authored papers and written (as opposed to edited) books that are broadly read and highly regarded. However, as academic medicine, finally, is recognizing the importance of the clinical care and educational infrastructures that support medical research, other types of publications and communications also have become important in recently initiated teacher-clinician, clinician-scholar, or other promotion tracks for full-time faculty not focused on research. Such communications include innovative program descriptions, review articles, chapters in books, edited books, continuing education materials, policy and procedure manuals, quality assurance and improvement materials, patient education materials, and so on. Regardless of the track, however, to build an academic psychiatry career some level of publication of one's findings, activities, programs, policies, and teaching materials is usually necessary for advancement.

The goal of this chapter is to help the reader become a better, smarter, more successful writer for publication in the professional literature. Although much of the focus is on writing articles for peer-reviewed journals, the same principles of writing, organization, and review generally pertain to most kinds of written communications in the field. I intend this chapter to be helpful to neophyte writers in getting "over the hump" and completing an article, submitting it, and revising their initial manuscripts into publishable form. Many junior faculty get "stuck" while writing their first papers, as they realize that their work is imperfect and fear it is not good enough to avoid criticism from reviewers. Experienced authors recognize that all research is incremental, all studies and the papers reporting them are imperfect, and critique in the review process can be helpful rather than devastating.

Why Write?

One obvious answer to the question "Why write?" is that, as mentioned in the last section, in many settings publishing is a prerequisite for academic advancement. However, an academic psychiatrist will want to learn to write for publication for many other important reasons. If you value the programs you design and implement, the ideas and understandings you gain from your clinical experiences, and any formal research studies you have undertaken, you will want to share these products of your creativity and hard work with others in the field. The broadest way to disseminate your ideas is through written materials that others near and far can read and apply to their own settings or experiences. Writing provokes feedback about your ideas, findings, and programs that can stimulate you to think further, learn more, and investigate in greater depth in light of the additional perspectives gained from others. In submitting a paper for publication, you will get feedback both from expert peer reviewers and, eventually, from peer readers who will compare your ideas against their experiences. Disseminating your ideas that corroborate or dispute others' work will lead, incrementally and cumulatively, to greater knowledge in our field.

A basic tenet in writing a paper is that it has to start with a good idea about an area, issue, or problem in which the writer is invested (Kahn 1994). Such investment stimulates the writer to study the area, implement a program, or delineate a process, the results of which are reported in a publication. If the problem, program, or process doesn't really matter to the writer, it will be hard to convey convincingly its worth to reviewers, the editor, and readers in a way that will likely have much impact. Writers may get "cold feet," feel lost, wonder how to organize their data, and question what possible value their findings could have to others at several phases in the course of research or program innovation. At such moments an author must press forward, trusting that if the study or program was important enough to do, other academic psychiatrists will benefit from hearing of and building on the author's experience.

How Are Papers Organized?

Papers in the medical and psychiatric literature follow a logical structure and often the same basic formula, which presents, in sequence, sections that introduce the area, describe the methods used, delineate the results found, and discuss the meaning of the findings (International Committee of Medical Journal Editors 1997). In addition, almost all journals require an abstract that summarizes the article's sections in a limited number of words.

The Introduction

The initial portion of the paper introduces the reader to the area in which the author is working. This usually includes a review of the relevant literature that leads up to and "sets the stage" for the study, program, or process that will be the focus of the report. This literature review points out gaps in the literature and explains where the author's contribution will fit. The introduction section usually ends with a statement of why the study is a next step in the literature and what it proposes to add to the knowledge base.

Methods

The methods section provides the reader with vital basic information about the setting of the study or program, the sample studied, the time frame in which the study occurred, the measures used to evaluate the issue being studied or to implement the process or program being described, the outcomes targeted, and the plan for analyzing the data obtained. The reader needs all of this information to evaluate how much credence to give the author's findings and to decide how far the data can be generalized to other settings and their own experience. A cardinal rule in undertaking psychiatric research is that it is always best to consult with a biostatistician and/ or psychometrician before undertaking a study to ensure that you investigate the most appropriate sample, use relevant measures, collect data that can be analyzed, and have a data analysis plan with the potential to find significant results. Most academic psychiatrists have had the disquieting experience early in their career of realizing that such consultation about methodological issues before conducting a study would have avoided their later being stuck with large amounts of extraneous data that they did not know how to analyze.

Results

In the results section the author describes the findings of the study, often through a combination of description in the text that highlights the prominent positive and negative findings, and tables that display a larger amount of the data than can be described in the text. Tables are an especially economical way to provide the breadth of information the reader will require to evaluate the findings and assign meaning to them. Tables also are helpful places to present nonsignificant findings that, in the long run, may be important to the advancement of the field.

Case reports, literature reviews, and conceptual papers often have a different "middle section" that substitutes for the formal methods and results sections of data-based papers. After a stage-setting introduction, this middle section describes the details of the case, synthesizes the findings of the literature, or explicates the conceptual hypothesis being proposed, which are the data and findings of such papers.

Discussion

In the discussion section the author summarizes the important findings and provides an understanding of what the data mean. This section describes what the findings add to the literature reviewed in the introduction, and the study's significance. Since all studies and papers are imperfect, the author will be wise to acknowledge the study's limitations to avoid overgeneralization of its significance and "head off" negative criticism by reviewers about these limitations. Most papers end with a delineation of the next steps necessary to build on the reported findings.

Building Your Case

Both in papers about empirical research studies as well as in more descriptive reports about programs, issues, or theories, the author structures the paper as described in the last section to lead logically up to what the findings mean and why they are important. Writing a paper is always a step-by-step "building project" intended to convince readers that they have made a good investment of their time in reading the paper because it incrementally advances their knowledge base. Providing frequent subheadings helps guide the reader and build the argument to show the logical progression of what is reported.

How and Where Should You Aim Your Paper?

Before you write the paper, you should come to a preliminary decision about where you would like it to be published and then "aim" it toward the appropriate journal. To do this intelligently you should first explore the wide variety of journals in psychiatry to know which are interested in the type of data you plan to report in your paper, whether they have published a similar paper in your area recently, and what are their publication requirements and style. If you send a descriptive article to a journal that only publishes manuscripts with "hard data" and p values, you are assuring yourself an unnecessary rejection (and every writer will experience more rejections than desired without purposely walking up blind alleys). Once you have decided which journal to submit to, you should carefully read the Information for Contributors guidelines (which every journal publishes at least once per year) to help prepare your article and references in the journal's preferred style.

A helpful way to get to know a journal is to review the abstracts in several issues to see what kinds of articles it takes, what content areas it is interested in, what methodologies it requires, and whether it has recently published something about your topic that would either make your paper a helpful next step or redundant. The American Psychiatric Association (APA) has published a helpful synopsis of much of this information for many of the major psychiatric journals (Psychiatric Research Reports 1997) (see Appendix 2–A). Doing this homework before submitting a paper can avoid unnecessary disappointment; some journals will automatically return papers without review that are not in their area of focus or that exceed the length expectations described in their Information for Contributors guidelines.

This exploration is important not only for selecting your first choice journal; if you are resubmitting a previously rejected article, it is vital that you read and revise your manuscript according to the second journal's Information for Contributors. Seeing an article clearly written in another journal's style tells the editor that his or her journal was (at least) your second choice. Different journals, for example, have different ways they wish to have references cited in the text (some use numbers, some use author names) and listed on the reference page, and a sure giveaway that either the author has not read the Information for Contributors or not bothered to change the manuscript when resubmitting it to a second, third, or fourth journal is that the references are incorrectly formatted.

There are additional reasons to carefully consider which journal you wish to aim your manuscript toward (Frank 1994). Journals have different academic rankings, and successful publication in some will give you more "credit" with promotions committees than others. These rankings are based on the perceived quality of the articles the journals publish, the breadth and size of their readership, the difficulty involved in having an article published in them (including their rejection rate), and the likelihood that an article published in a specific journal will be read and cited by others to make further scientific advancements. Some journals have specialized readerships in specific areas; you may choose to aim toward an audience you're particularly interested in reaching rather than a broader audience less focused on your area. In addition, journals have different review "habits," with some featuring speedy review while others may hold your manuscript literally for years before providing you feedback. Some journals will provide authors with multiple detailed critiques of the manuscript; others will provide almost no helpful feedback. A senior colleague should be able to help you aim your manuscript by providing advice about the academic ranking and usual review habits of particular journals. I recommend that authors submit first to the journal with the largest readership in the area that their manuscript describes, that is, "aim high rather than low." A rejection from an excellent journal that provides you with helpful reviews or, better yet, a request to revise with suggestions on how to improve the paper is a better investment for an author than acceptance in a bottom-tier journal that few people read and that will garner little academic credit. The only caveat is that submission to a prestigious journal that is unlikely to publish your article and has a lengthy review process may cause an inordinate delay in your resubmission to another journal in which you have a greater likelihood of publication; happily, many of the best journals provide rapid, detailed review.

The Review Process

After writing your paper in the style of the journal for which you are aiming, it is essential that you "prereview" your own manuscript. You and someone else you trust should carefully proofread the manuscript before it is submitted. Few things irritate reviewers more than being asked to read a manuscript with multiple typos and obvious errors that careful proofreading would have avoided. Finding such errors stimulates the reviewer to wonder whether you were similarly careless in conducting the study and analyzing the data. If you are a new writer, it will also help to have a more senior colleague review and edit your paper before you submit it. We all become enamored with the precious words to which we give birth, and it is difficult to see how our thesis could be stated in any other way; however, space in journals is precious, and editors always press to find the most economical way to present information. Although every writer should make an article as brief as possible to communicate important findings, a more-seasoned colleague often can help edit your manuscript to a point where it is more likely to be favorably received by the reviewers and editor. Finally, when you submit your manuscript, it should be accompanied by a cover letter to the editor that states the basic thesis of the article. This gives the editor an insight into your topic area and helps him or her select appropriate reviewers.

What Do Reviewers Look For?

When your article arrives at the journal, the editor will assign peer reviewers who, it is hoped, have both knowledge and experience in the area described in your manuscript. Journals have various ways of recruiting reviewer panels, but all ask their reviewers to designate specific content areas in which they have the expertise to knowledgeably review a paper. When reviewers are sent a manuscript, they are asked to disqualify themselves if they have any connection to the author or if they have any other conflict of interest in impartially reviewing a paper. Many journals provide "blind review," in which the authors' names, and all parts of the paper that might identify the authors to reviewers, are deleted. Blind review is an attempt to further decrease the likelihood that the authors' identities, rather than the article's scientific content and communicativeness, will sway the reviewers' evaluation of the article (Fisher et al. 1994; Laband and Piette 1994). In reality, no review is completely blind, because reviewers expert in a topic area usually know who else is working in that area, and careful scrutiny of the references often reveals, or narrows down, the identity of the authors. The editor, never blind to the author's identity, ultimately decides how much the author's reputation and past performance adds to (or detracts from) the credence of the results reported in a particular manuscript.

Reviewers look at an article both as a whole and through its component parts (Cotton 1993). They determine whether the information presented makes sense and adds to the area being studied (Abby et al. 1994; Kassirer and Campion 1994). They consider if the information is presented logically, the article is well organized, the content is interesting and meaningful, the points are clearly presented with a minimum of jargon, the method is clearly outlined and the results clearly stated, the analysis is appropriate to the data available, the generalizations fit the findings and do not go beyond the data displayed, the article answers the questions it purports to study, and so on. Reviewers also will determine whether the data in the text and tables are similar, and if the numbers in the table "add up"; they will ascertain whether the sample studied can appropriately produce the findings presented and justify the generalizations made from these findings; they will see whether the author goes beyond the data in making claims for the meaning of the study. It is helpful to ask senior colleagues who have served as reviewers to show you the review forms they are asked to complete for various journals to give you an idea of the areas on which your submission will be evaluated and the types of feedback requested of reviewers.

Reviews vary in their content and helpfulness to authors, and different journals require different types of feedback to authors. I believe that a journal can be most helpful to authors by providing detailed, positively and negatively critical reviews of each manuscript. Reviews that simply transmit positive or negative publication decisions are not helpful to the author, and since no paper is "perfect," all reviews should be able to describe ways the paper could be improved.

How Are Publication Decisions Made?

The actual publication decision is not in the hands of the reviewers but is the responsibility of the journal editor (Fletcher and Fletcher 1993). Reviewers are specifically instructed not to comment on the publishability of the paper in their feedback to authors, because, frequently, different reviewers have differing opinions on this point. Reviewers often transmit their thoughts about publication on a separate review page for the editor's eyes only; however, the editor must read the paper and, taking into account the comments of all reviewers, make the ultimate publication decision.

The editor has three choices: accept the manuscript as is, request revision, or reject the paper. Initial acceptance without revision is a rare editorial decision in good journals, and initially even the best papers usually receive conditional acceptance accompanied by a request that the authors carefully read the reviewers' feedback and integrate what they believe helpful into the final draft. Initial rejection is a more frequent decision for papers that do not meet the journal's basic standards of scientific acceptability, content relevance, or importance and significance. Every author must keep in mind that most journals ultimately reject more than 50% of all submissions and that the "most desirable" journals with the greatest number of submissions for always limited space have much higher rejection rates. A third initial editorial decision is to give the author the opportunity to revise or modify the paper in light of the reviewers' and editor's comments. The revision requested can be for a minor modification of a basically acceptable paper, or a major modification, without promise of publication, that includes requirements the author may or may not be able to meet, that is, to provide additional data, do additional analyses, and so on.

The Author's Response to the Initial Review Decision

The invitation to revise a paper should always be seen as an opportunity to learn from the reviews and resubmit a better paper. It is vital that authors carefully read the letter that comes from the editor, and the reviewers' comments, before deciding whether and how to respond. The editor's letter will indicate the reasons for a particular decision and, in the case of a request for revision, will often indicate the extent of the revision expected. A request to revise in no way implies a guarantee of publication, but it does suggest that the editor and reviewers feel that the paper, if properly revised, could be a credit to the journal. A request for revision is a sign that the journal is willing to work with you if you are willing to do the work it requests. Carefully reading an editor's letter and the reviewers' comments will also, hopefully, give you some idea why a manuscript was rejected. On rare occasions the author may feel that the reasons for rejection are totally without merit and/or demonstrate the reviewers' lack of expertise. In such cases it is helpful to have a senior colleague read the comments to see if he or she agrees; if so, it is worthwhile corresponding with the editor and, in a polite and detailed way, pointing out why you believe the review of your rejected manuscript was inaccurate or uninformed. If you can convince the editor, you may get a fresh evaluation by new reviewers.

If you have been asked to revise a manuscript, carefully respond in the text as best you can to *every* reviewer and editor suggestion if you believe they will improve the paper (Roberts et al. 1994). Then write a cover letter to the editor describing which suggestions you incorporated and which you did not, detailing your reasons for not heeding some of the reviewers' recommendations. For example, reviewers may have requested that you provide data that you have not collected or that you do a different study (often the one that would logically follow the one you've done). Pointing out that one cannot collect new data for this study but that the reviewer was helpful in describing logical steps for the next study will show the editor (and the reviewers, who, in many journals, eventually see your response) that you have attended to the comments even though you feel some requested changes cannot be made in this article.

Having one's manuscript not receive immediate acceptance is a narcissistic blow to even the most-experienced author. If you have been invited to revise the paper, put it at the *top* of your priority list, and make the revision as soon as possible. Revisions do not get easier with time, and, in fact, authors often feel more discouraged and see the review as more devastating the longer they wait before working again on the paper. Most requests for revision include some expectations you can meet and others you cannot, and the quicker you incorporate those which are possible to improve the paper, detail why you cannot incorporate the rest, and return the paper to the editor, the better chance you have of it not getting lost on your desk and losing an opportunity for publication.

It is important to realize that a rejection of your manuscript is not a rejection of you as an author. Every author has invested an enormous amount in undertaking a study, implementing a program, or analyzing a process, and then doing the hard work of communicating these efforts in journal article form for readers elsewhere. Getting feedback that a paper was not accepted can lead some authors to abandon important work, when the rejection occurred not because the paper's information was unimportant but because the paper was misaimed or had a peculiar review. If your article is rejected, carefully read through the comments, think about them as though you've been asked to revise the paper, incorporate into the manuscript those comments you believe will improve it, and then decide which journal to submit the article to next. In general, if you think that you have something interesting to convey, it is worthwhile to submit an article until you find a journal that will publish it. If, however, the reviews show you that what you have submitted is inevitably flawed and of lesser importance than you thought, and if your senior colleagues concur, move on to your next manuscript.

Consultation

Most academic departments have many seasoned writers with whom to consult, and I believe it is the responsibility of senior academics to teach junior faculty about writing, to review and critique their manuscripts in a helpful way, and to help them understand the "politics" of getting published. Many departments, including my own, have writing seminars in which faculty and trainees critique one another's manuscripts before submission and in response to feedback from reviewers, together learning to become better and more successful authors. Although at first it may seem daunting to expose a close to final draft to peers in your department, it is much better to get friends' critiques and incorporate them into an improved final product than to receive the same criticism from a journal's reviewers accompanied by an unfavorable editorial decision. It is also helpful for junior faculty to see that senior, experienced writers also get rejections, requests for revision, and so on and to see that they can be helpful in providing perspective and ideas that improve even "the professor's" papers. Some institutions also provide editorial services to help faculty authors organize, draft, and polish their manuscripts to produce clear and consistent prose, correct grammar and syntax, and clarity in communication of ideas.

Authorship

Institutions and journals have various rules governing issues of authorship. When many people work on a study, the thorny issue of multiple authorship arises, which can be the source of great conflict. I have delineated a set of rules for my department to try to avoid authorship warfare before it begins. I call my first rule of multiple authorship, having to do with the order of author citation (especially who will be the first author of any paper), "The Little Red Hen Rule"; the first author is the individual who has done the most work in conceiving and performing the study and takes the lead in writing up the results for publication. As in the children's tale, the person who has done the most work gets the greatest reward, first authorship, at "harvest time"; this is the person—who may not be the most academically senior member of the investigative team—who had the idea, formed the hypothesis, organized the study, analyzed the data, and took the lead in the successful completion of the study being reported. The first author has the responsibility for writing all drafts of the paper, incorporating feedback from coauthors who review the paper, and determining the final content and style of the paper to be submitted for publication. First authors are ultimately responsible for what gets submitted and have the right to accept or reject suggestions from coauthors; if coauthors have strong objections to the first author's final draft of the manuscript, they can delete their names from authorship. Unfortunately, there are still some laboratories and departments in which the most senior faculty member is automatically the first author, despite the fact that the person may not have taken the lead in producing the information reported by the manuscript; I believe that this practice is unfair and exploitive of junior faculty. Happily, most senior faculty are sufficiently generative to not appropriate the work of their junior colleagues and are satisfied to have their contribution noted elsewhere in the authorship line. It is also my belief that the order of additional authors should be determined by the amount of work each has done to complete the study and produce the submitted manuscript.

Such authorship issues are always best decided before the first word is written. Often large studies will provide many types of data that appropriately can be reported in more than one article; which of the investigators will take the lead and therefore be the first author on manuscripts reporting each part of the data should be decided early on, as should the likely order and inclusion of coauthors, because it is very difficult after the fact to determine appropriate authorship order.

The second rule I insist on is that an individual should only be an author on a manuscript describing work to which the person has made a substantive contribution; that is, the person has helped design the study or program, been part of the investigative team, and contributed to the manuscript by providing detailed review and critique of each draft prior to submission. Simply providing the setting for a study (e.g., being the clinical service chief or head of a laboratory) but having no clear involvement with the particular investigation reported does not merit authorship, nor does review and critique of an article by a senior faculty member who has not been involved in the study itself. Although both of these activities may contribute to the ultimate publication of an article, they do not deserve authorship.

How many authors should a paper have? Some journals set limits on the number of authors they will allow on any paper, and all attempt to eliminate "honorary authorships." A recent study questioned first authors of papers in leading journals about the contributions of their coauthors (Shapiro et al. 1994). This study found that 30% of clinical authors and

21% of basic science authors made no contributions to the intellectual tasks of research (conception, design, analysis and interpretation, and writing revisions). It must be remembered that being an author on a paper not only implies credit but also responsibility for what is submitted and published, and recent scandals of fraudulent research have led to retraction of articles, scientific humiliation, and public reprimand (Whitely et al. 1994). Never allow your name to be on an article in which you do not have the highest confidence of its scientific or programmatic merit and clear knowledge of its methodology, content, and appropriateness.

Books and Chapters

There are both advantages and disadvantages in writing books. As already discussed, most academic centers put the highest premium on peer-reviewed articles in prestigious and broadly read journals. However, writing for journals requires following a preset format and communicating ideas in very limited space. Writers may believe they have important ideas or findings that require much greater space than is available in a journal article, and therefore they decide to write a book. Book authors should remember that few books are best-sellers, and fewer yet are actually read. Unlike publications such as the *DSM* or successful multiauthored textbooks, most single-authored books in psychiatry sell only a few thousand copies, and many of the sold copies remain unread on bookshelves. The enormous amount of work required to write, edit, and revise a book must be measured against the likely influence it will have on the profession and reading public. In addition, unless a book has a pivotal influence on the field, it is not often given much importance by academic promotion committees. Early in my career a senior mentor advised me to not write a book until I was a full professor and to instead put my energies into writing journal articles and editing, activities more highly regarded academically within my university.

Edited books may seem easier than ones you write yourself, but they may not be. As editor, one asks others to contribute chapters, but it is the editor's responsibility to carefully mold these chapters into a readable text, eliminating redundancy, tightening the writing of all authors, and weaving the articles together into a cohesive whole. This can be a very time-consuming, and in many ways unrewarding, task. Edited textbooks are only profit makers if they fill a specific unmet need in the field and if they are well done and tightly edited.

Most faculty are called on to write chapters for edited books being put together by colleagues or senior leaders in the field. Unlike journal articles, which often focus on the addition of new knowledge to the field, book chapters are usually reviews of a topic area that integrate findings from many studies to provide the reader with the current state of an area. Book chapters require collation of others' work, synthesis of findings, and usually some comment on where the field is and where it will move next. Such reviews in top-line textbooks are frequently well read by students and trainees and often provide the writer with exposure and some prominence; however, contribution of chapters to less-read books only assure the writer of another citation on his or her curriculum vita and usually gather dust on bookshelves and remainder bins.

There are many considerations in deciding whether to write a chapter. A contribution to a well-read textbook in psychiatry may be worth the author's efforts, denoting the author as a national expert in a particular area. In addition, political considerations often convince a junior faculty member to write a chapter for an editor who can be helpful to one's academic career by, for example, writing a letter of recommendation at promotion time citing the author's important contribution to the prominent text. Since chapters in books rarely "count" as much as journal articles, authors must question the trade-off expending always limited time and writing energies on publications that will be less widely read and provide less credit for one's academic career.

Finally, in psychiatry as in other fields of medicine, there are a category of publications known as "throwaways." These include pseudojournals, monographs, or other publications sponsored by pharmaceutical companies, and newspapers or magazines printed for their advertising revenue. None are peer reviewed, and therefore they will not garner any academic credit for the writer. Although some throwaways will pay you for your writing, it is my experience that the monetary recompense is never worth the time and energy such publications remove from other writing endeavors.

Reviewing

A few words should be said about the learning opportunities available as a journal reviewer. Young writers will gain an immense amount if they have the opportunity to review others' papers. They will learn from other author's blind spots, writing problems, and methodologic deficits and can apply this learning to their own investigative and writing efforts. You can ask a senior colleague who reviews frequently to allow you to coreview an article to see how your review and theirs stack up. Many journals are looking for additional reviewers, and junior faculty should consult their senior colleagues to ascertain how to volunteer to be on a reviewer panel. Just as reviewing grant applications teaches the reviewer how to write a better grant, the opportunity to review manuscripts will provide the neophyte writer with a better understanding of the review process and how to write effectively.

References

Abby M, Massey MD, Galandiuk S: Peer review is an effective screening process to evaluate medical manuscripts. JAMA 272:105–107, 1994

American Psychiatric Association: Program profile: information on selected journals. Psychiatric Research Report of the American Psychiatric Association 13(3):2–7, Summer 1997

Batshaw ML, Plotnick LP, Petty BG, et al: Academic promotion at a medical school. Experience at Johns Hopkins University School of Medicine. N Engl J Med 318:741–747, 1988

Cotton P: Flaws documented, reforms debated at congress on journal peer review. JAMA 270:2775–2778, 1993

Fisher M, Friedman SB, Strauss B: The effects of blinding on acceptance of research papers by peer review. JAMA 272:143–146, 1994.

Fletcher RH, Fletcher SW: Who's responsible? Ann Intern Med 118:645–646, 1993

Frank E: Authors' criteria for selecting journals. JAMA 272:163–164, 1994

International Committee of Medical Journal Editors: Uniform requirements for manuscripts submitted to biomedical journals. Ann Intern Med 126:36–47, 1997

Kahn CR: Picking a research problem. N Engl J Med 330:1530–1533, 1994

Kassirer JP, Campion EW: Peer review: crude, and understudied, but indispensable. JAMA 272:96–97, 1994

Laband DN, Piette MJ: A citation analysis of the impact of blinded peer review. JAMA 272:147–149, 1994

Roberts JC, Fletcher RH, Fletcher SW: Effects of peer review and editing on the readability of articles published in Annals of Internal Medicine. JAMA 272:119–121, 1994

Shapiro DW, Wenger NS, Shapiro MF: The contributions of authors to multi-authored biomedical research papers. JAMA 271:438–442, 1994

Whitely WP, Rennie D, Hafner AW: The scientific community's response to evidence of fraudulent publication. JAMA 272:170–173, 1994

APPENDIX 3-A

*Those journals with an asterisk are indexed in *Index Medicus.*

Academic Medicine*
Association of American Medical Colleges
Aden S. Caelleigh, Editor
2450 N Street, N.W.
Washington, DC 20037
(202) 828–0590

Academic Psychiatry
American Association of Directors of Psychiatric Residency Training and
    Association for Academic Psychiatry
Sam Keith, M.D., Editor
American Psychiatric Press, Inc.
1400 K Street, N.W.
Washington, DC 20005
(202) 682–6310

Acta Psychiatrica Scandinavica*
Prof. Jan-Otto Ottosson, Editor
Department of Psychiatry
Sahlgrenska Hospital
S-41345 Gothenburg, Sweden
011–45–33–127030

Addictive Behaviors: An International Journal*
Dr. Peter M. Miller, Editor-in-Chief
Hilton Head Institute
Valencia Road In Shipyard Plantation
P.O. Box 7138
Hilton Head Island, SC 29938
(803) 785–7292

Reprinted from "Program Profile: Information on Selected Journals." *Psychiatric Research Report of the American Psychiatric Association* 13(3):2–7, Summer 1997. Used with permission.

Administration and Policy in Mental Health
Dr. Saul Feldman, Editor
Bay Area Foundation for Human Resources
850 California Street
San Francisco, CA 94108
(415) 652–1402, ext. 219

American Journal of Drug and Alcohol Abuse*
Edward Kaufman, M.D., Editor-in-Chief
33971 Selva Road, Suite 125
Dana Point, CA 92629
(914) 796–1919

American Journal of Forensic Psychiatry
American College of Forensic Psychiatry
Debra Miller, Editor
P.O. Box 5870
Balboa Island, CA 92662
(714) 831–0236

American Journal of Geriatric Psychiatry
American Association for Geriatric Psychiatry
Gene D. Cohen, M.D., Ph.D., Editor
American Psychiatric Press, Inc.
1400 K Street, N.W.
Washington, DC 20005
(202) 682–6336

American Journal of Law & Medicine*
American Society of Law & Medicine and Boston University School of Law
Frances H. Miller, J.D., Faculty Editor-in-Chief
765 Commonwealth Avenue, Suite 1672
Boston, MA 02215
(617) 353–2912

American Journal of Neuroradiology*
Juan M. Taveras, M.D., Editor
Department of Radiology
55 Fruit Street
Boston, MA 02114
(630) 574–0220

American Journal of Orthopsychiatry*
American Orthopsychiatric Association
Ellen L. Bassuk, M.D., Editor

330 Seventh Avenue, 18th Floor
New York, NY 10001
(212) 564–5930

American Journal of Psychiatry*
American Psychiatric Association
Nancy C. Andreasen, M.D., Ph.D., Editor
1400 K Street, N.W.
Washington, DC 20005
(202) 682–6020

American Journal of Psychoanalysis*
Association for the Advancement of Psychoanalysis
Douglas H. Ingram, Editor
329 East 62nd Street
New York, NY 1002
(212) 838–8014

American Journal of Psychotherapy*
Association for the Advancement of Psychotherapy
T. Byram Karasu, M.D., Editor-in-Chief
Belfer Center, Room 402
1300 Morris Park Road
Bronx, NY 10461
(212) 823–7754

American Journal of Public Health*
American Public Health Association
Mervyn Susser, Dr.P.H., Editor
1015 15th Street, N.W.
Washington, DC 20005
(202) 789–5661

American Journal on Addictions
American Academy of Psychiatrists in Alcoholism and Addictions
Sheldon I. Miller, M.D., Editor
American Psychiatric Press, Inc.
1400 K Street, N.W.
Washington, DC 20005
(202) 682–6310

American Psychologist
American Psychological Association
Raymond D. Fowler, Editor
750 First Street, N.E.

Washington, DC 20002–4242
(202) 336–6011

Annals of Clinical Psychiatry*
American Academy of Clinical Psychiatrists
Charles L. Rich, M.D., Editor-in-Chief
Department of Psychiatry
University of South Alabama
3421 Medical Park Drive West, Suite 2
Mobile, AL 36693
(212) 620–8466

Annals of Internal Medicine*
American College of Physicians
The Editor
Independence Mall West
Sixth Street at Race
Philadelphia, PA 19106–1572
(215) 351–2629

Anxiety*
Thomas Unde, Editor
605 3rd Avenue
New York, NY 10021
(212) 850–6645

Archives of General Psychiatry*
American Medical Association
Jack D. Barchas, M.D., Chief Editor
Department of Psychiatry
Cornell Medical Center
525 East 68th Street, Box 171
New York, NY 10021
(212) 746–3771

Archives of Neurology*
American Medical Association
Robert J. Joynt, M.D., Editor
University of Rochester School of Medicine
601 Elmwood Avenue
Rochester, NY 14642
(312) 464–5000

Australian and New Zealand Journal of Psychiatry*
Royal Australian and New Zealand College of Psychiatrists
Associate Prof. Sydney Bloch, Editor

Editorial Office
P.O. Box 378
Carlton, Victoria 3053
Australia
011–61–3-3470300

Behavioral Science: Journal of the International Society for the Systems Sciences*

International Society for the Systems Sciences and Institute of Management
    Sciences
James Grier Miller, Editor
P.O. Box 8369
La Jolla, CA 92038–8360
(619) 450–9163

Biological Psychiatry: A Journal of Psychiatric Research*

Society of Biological Psychiatry
Wagner Bridger, M.D., Editor-in-Chief
Medical College of Pennsylvania, EPPI
3200 Henry Avenue
Philadelphia, PA 19129–1137
(215) 842–4146

BMJ: British Medical Journal*

British Medical Association
Richard Smith, Editor
Tavistock Square
London WC1H 9JR, UK
071–387–4499

Brain and Cognition*

Harry A. Whitaker, Jr., M.D., Editor
525 B Street, Suite 1900
San Diego, CA 92101–4495
(407) 345–4100

Brain and Language*

Harry A. Whitaker, Jr., M.D., Editor
525 B Street, Suite 1900
San Diego, CA 92101–4495
(407) 345–4100

British Journal of Psychiatry*

Royal College of Psychiatrists
The Editor

17 Belgrave Square
London SW1X 8PG, UK01–235–8857

Bulletin of the American Academy of Psychiatry and the Law*
American Academy of Psychiatry and the Law
Seymour L. Halleck, M.D., Editor-in-Chief
Department of Psychiatry
University of North Carolina, CB 7160
Medical School Wing D
Chapel Hill, NC 27514
(410) 539–0379

Bulletin of the History of Medicine*
American Association for the History of Medicine and John Hopkins Institute
    of the History of Medicine
Gert H. Brieger and Jerome J. Bylebyl, Editors
1900 East Monument Street
Baltimore, MD 21205
(410) 955–3179

**Bulletin of the Menninger Clinic: A Journal for the Mental Health
Professions***
Menninger Clinic
Philip R. Beard, M.Div., M.A., Managing Editor
P.O. Box 829
Topeka, KS 66601–0829
(913) 273–7500

Canadian Journal of Psychiatry*
Canadian Psychiatric Association
Edward Kingstone, Editor
Suite 200, 237 Argyle Street
Ottawa, Ontario K2P 1B8
Canada
(613) 234–2815

Cerebal Cortex*
P.S. Goldman-Rakic or P. Rakic, Co-Editors
Section of Neurobiology
Yale University School of Medicine, SHM
P.O. Box 208001
New Haven, CT 06520–8001
(919) 677–0977

CMAJ: Canadian Medical Association Journal*
Canadian Medical Association
John Hoey, M.D., Editor-in-Chief
1867 Alta Vista Drive
Ottawa, Ontario K1G 3Y6
Canada
(613) 731–9331

CNS Spectrums: The International Journal of Neuropsychiatric Medicine
Eric Hollander, M.D.
Mt. Sinai School of Medicine
Box 1230
One Gustave Levy Place
New York, NY 10029
(212) 241–3623

Community Mental Health Journal*
National Council of Community Mental Health Centers
David L. Cutler, M.D., Editor
Department of Psychiatry OPO2
Oregon Health Sciences University
3181 Sam Jackson Park Road
Portland, OR 97201
(212) 620–8461

Comprehensive Psychiatry*
American Psychopathological Association
David L. Dunner
University of Washington
Outpatient Psychiatry Center
4225 Roosevelt Way, N.E., Suite 306
Seattle, WA 98105
(206) 543–6768

Convulsive Therapy*
Jill Filler, Administrating Editor
1803 Research Boulevard, Suite 300
Rockville, MD 20850
(803) 792–0053

Corrective and Social Psychiatry and Journal of Behavior Technology Methods and Therapy
American Association of Mental Health Professionals in Corrections
Clyde V. Martin, M.D., M.A., J.D., Editor
Martin Psychiatric Research Foundation

P.O. Box 3365
Fairfield, CA 94533
(707) 864–0910

Culture, Medicine and Psychiatry*
Byron J. Good, Ph.D., and Mary-Jo DelVecchio Good, Ph.D., Editors-in-Chief
Department of Social Medicine
Harvard Medical School
641 Huntington Avenue
Boston, MA 02115
(617) 432–0716

Depression*
Charles B. Nemeroff, M.D.
Department of Psychiatry and Behavioral Sciences
Emory University School of Medicine
1639 Pierce Drive, Suite 4000, Drawer AF
Atlanta, GA 30322–4990
(404) 727–5881

Dreaming: Journal of the Association for the Study of Dreams
Association for the Study of Dreams
Earnest Hartmann, M.D., Editor
Tufts University School of Medicine
27 Clark Street
Newton, MA 02159–2425
(617) 965–5872

European Journal of Psychiatry
Prof. A. Swva, Editor-in-chief
P.O. Box 6029
50080 Saragosse, Spain
976–279402

Family Process*
Peter Steinglass, M.D., Editor
149 East 79th Street
New York, NY 10021
(201) 764–1026

General Hospital Psychiatry: Psychiatry, Medicine and Primary Care*
Don R. Lipsitt, M.D., Editor-in-Chief
Department of Psychiatry
Mount Auburn Hospital

330 Mt. Auburn Street
Cambridge, MA 02238
(617) 499–5008

Harvard Review of Psychiatry*
Shelley F. Greenfield, M.D., Deputy Editor
McLean Hospital
115 Mill Street
Belmont, MA 02178
(617) 855–3396

Hastings Center Report*
Hastings Center
Bette-Jane Crigger, Editor
255 Elm Road
Briarcliff Manor, NY 10510
(914) 762–8500, ext. 222

Health Services Research*
American College of Healthcare Executives
Sheryl Lilke, Editor
One North Franklin Street, Suite 1700
Chicago, IL 60606
(312) 424–2800, ext. 3000

Hospital & Health Services Administration
Foundation of the American College of Healthcare Executives
Richard S. Kurz, Editor
3663 Lindell Boulevard
Saint Louis University School of Public Health
Saint Louis, MO 63108–8684
(314) 577–8682

Infant Mental Health Journal
International Association for Infant Mental Health, World Association for
    Infant Psychiatry and Allied Disciplines, and Michigan Association for
    Infant Mental Health
Joy D. Osofsky, Ph.D., Editor
Louisiana State University Medical School
1542 Tulane Avenue
New Orleans, LA 70112–2822
(203) 868–7585

International Journal of Group Psychotherapy*
American Group Psychotherapy Association
William E. Piper, Ph.D., Editor

25 East 21st Street, 6th Floor
New York, NY 10010
(212) 477–2677

International Journal of Law and Psychiatry*
International Academy of Law and Mental Health
David N. Weisstub, Editor-in-Chief
Université de Médicine, C.P. 6128
Succursale A
Montreal, Quebec H3C 3J7
Canada
(514) 343–5938

International Journal of Psychiatry in Medicine: Biopsychosocial Aspects of Primary Care*
Thomas E. Oxman, M.D., Editor
Department of Psychiatry
Dartmouth-Hitchcock Medical Center
One Medical Center Drive
Lebanon, NH 03756
(516) 691–1270

International Journal of Psycho-Analysis*
Institute of Psycho-Analysis
for submissions from the U.S.:
Arnold Cooper, M.D.
50 East 78th Street, Suite 1C
New York, NY 10021
(212) 879–7182
for submissions from outside the U.S.:
David Tuckett, Editor
63 New Cavendish Street
London W1M 7RD, UK
011–44–171–5804952

Journal of the American Medical Association*
American Medical Association
George D. Lundberg, M.D., Editor
515 North State Street
Chicago, IL 60610
(312) 464–2400

Jefferson Journal of Psychiatry: A Resident Publication
Residency Training Program of the Department of Psychiatry of Jefferson
Medical College and the Committee of Residents and Fellows of the APA

Carmen Z. Harlan, M.D., Chief Editor
1025 Walnut Street, Third Floor
Philadelphia, PA 19107

Journal of Abnormal Psychology*
American Psychological Association
Milton E. Strauss, Incoming Editor
Department of Psychiatry
Case Western Reserve University
10900 Euclid Avenue
Cleveland, OH 44106–7123
(216) 336–5600

Journal of Affective Disorders*
Prof. H. S. Akiskl, Editor-in-Chief
University of California at San Diego
VA Medical Center-Psychiatry (116A)
3350 La Jolla Village Drive
San Diego, CA 92161

Journal of Applied Behavioral Science
NTL Institute for Applied Behavioral Science
Clayton P. Alderfer, Editor
Rutgers Graduate School of Applied and Professional Psychology
P.O. Box 819
Piscataway, NJ 08855–0819
(805) 499–0721

Journal of Behavior Therapy and Experimental Psychiatry*
Behavior Therapy and Research Society
Joseph Wolpe, M.D., Editor
Department of Psychology
Pepperdine University
Graduate School of Education and Psychology
400 Corporate Pointe
Culver City, CA 90230
(310) 568–5753

Journal of Cerebral Blood Flow and Metabolism*
Dr. Myron D. Ginsberg, Editor
Department of Neurology (D4–5)
University of Miami School of Medicine
P.O. Box 016960
Miami, FL 33136
(215) 238–4200

Journal of Child and Adolescent Psychopharmacology
Charles W. Popper, M.D., Editor
McLean Hospital
115 Mill Street
Belmont, MA 02178–9106
(617) 855–2843

Journal of Child Psychology and Psychiatry and Allied Disciplines*
Association for Child Psychology and Psychiatry
Judith L. Rapoport, Corresponding Editor
Child Psychiatry Branch
NIMH, Bldg. 10, Rm. 6N240
9000 Rockville Pike
Bethesda, MD 20892

Journal of Clinical Psychiatry*
American Academy of Clinical Psychiatrists
Physician Postgraduate Press
P.O. Box 752870
Memphis, TN 38175–2870
(901) 682–1001

Journal of Clinical Psychoanalysis
New York Psychoanalytic Institute and Society
Herbert M. Wyman, M.D. and Stephen M. Rittenberg, M.D., Co-Editors
200 East 59th Street
New York, NY 10128
(212) 534–5565

Journal of Clinical Psychology*
Kenneth J. Howard, Co-Editor
Department of Psychology
Northwestern University
Evanston, IL 60208
(212) 850–6645

Journal of Clinical Psychopharmacology*
Richard I. Schader, M.D., Editor-in-Chief
Department of Pharmacology and Experimental Therapeutics
Tufts University School of Medicine
136 Harrison Avenue
Boston, MA 02111
(617) 956–0178

Journal of Consulting and Clinical Psychology*
American Psychological Association
Philip C. Kendall, Editor
Department of Psychology
Weiss Hall
1701 North 13th Street
Temple University
Philadelphia, PA 19122–6085
(202) 336–5600

Journal of Contemporary Psychotherapy
Long Island Institute for Mental Health
Erwin R. Parson, Ph.D., Editor-in-chief
P.O. Box 62
Perry Point, MD 21902–0062
(212) 620–8000

**Journal of Geriatric Psychiatry and Neurology: An
Interdisciplinary Forum for Clinicians and Scientists***
Alzheimer's Foundation
Michael A. Jenike, M.D.
Massachusetts General Hospital East
13th Street, Bldg. 149, Ninth Floor
Charlestown, MA 02129
(617) 726–2998

Journal of Group Psychotherapy, Psychodrama and Sociometry
American Society of Group Psychotherapy And Psychodrama
Helen Kress, Managing Editor
HELDREF Publications
1319 18th Street, N.W.
Washington, DC 20036–1802

Journal of International Medical Research*
R.J. Kasprowicz, European Coordinator
Wicker Hours
High Street
Worthington, West Sussex
BN11 1DJ, UK
01–903–205884

Journal of Marital and Family Therapy
American Association for Marriage and Family Therapy
Froma Walsh, Ph.D., Editor-Elect
Center for Family Health

University of Chicago
969 East 60th Street
Chicago, IL 60637
(202) 452–0109

Journal of Marriage and the Family
National Council on Family Relations
Robert Milardo, Editor
Human Development and Family Studies
30 Merrill Hall
University of Maine
Orono, ME 04469–5749
(207) 581–3103

Journal of Mental Health Administration
Association of Mental Health Administrators
Bruce Lubotsky Levin, Dr.P.H., FAMHA, Editor
Mental Health Institute
University of South Florida
13301 Bruce B. Downs Boulevard
Tampa, FL 33612–3899
(813) 974–6400

Journal of Nervous and Mental Disease*
Eugene B. Brody, M.D., Editor-in-Chief
Sheppard and Enoch Pratt Hospital
6501 North Charles Street
Baltimore, MD 21285–6815

Journal of Neurology, Neurosurgery and Psychiatry*
British Medical Association
Prof. C. Kennard, Editor
Charing Cross Hospital
Fulham Palace Road
London W6 8RF, UK
0181–846–1213

Journal of Neuropsychiatry and Clinical Neurosciences*
American Neuropsychiatric Association
Stuart C. Yudofsky, M.D., Editor
American Psychiatric Press, Inc.
1400 K Street, N.W.
Washington, DC 20005
(202) 682–6310

Journal of Neuroscience*
David C. Van Essen, M.D., Editor-in-Chief
Box 8108
Washington University School of Medicine
660 South Euclid Avenue
St. Louis, MO 63310

Journal of Pastoral Care
Orlo Strunk, Jr., Managing Editor
1068 Harbor Drive, S.W.
Calabash, NC 28467
(404) 320–1472

Journal of Practical Psychiatry and and Behavioral Health
John M. Oldham, M.D., Editor
Department of Psychiatry
Columbia University
New York State Psychiatric Institute
722 West 168th Street
New York, NY 10032
(212) 960–2300

Journal of Preventive Psychiatry and Allied Disciplines
Center for Preventive Psychiatry
Gilbert W. Kliman, M.D., Editor-in-Chief
Psychological Trauma Center
Preventive Psychiatry Associates Medical Group, Inc.
1010 Sir Francis Drake Boulevard
Kentfield, CA 94904

Journal of Psychiatric Research*
John F. Greden, M.D., and Florian Holsboer, M.D., Ph.D., Editors-in-Chief
Department of Psychiatry
University of Michigan
1500 E. Medical Center Drive, B2964/0704
Ann Arbor, MI 48109–0704
(313) 763–9629

Journal of Psychiatry and Law
Dianne Nashel, Managing Editor
149 Oak Street
Tenafly, NJ 07670
(201) 569–5332

Journal of Psychiatry & Neuroscience*
Canadian College of Neuropsychopharmacology
Editorial Office
237 Argyle Avenue, Suite 200
Ottawa, Ontario K2P 1B8
Canada
(613) 234–2815

Journal of Psychotherapy Practice and Research*
Jerald Kay, M.D., Editor
American Psychiatric Press, Inc.
1400 K Street, N.W.
Washington, DC 20005
(202) 682–6310

Journal of Studies on Alcohol*
Center of Alcohol Studies, Rutgers University
Patricia Castellano, Editorial Secretary
P.O. Box 969
Piscataway, NJ 08855–0969
(908) 932–2190

Journal of Substance Abuse Treatment*
North Shore University Hospital-Cornell University Medical College
John E. Imhof, Ph.D., Editor-in-Chief
Division of Addiction Treatment Services
Department of Psychiatry
400 Community Drive
Manhasset, NY 11030
(516) 562–3008

Journal of the American Academy of Child and Adolescent Psychiatry*
American Academy of Child and Adolescent Psychiatry
Mina Dulcan, M.D., Editor
Children's Memorial Hospital
2300 Children's Plaza #156
Chicago, IL 60614–3394
(410) 528–4000

Journal of the American Academy of Psychoanalysis*
American Academy of Psychoanalysis
Jules R. Bemporad, M.D., Editor
47 East 19th Street, 6th Floor
New York, NY 10003
(212) 475–7980

Journal of the American Geriatrics Society*
American Geriatrics Society
William B. Applegate, M.D.
66 North Pauline, Suite 633
Memphis, TN 38105
(901) 448-5567

Journal of the American Medical Women's Association*
American Medical Women's Association
Wendy Chavkin, M.D., Editor-in-Chief
Chemical Dependency Institute
Beth Israel Medical Center
215 Park Avenue South
New York, NY 10003
(703) 838–0500

Journal of the American Psychoanalytic Association*
Anerican Psychoanalytic Association
Arnold D. Richards, M.D., Editor
200 East 89th Street
New York, NY 10128–4300
(203) 245–4000

Mental Retardation*
American Association on Mental Retardation
Steven J. Taylor, Editor
Center on Human Policy School of Education
Syracuse University
200 Huntington Hall
Syracuse, NY 13244–2340
(516) 482–0341

Molecular Psychiatry*
Julio Lucinio
CNE, NIMH, NIH
Building 10, Room 2046
10 Center Drive MSC 1284
Bethesda, MD 20892–1284
(301) 496–6885

Nature*
Editor
968 National Press Building
Washington, DC 20045–1938
(212) 726–9200

Neuropsychiatric Genetics*: A Section of the American Journal of Medical Genetics*
MingT. Tsuang, M.D., Ph.D., Section Editor
1280-A Belmont Street, Suite 192
Brockton, MA 02401
(508) 582–4500, ext. 729

Neuropsychopharmacology*
American College of Neuropsychopharmacology
H. Christian Fibiger, Ph.D., Co-Editor-in-Chief
Department of Psychiatry
Division of Neurological Sciences
University of British Columbia
2255 Westbrook Mall
Vancouver, British Columbia V6T 1Z3
Canada
(212) 633–3950

New England Journal of Medicine*
Massachusetts Medical Society
Jerome D. Kassirer, M.D., Editor-in-Chief
10 Shattuck Street
Boston, MA 02115–6094
(617) 734–9800

New Trends in Experimental and Clinical Psychiatry
Prof. Giordano Invernizzi
Institute of Psychiatry
Policinico-Pad. Guardia 2
Via Francesco Sforza 35
20122, Milan, Italy
011–39–6–8412673

Occupational Therapy in Mental Health
Marie-Louise F. Blount, Co-Editor
New York University
Department of Occupational Therapy
35 West Fourth Street, 11th Floor
New York, NY 10012–1172
(607) 722–2493

Psychiatric Bulletin of the Royal College of Psychiatrists
Royal College of Psychiatrists
Dr. Alan Kerr, Editor
17 Belgrave Square
London SW1X 8PG, UK
071–408–2119

Psychiatric Genetics*
International Society of Psychiatric Genetics
John. I. Nurnberger, M.D., Ph.D., Editor
Institute of Psychiatric Research 791 Union Drive
Indiana University Medical Center
Indaianapolis, IN 46202–4887
(317) 274–8382

Psychiatric Services*
American Psychiatric Association
John A. Talbott, M.D., Editor
1400 K Street, N.W.
Washington, DC 20005
(202) 682–6070

Psychiatric Quarterly*
Stephen Rachlin, M.D., Editor-in-Chief
P.O. Box 117H
Scarsdale, NY 10583
(212) 620–8000

Psychiatry: Interpersonal and Biological Processes*
Washington School of Psychiatry
David Reiss, M.D., Editor
Department of Psychiatry and Behavioral Sciences
George Washington University Medical Center
2300 Eye Street, N.W.
Washington, DC 20037
(202) 994–2636

Psychiatry Research* and Psychiatry Research: Neuroimaging*
Monte S. Buchsbaum, M.D., Editor-in-Chief
Department of Psychiatry
Munt Sinai School of Medicine
P.O. Box 1505
One Gustave L. Levy Place
New York, NY 10029–6574

Psychoanalytic Study of the Child*
Albert J. Solnit, M.D., Managing Editor
Yale Child Study Center
P.O. Box 3333
New Haven, CT 06510
(203) 785–2518

Psychological Medicine: A Journal for Research in Psychiatry and the Allied Sciences*
Prof. Eugene Paykel
Department of Psychiatry
University of Cambridge
Addenbrooke's Hospital
Cambridge, CB2 2QQ, UK

Psychological Record
Kenyon College
Charles E. Rice, Editor
Gambier, OH 43022
(614) 427–5377

Psychoneuroendocrinology*
Dr. Ned H. Kalin
Department of Psychiatry
Suite 1224
University of Wisconsin Medical School
6001 Research Park Boulevard
Madison, WI 53719

Psychomatic Medicine*
American Psychosomatic Society
Joel E. Dimsdale, M.D., Editor-in-Chief
University of California, San Diego
9500 Gilman Drive
La Jolla, CA 92093–0804
(619) 543–5468

Psychosomatics: The Journal of Consultation and Liaison Psychiatry*
Academy of Psychosomatic Medicine
Thomas N. Wise, M.D., Editor-in-Chief
American Psychiatric Press, Inc.
1400 K Street, N.W.
Washington, DC 20005
(202) 682–6336

Schizophrenia Bulletin*
National Institute of Mental Health
John K. Hsiao, M.D., Editor-in-Chief
Parklawn Building, Room 18C-06
5600 Fishers Lane
Rockville, MD 20857
(202) 275–3328

Schizophrenia Research*
for submissions from the Americas:
Prof. H. A. Nasrallah, Co-Editor
Department of Psychiatry
OSU College of Medicine
473 West 12th Avenue
Columbus, OH 43210–1228
(614) 293–8283
for submissions from outside the Americas:
Dr. L. E. DeLisi, Co-Editor
Department of Psychiatry
School of Medicine
Health Sciences Center, SUNY
Stony Brook, NY 11794

Science*
American Association for the Advancement of Science
Floyd Bloom, Editor-in-Chief
1333 H Street, N.W.
Washington, DC 20005
(202) 326–6501

Treatment
The American Psychological Association and the American Psychiatric
    Association
Donald F. Klein, M.D., and Martin P. Seligman, Ph.D., Editors
www.journals.apa.org/treatment

4

Women in Academic Psychiatry

Ellen Leibenluft, M.D.

Psychiatrists who choose to embark on an academic career face many challenges; which of these challenges are unique, or especially burdensome, for women? This chapter will attempt to answer this question and to outline individual and collective strategies that women (and the men who support their efforts) can use to confront the obstacles and barriers that they face.

Challenges Facing Women in Academic Psychiatry: The Data

These are difficult times for all academic physicians. When a female academic psychiatrist encounters adverse events, how can she distinguish those caused by her gender from the usual lumps and bumps of academic life? Group data can help to answer this question, and so the chapter begins with a brief review of the available data concerning gender differences in academic careers. However, it must be acknowledged that these data have significant limitations. Studies of gender differences in academic careers are aimed at a moving target, because momentous changes are occurring now in both academic medicine and in societal attitudes about gender roles. In addition, it is easier to describe a phenomenon than to learn why it occurs. Thus, the data can help to define problem areas, but we will have to overstep it when we discuss strategies for success.

In reviewing the available data, it is helpful to examine seven areas: recruitment, retention, research and publications, rank, the glass ceiling, salary, and sexual harassment (Table 4–1). Beginning with recruitment, the most recent cross-sectional study of psychiatrists' professional activities found that the number of female psychiatrists on university and medical school faculties is 77% of what would be expected if women were represented proportionately in these settings (Dial et al. 1994). However, if one examines younger cohorts of faculty, the proportion of female academic psychiatrists more nearly reflects the proportion of female psychiatrists. For example, in a recent survey of psychiatric faculty, 26% of the psychiatric faculty who had graduated medical school between 1976 and 1985 were female (Leibenluft et al. 1993a), compared with 27% of all the psychiatrists who graduated medical school in those years (APA, unpublished data). Therefore, it appears that women are now being recruited into academic psychiatry in representative numbers.

Once women are hired onto a faculty, how do their career paths differ from those of their male peers? A preliminary study of retention found that female psychiatrists who had first been hired in 1978 were less likely than their male peers to still be on faculty in 1989, but the sample was small and the difference was not statistically significant ($p = 0.12$) (Leibenluft et al. 1993b). In terms of their academic activities while on faculty, it is clear that women in academic psychiatry are less likely than men to do research or to have peer-reviewed grants, and that women publish fewer papers than men (Leibenluft et al. 1993a). Further, these gender differences exist in cohorts of relatively young faculty, despite the fact that the women in the young cohorts are as likely as the men to have had research training. Among psychiatric faculty who do not do research, women were more likely than men to cite "lack of time" and "lack of a mentor" (but not "lack of interest") as reasons for not doing research (Leibenluft et al. 1993a).

Table 4–1. Gender differences in academic psychiatry: variables of interest

1. Recruitment into academic careers
2. Retention in academia
3. Research activity and publications
4. Academic rank
5. "The glass ceiling"
6. Salary
7. Sexual harassment

An analysis of academic rank among psychiatric faculty shows marked and consistent gender differences across all cohorts, with men overrepresented at the professor and associate professor levels, and women overrepresented at the instructor and assistant professor levels (Leibenluft et al. 1993a). This cohort analysis, accounting as it does for seniority, demonstrates that the gender difference in rank is not simply the result of the recent influx of women into medicine.

An obvious question is whether the gender differences in research activities and publications account for the gender differences in rank; to the extent that they do not, this would be evidence of a "glass ceiling." Although it is extremely difficult to prove the existence of a glass ceiling because of the complexities involved in matching men and women on all of the variables that may affect career advancement (publications, institutional prestige, administrative experience, etc.), there is suggestive evidence that a glass ceiling may exist in academic psychiatry. In the previously mentioned survey of research activities among psychiatric faculty, individuals in the three oldest cohorts (those who graduated medical school before 1976) had been on faculty for a minimum of 13 years (Leibenluft et al. 1993a). In these cohorts, 15% of the respondents were women, and women constituted 10% of the individuals who met the study's criteria for "full" researchers. However, while these senior women were relatively productive in terms of research and publications, they constituted only 5% of the professors and 2% of the department chairs. This analysis is obviously quite preliminary, but it does suggest that the question of a glass ceiling in academic psychiatry merits further study.

With regard to salary, a recent multivariate analysis of data from the APA Biographical Survey found that, after a number of relevant variables were controlled, the salary difference due to gender among psychiatrists overall was $15,000 (with women receiving less pay) (Dial et al. 1994). A gender analysis of academic psychiatrists' salaries has not been done, and studies that show lower pay among female than male physicians are generally confounded by differences in specialty, seniority, and hours worked. Nonetheless, a number of studies in various professions, including science, show that women are generally paid less than men doing comparable work.

Similarly, there are no published studies of sexual harassment in academic psychiatry. However, a number of studies of female medical students, residents, and faculty have reported high rates of sexual harassment and discrimination (Charney and Russell 1994). In a survey of female physicians at all levels of training and in practice, female psychiatrists reported experiencing lower levels of harassment than other female physicians, although the numbers were still considerable. Twelve percent (12%) of female psychiatrists reported experiencing harassment, compared with 50% of female surgeons, 37% of internists, and 25% of pediatricians and obstetrician-gynecologists (Lenhart et al. 1991).

In sum, this review indicates that a woman graduating psychiatric residency today is probably as likely as a male colleague to be offered an academic position. However, she is less likely than her male peer to advance through the academic ranks, and she is less likely to participate in research and publishing, the academic activities that, at least historically, have been most highly rewarded. It may be particularly difficult for her to enter the highest echelons of the profession. Further, at each stage in her career, she may encounter sexual harassment, and she would be wise to ascertain that she is receiving pay comparable to that of her male peers.

These data for academic psychiatry are similar to those that have been published in many other academic and scientific fields. In general, studies show a lack of gender equity in rank and pay, and decreased research activity and publications among women, compared with men. In attempting to understand these gender disparities, investigators have contrasted the "deficit" and "difference" models (Sonnert and Hofton 1995). Whereas the deficit model emphasizes external obstacles confronting women (women don't succeed because they are treated differently), the difference model emphasizes characteristics of women's behavior that hamper success (women don't succeed because they act differently). Of course, both internal and external factors can be active at the same time, and we know that women who are treated differently will eventually act differently (that is, after all, what we call socialization). Nonetheless, a woman confronting difficulties in her career may find it helpful to analyze her dilemma in terms of the relative contributions of "deficit" (the treatment she's receiving) and "difference" (her own behavior).

Confronting the Challenges: Individual Strategies

What steps can an individual woman take to increase her chances for academic success? This discussion focuses on five action-oriented strategies (Table 4–2): (1) giving serious consideration to acquiring research training and experience; (2) developing a focus and setting priorities; (3) think-

Table 4–2. Strategies for success

---

1. Consider acquiring research training and experience.
2. Develop a focus and use it to set priorities.
3. Analyze how you and your colleagues express (and respond to) aggression, competition, and self-doubt.
4. Develop relationships with role models and mentors.
5. Be a creative problem solver.

---

ing through issues concerning aggression, competitive drive, and self-confidence; (4) developing relationships with role models and mentors; and (5) engaging in creative problem solving.

Research Training and Experience

Historically, the criteria for academic promotion have centered on research activities and publications; as we have seen, women are less likely than men to be successful when judged by these criteria. It is possible that the importance of research and publications in an academic career may diminish as academic medical centers derive a greater proportion of their income from patient care and a smaller percentage from grant funding. However, despite these financial shifts, it is likely that research productivity will always be an important factor in promotion decisions, especially to the more prestigious and powerful positions.

Studies show that research training is generally the most important predictor of research productivity (Pincus et al. 1993); however, for women, research training appears to be a necessary but not sufficient condition for success. That is, women with research training still lag behind men with the same training in terms of rank, grants, number of publications, and so on. To explain findings such as these in academic psychiatry and other fields, investigators have developed a number of hypotheses; for example, the existence of an "old-boy" network in research deprives women of effective mentoring and excludes them from opportunities; the responsibilities of home and children have a greater impact on women's careers than on men's; there is a mismatch between aggressive, competitive research environments and women's socialization. Strategies to address each of these potential problems will be offered in the following sections, when we discuss setting priorities, dealing with competition, and acquiring mentors. In addition, other chapters in this *Handbook* outline actions both men and women can take to establish a research career. Our purpose here is simply to encourage women to acquire research training, to place a high priority on research activities, and to address actively any barriers to research productivity that they may experience. Although it may be possible to succeed in academia without research training or experience, it is certainly easier to do so with that training and experience.

Develop a Focus and Set Priorities

Both male and female faculty members experience anxiety and burnout from feeling pulled in too many directions. However, most observers believe that this problem is particularly acute for women because, in most families, women still assume primary responsibility for child care and housekeeping responsibilities. Many investigators have examined whether marriage and children decrease a woman's research productivity, and their results have been consistently negative (Zuckerman 1991). Nonetheless, both these investigators and women scientists themselves have noted that simple univariate analyses of, for example, numbers of publications and marital status, do not do justice to the complexity of the issue. It is possible (if not likely) that marriage and children have an impact on both men's and women's careers, but the precise nature of the impact probably depends on several factors, such as the demands of the spouse's work, availability of financial resources, the negotiation of shared responsibilities, children's needs, and so on.

Certainly, when academic women gather, the talk frequently turns to balancing the demands of career and family, and most successful women appear to be both very energetic and frequently fatigued. In discussing coping mechanisms, several themes emerge (Table 4–3). The first of these is the need to relinquish the fantasy that you can meet all of the competing demands that one faces, and instead to establish priorities that will allow

Table 4–3. Setting (and living by) your priorities

1. Accept that you can't do it all.
2. Define your long-term goals.
3. Adopt a developmental perspective.
4. Scrutinize your weekly schedule.
5. Negotiate to make your job description more efficient.
6. Learn when and how to say "no."

you to choose among them. Define your long-range professional goals (as you currently see them), and decide what should you be doing now to advance your progress toward those goals. Adopt a developmental perspective when making these decisions, acknowledging that your priorities are likely to change over time. Activities that are high priority when your children, or your career, are at a certain developmental stage may no longer be so at a later time. Also, it is most important to determine what, for you, is the proper balance between career and family, and how you might shape your life to more closely approximate it.

After a careful analysis of your schedule, you may find that your weekly time allocation is not congruent with either your long- or short-term goals. Then, of course, you must face the challenge of redressing mismatches between your priorities and your schedule. It is important to delegate wherever possible and to maximize efficiency by choosing high-impact tasks that serve more than one goal. For example, if you have placed a priority on research but need to fund a part of your salary with clinical work, you can start (or work in) a clinic for patients who have the illness that you wish to study; the clinic then becomes the basis for both your research projects and your clinical responsibilities. Efficiency is in the department's interest, as well as your own, so you can negotiate for changes in your job description that will simultaneously further both your and the department's goals.

It is crucial to learn how and when to say no. Some committees will be worth your time, either because they will increase your contacts or because the committee's work will affect (or overlap) your primary area of responsibility. Other committees will not be worth your time, and it is important to learn how and when to turn down these and other invitations. Although saying no has its price, that price will sometimes be worth paying. The more clearly you have defined your priorities, the easier it will be to make these decisions.

Aggression, Competitive Drive, and Self-Confidence

Academic settings, particularly those focused on research, are usually highly competitive. Although some women are comfortable competing and acknowledging their aggression (and some men are not), generally this issue poses more conflict for women than men. Data indicate that, compared with men, women may be less comfortable in competitive environments and more likely to withdraw from them. Studies of high school math classes show that "girl-friendly" classes (as defined by the girls' satisfaction and by their likelihood to elect subsequent math classes) differ from "girl-unfriendly" ones in having a more cooperative, rather than competitive, culture, with less emphasis on individual, public performance (Eccles 1985). A woman who finds herself in a "girl-unfriendly" environment may thus feel uncomfortable and may doubt her ability to succeed. In addition, many observers have noted that women in academia (and many other work settings) may be in a classic double bind with respect to aggression. That is, at the same time that the work culture may both expect and reward aggressive competition, such behavior may be poorly tolerated when it is exhibited by a woman.

Thus, a woman entering a competitive work environment struggles with both "deficit" and "difference." She may recognize that a low-key approach is unlikely to be successful, yet unmodulated aggression may be ambivalently received when it comes from a woman. Women may also feel disapproving of a workplace's competitive culture. They may question whether they want to become acculturated to it; to the extent that they do want to fit in, they may be unsure how to.

Similarly, many women are socialized to be uncomfortable with overt self-promotion, although the ability to advertise one's talents and accomplishments is frequently rewarded with resources and honors. Like aggression, self-promotion spans a spectrum from the functional to the obnoxious and unhealthy. Each individual must consider her (or his) position on the spectrum, and whether that position works well in terms of acquiring the resources and credit needed for success. If not, then the individual must consider how she would change her position on the spectrum, and whether she wants to.

Lurking behind these dilemmas about aggression and self-promotion is, of course, the issue of self-confidence; it is easier to promote your own interest when you are firmly convinced of your value. Studies show that high-achieving girls are usually less confident in their abilities than high-achieving boys (Dweck 1986). Faced with failure, girls often begin to doubt themselves, and their performance declines. Boys, on the other hand, tend to attribute their failure to external factors and to redouble their efforts to succeed. Similarly, women exposed to the inevitable downturns of academic life (e.g., rejections of papers and grant proposals) may be more likely than men to suffer self-doubt and may be less likely to persist and succeed.

These considerations can have concrete consequences when, for example, a junior faculty member is negotiating for her salary or resources.

Anecdotally, female deans and chairs report that female faculty may be less likely than their male colleagues to come to these negotiations with a clear argument outlining what they would like and why they should be given it. Furthermore, these senior women say, women may tend to ask for less. Although there is no doubt that women are sometimes denied equal pay because of bias, "differences" in behavior may compound "deficits" due to discrimination. Such gender differences may be most evident in the early stages of an academic career, when female faculty are least likely to feel self-confident, but gender differences in behavior at that time may have long-range effects. Scientists have noted the phenomenon of "cumulative advantage," in which the availability of resources at the beginning of a scientist's career facilitates achievements that increase the probability of acquiring more resources later. Thus, small differences between male and female scientists early on become magnified over time. This phenomenon is then compounded by the "Matthew effect," in which a recognized scientist's contribution to a project is overemphasized, whereas a junior collaborator's contribution is minimized or overlooked. In academia as in other areas of life, them that has, gits.

These complex dilemmas do not have simple solutions. Each faculty member must discover where he or she is, and where he or she wants to be, on the spectra of competitiveness, aggression, and self-confidence. Faculties as well as individuals vary in these characteristics, and mismatches do occur. In thinking through these issues, junior faculty can get assistance from mentors and role models, the topic to which we turn next.

Role Models and Mentors

Compared with men, women in science and academia are more likely to report that a lack of role models and mentors has been an obstacle to their achieving success. A mentor is generally defined as someone who provides substantive support, such as resources or expertise, while a role model is, obviously, an individual on whom one wishes to model oneself. Drawing this distinction highlights the fact that a single senior faculty member is unlikely to fulfill all of these functions for a junior colleague. For example, a junior faculty member might have two male mentors with whom she works on research projects. One of these mentors might also serve as a role model, and the junior faculty member might then have an additional, female role model who works in a different subspecialty area. Recognizing that one person is unlikely to fill all of these roles helps the junior faculty member avoid disappointment. In addition, junior faculty who are aware of deficits in a mentoring relationship can look to other individuals to provide some of what is lacking.

Lack of mentors and role models may take several forms. Sometimes, women feel shut out of an "old-boy" network, such as lunches where department business is discussed, or meetings where research ideas are exchanged. Women may also experience the mentoring that they receive as "girl-unfriendly," with a rigid style that emphasizes competitiveness. Finally, although mentors can be of either gender, it is desirable for a woman to have one or more female role models; given the dearth of senior women in academic psychiatry, this can be a difficult goal to achieve.

In suggesting strategies to approach these problems, we will draw on the preceding discussions concerning priorities and aggression. The junior faculty member should define what she wishes to achieve in one or more mentoring relationships and should then pursue these goals. Sometimes a direct approach is desirable, such as asking to be included in certain meetings or gatherings. At other times, it can be helpful to negotiate a "mentoring contract" that specifies what each individual will contribute to, and derive from, the relationship (e.g., the junior faculty member will provide clinical services for a study in return for coauthorship on the main project and supervision and first authorship on a spin-off project). Female academic psychiatrists often find role models at other institutions or even in other cities; many find that national meetings provide excellent opportunities to develop relationships with female peers and role models.

Be Creative

Because most faculties have already had their first female member, and most national psychiatric organizations have had their first female president, female academic psychiatrists generally believe that the era of "pioneers" is past. Although this belief is partially valid (the success of these "firsts" has proven that women are as capable as men in these roles), it is also a misperception. A female faculty member may discover that her department has had female members before, but none of them wanted to join the department's research team. In many departments, it is still possible to be the first female service chief, residency training director, or certainly the first female chair. It is also still possible to be a member of the first group of women to comprise a significant proportion of the faculty, for example, 25% or 30%. And women wishing to take a maternity leave, or to remain on the core faculty but reduce their hours to accommodate family responsibilities, may well be surprised to learn that they are the first to make these requests.

Times have not only changed, they are still changing. It is therefore important to allow oneself the freedom of ideas that comes from considering yourself a trailblazer. In some circumstances, this may entail advocating for systemic change, a topic we discuss in greater detail in the next section. In other circumstances, it may involve suggesting a job description that is unconventional but fits both your and the department's needs well. In these circumstances, it is essential to determine the intersection between the department's interest and your own, and to analyze the impact of your request on the department's bottom line. For example, a woman whose children are very young and whose spouse works weekdays may prefer to work some weekend hours, when the department needs additional coverage. However, be aware that innovative suggestions may elicit negative responses based on bias or untested assumptions. For example, some department chairs assume that part-time faculty are unlikely to be academically productive, based on their experience with (mostly male) faculty members who combined part-time work in the department with part-time (or even full-time) private practice. However, these faculty members' commitment to the department's mission and their availability for work outside scheduled hours may be different from that of others who choose to work part-time because of family responsibilities. A woman asking for a flexible schedule would need to be aware of such biases and to make effective counterarguments.

Confronting the Challenges: Collective Strategies

As already noted, some of the challenges faced by women in academic careers stem from "difference," but others stem from "deficit." Many (if not most) administrative structures in academia date from a time when two-career families were an anomaly, and many of these structures and policies are not "family-friendly." Some have argued, for example, that the traditional seven-year, up-or-out tenure policy has a disproportionately adverse impact on women, because the seven years in question were likely to overlap with prime childbearing years. Therefore, both male and female academics may encounter situations where the wisest course of action is to advocate for change in, for example, leave or tenure policies. Indeed, many academic medical centers are in the process of revising their tenure policies because of changing fiscal pressures, and some of this increased flexibility can work to the advantage of female faculty.

Of course, it is difficult for an individual acting alone to advocate effectively for systemic change. This is one of several reasons why it is advantageous for women in academic settings to establish networking opportunities both within and between departments. Such opportunities help to decrease the isolation that many women feel when working in a historically male-dominated environment and to increase their chances of finding a compatible role model. In many medical schools, networking opportunities (and many other relevant activities) are organized by an office charged with fostering the career development of female students and faculty. The effectiveness of many of these offices demonstrates the utility of having an administrative structure dedicated to the advancement of women's careers at both school and departmental levels. For example, staff from the women's office may suggest to departments the names of prominent women in their field who can be brought to the campus to lecture and give seminars. In addition, representatives of the women's office may monitor the activity of important search committees to ensure that the nominations of qualified women are sought and given serious consideration. It is important to note the distinction between appointing a woman to be a member of a search committee, on the one hand, and ensuring that someone charged with the furtherance of women's careers is involved with the search process, on the other, since the two are not necessarily synonymous.

Indeed, search committees and appointments to powerful positions are important areas of concern now that women in most fields (including psychiatry) are represented proportionately in entry-level positions but may still face a glass ceiling. Many observers believe that the major challenges facing women in science and academic medicine currently involve achieving equity at the top and attaining critical mass. That is, the experience of both men and women in a department differs depending on whether the women on the faculty number one, a small minority, or a significant proportion that includes some in leadership positions. Many believe that women must achieve a critical mass for deficits to be redressed and differences to diminish as both men and women become knowledgeable about, and supportive of, diversity in the workplace.

Conclusion

For both women and men, a career in academic psychiatry offers exciting opportunities as well as painful challenges. For women in particular, there may be times when it is difficult to maintain one's sense of equilibrium and optimism. At such times, it is important to reevaluate one's priorities, behavior, and environment to determine the best course of action. It can be helpful to confer with colleagues, mentors, role models, and friends, as well as to adopt a long-range, historical perspective. The first women to graduate medical school, and to join medical faculties, did so only a relatively short time ago. Women who aspire to a successful academic career, and to a life meshing career and children, are striving toward a goal that few have attained. Perhaps it is not surprising, therefore, if these women face setbacks and struggles along the way. But they can take solace in knowing that they face fewer barriers than the women before them and that, hopefully, their (and others') daughters will face fewer barriers still.

References

Charney DA, Russell RC: An overview of sexual harassment. Am J Psychiatry 151:10–17, 1994

Dial TH, Grimes PE, Leibenluft E, et al: Sex differences in psychiatrists' practice patterns and incomes. Am J Psychiatry 151:96–101, 1994

Dweck CS: Motivational processes affecting learning. Am Psychologist 41:1040–1048, 1986

Eccles JS: Bringing young women to science, in Psychology and Gender. Edited by Sonderiggers T. Lincoln, University of Nebraska Press, 1985, pp 97–132

Leibenluft E, Dial TH, Haviland MG, et al: Sex differences in rank attainment and research activities among academic psychiatrists. Arch Gen Psychiatry 50:896–904, 1993a

Leibenluft E, Haviland MA, Dial TH, et al: Sex differences in faculty retention and rank attainment in academic departments of psychiatry. Academic Psychiatry 17:73–76, 1993b

Lenhart SA, Klein F, Falcao P, et al: Gender bias against and sexual harassment of AMWA members in Massachusetts. JAMWA 46:120–125, 1991

Pincus HA, Dial TH, Haviland MG: Research activities of full-time faculty in academic departments of psychiatry. Arch Gen Psychiatry 50:657–664, 1993

Sonnert G, Hofton G: Gender Differences in Science Careers. New Brunswick, NJ, Rutgers University Press, 1995

Zuckerman H: The careers of men and women scientists: a review of current research, in The Outer Circle: Women in the Scientific Community. Edited by Zuckerman H, Cole JR, Bruer JT. New York, WW Norton, 1991, pp 3–45

5

Minorities in Academic Psychiatry

Francis G. Lu, M.D., Kewchang Lee, M.D., and Sudha Prathikanti, M.D.

As the U.S. population changes to include an increasingly culturally diverse population, academic psychiatry faces the ongoing challenge of training practitioners, teachers, and researchers who can address the cultural issues of these populations as well as reflect the diversity of these populations. Although the term *cultural diversity* includes characteristics beyond that of ethnicity (i.e., race, language, age, country of origin, sexual orientation, religion/spiritual beliefs, social class, and physical disability), we focus in this chapter on ethnic minorities, gays, and lesbians in academic psychiatry. First, a rationale is provided for the importance of valuing cultural diversity in academic psychiatry. Second, strategies for both mentorship of individual faculty and institutional/organization change concerning ethnic minority faculty are discussed. Finally, the chapter concludes with a discussion of gays and lesbians in academic psychiatry.

Rationale for Valuing Cultural Diversity

The rationale for valuing cultural diversity in academic psychiatry includes the importance of a diverse workforce that (1) is proportionate with the population, (2) will serve underserved ethnic minorities in clinical care, (3) will help recruit and role-model for increasingly large ethnic minority medical student and residency classes, and (4) will help educate all residents in the cultural aspects of clinical care (what has been termed *cultural competence*).

Recent data from the Association of American Medical Colleges (AAMC 1995) and the American Psychological Association (Murray 1996) demonstrate a vast underrepresentation of Black, Hispanic, and Native Americans among the faculties of U.S. medical schools, departments of psychiatry and graduate departments of psychology (see Table 5–1). For example, whereas blacks constitute 12.7% of the population, they represent only 2.5% of the medical school faculty, 3.5% of the psychiatry faculty, and 4.0% of the psychology faculty. For Hispanics, although being 8.9% of the population, their respective percentages are 2.9%, 3.5%, and 2.0%. Especially underrepresented are Mexican Americans; whereas they are 6% of the population, they constitute only 0.3% of the medical school faculty and 0.45% of the psychiatry faculty. While 0.75% of the population is Native American/Native Alaskan, they represent only 0.1% of medical school faculty, 0.14% of psychiatry faculty and less than 1% of psychology faculty. These three ethnic minority groups have been designated under-

Table 5–1. Percentage of the Distribution of U.S. population and selected faculty by ethnicity

	Black	Hispanic	Native American	Asian	White
1994 U.S. Population[1]	12.7	8.9	0.75	3.0	175.0
		(6% Mexican)			
2000 U.S. Population[1] (Estimated)	13.0	11.0	<1.0	4.0	72.0
1995 U.S. Medical School Faculty[2]	2.5	2.9	0.10	8.6	79.9
		(0.3% Mexican)			
1995 U.S. Department of Psychiatry Faculty[2]	3.5	3.5	0.14	6.0	84.4
		(0.45% Mexican)			
1995 U.S. Graduate Departments of Psychology Faculty[3]	4.0	2.0	<1.0	1.0	92.0

[1]U.S. Bureau of the Census. *Current Population Reports, Series P23-189 Population Profile of the United States: 1995.* U.S. Government Printing Office, Washington, DC, 1995.

[2]Association of American Medical Colleges. *U.S. Medical School Faculty, 1995.* AAMC, Washington, DC, 1995.

[3]American Psychological Association. *Survey of Graduate Departments of Psychology.* Washington, DC, 1995.

represented minorities by the AAMC (for the Hispanic group, Mexican Americans and mainland Puerto Ricans only). Data about faculty of medical schools and graduate schools of psychology are included to show that academic psychiatry is not alone in this underrepresentation trend.

The AAMC has initiated two major programs to reverse this underrepresentation. To increase minority representation in medical school enrollment, the AAMC in 1990 embarked on "Project 3000 by 2000" to double the number of matriculants of underrepresented minority groups from 1,500 to 3,000 by the year 2000. Gains realized during the period from 1990 to 1995 included a 37% increase in matriculants and a 62% increase in applicants from underrepresented minorities (AAMC 1996b). It is hoped this effort will also improve representation among the medical school and psychiatric faculties in the long run. Second, in August 1996, the AAMC initiated the Health Professionals for Diversity coalition, which now includes 44 medical associations to support affirmative action in health professional education.

A similar significant trend in underrepresentation of these three ethnic groups exists at the practitioner level for all three fields. For example, only 4% of physicians are Hispanic and 5% are black. In 1996, membership in the American Psychiatric Association was 2.1% black, 4.2% Hispanic, and 0.06% Native American. Three recent studies (Cantor 1996; Komaromy et al. 1996; Moy and Bartman 1995) examined the relationship between physician ethnicity and care of ethnic minority patients. The first study showed that "racial and ethnic minorities are more likely to receive care from non-White physicians. Low-income patients, Medicaid recipients, and the uninsured are more likely to receive care from non-White physicians. Individuals who receive care from non-White physicians are more likely to be in worse health, receive care in an emergency department, and be hospitalized" (Moy and Bartman 1995, p. 1520). The second study concluded that "black and Hispanic physicians have a unique and important role in caring for poor, black, and Hispanic patients in California. Dismantling affirmative-action programs, as is currently proposed, may threaten health care for both poor people and members of minority groups" (Komaromy et al. 1996, p. 1305). The third study found similar trends across disciplines. Furthermore, the AAMC survey of 1995 medical school graduates (AAMC 1996a) showed that 41.4% of blacks and 30% of other underrepresented minorities planned to practice in socioeconomically deprived areas. Even though additional specific studies involving psychiatrists have not been published to date, it can be reasonably hypothesized that increasing minority psychiatric faculty will help recruit and train psychiatrists who will work with these underserved populations.

A culturally diverse faculty will be needed to recruit and role-model an increasingly diverse medical student group. A dramatic shift has occurred in the U.S. medical student enrollment in the last decade (1985–1986 vs. 1995–1996). According to data from the Association of American Medical Colleges (AAMC 1996a), the Asian Pacific American group has increased from 6.4% to 17.0%, while underrepresented minorities—African Americans, Native Americans, mainland Puerto Ricans, and Mexican Americans/ Chicanos—increased from 8.5% to 12.0%. Stated differently, the white medical student enrollment has dropped from 81.6% in 1985–1986 to 66.6% in 1995–1996.

A culturally diverse faculty also will be needed to recruit and role-model an increasingly diverse psychiatric resident group. According to the APA Office of Education 1995–1996 Census of Residents (Scully and Jones 1996), the total number of residents in all classes has remained above 6,000 since 1988 despite the 41% drop in U.S. medical graduates entering through the Match from 1988 through 1994. The percentage of international medical graduate (IMG) residents has increased from 21.8% in 1989–1990 to 38.6% in 1995–1996. Moreover, in the PGY-1 (Post-Graduate Year 1) class in 1995– 1996, the percentage of IMGs was 43.7%. Another significant trend has been a decrease in the number of white residents from 76% in 1989–1990 to 60% in 1995–1996. From 1990–1991 to 1995–1996, Asian psychiatry residents have increased from 12.7% to 23.3%; Hispanic residents (including Mexican Americans, Puerto Ricans, and Spanish descendants) went from 6.5% to 8.7%; African Americans have increased from 5.3% to 6.1%; and Native American residents have remained constant (0.2%). The percentage of residents who are women has remained approximately 44% during the past six years.

The field of psychiatry can benefit by taking the opportunity to bridge the recruitment gap among U.S. medical graduates by recruiting more actively the best and the brightest among these minority U.S. medical graduates. For example, whereas in 1995–1996, 81.1% of the white psychiatric residents were non-IMGs, only 8% of the Asian/Indian, 8.7% of the Asian/ Filipino and 60.2% of the Asian/Oriental psychiatric residents were non-IMGs. This reflects not only the large number of IMGs entering psychiatry but also the relative weakness in recruiting non-IMG Asian residents, considering they constitute 17.0% of the total U.S. medical school enrollment.

A similar trend exists for black and Latino non-IMG resident recruitment (Scully and Jones 1996).

Finally, culturally diverse faculty will be needed to help teach future psychiatrists to provide culturally competent care to an increasingly culturally diverse population. The Accreditation Council for Graduate Medical Education Requirements for Residency Training in Psychiatry (effective January 1, 1995) included changes to provide greater specificity of instruction than in the previous requirements about the diverse cultures in the United States. The summary statement on this topic is as follows: "The residency program should provide its residents with instruction about American culture and subcultures, *particularly those found in the patient community associated with the training program. This instruction should include such issues as sex, race, ethnicity, religion/spirituality, and sexual orientation.*" (Changes are italicized.)

Taken as a whole these data point to an increasing service gap between rapidly growing underserved ethnic minority populations (Latinos, blacks, and Native American) for which academic psychiatry as well as medicine and psychology are not well prepared to narrow given the underrepresentation of practitioners and faculty. Organizations such as the AAMC have initiated programs to narrow this gap, which has increased the number of underrepresented ethnic minorities in medical school. Additionally, the Asian medical student group has already increased dramatically to 17%. Academic psychiatry will benefit by focusing efforts at recruitment of the best and the brightest of these medical students to bridge the recruitment downturn among U.S. medical graduates. These residents will be among the future academic psychiatrists.

Furthermore, dramatic shifts in ethnicity have already taken place among the psychiatry resident census: Only 60% of all residents in 1995–1996 were white. Academic psychiatry faces an enormous challenge to provide role modeling for these residents given the underrepresentation of ethnic minorities among our faculty.

Mentorship of Ethnic Minority Faculty

Women, ethnic minority, and lesbian/gay physicians face many obstacles to career advancement. In addition to the plethora of factual information and new skills/functions any entrant to a medical career track must rapidly master, physicians from marginalized groups often contend with additional external realities such as skepticism about competency, subtle forms of institutional discrimination, and the stresses of being newcomers to a field whose unspoken rules may be less familiar—and perhaps less acceptable —to them than to the majority counterparts. As a result, women and minority physicians may be more vulnerable to internal conflicts and distress over professional identity and role expectations, and they face the challenge of retaining their uniqueness and sense of self in a system that may stigmatize them for operating on cultural/behavioral paradigms different from the majority group.

Among the few recent articles on psychiatric faculty career development, two highlight the importance of mentorship. First, Gruber and Cherry (1996) describe concisely the gist of their department of psychiatry faculty handbook, which contains "grassroots" career development strategies. In addition to mentoring, they suggest networking with peers locally and nationally, establishing short- and long-term goals, documenting academic accomplishments in a professional curriculum vitae and career biography, and asking for a review toward promotion on a regular basis. Second, Baker (1993) provides a very personal description of her career development as a black woman academic psychiatrist. The roles of national mentors and national fellowships were critical in her career development from residency to the associate professor level. She also highlights how gender and race both have major consequences on interactions with peers and supervisors.

As Petersdorf et al. (1990) commented, "for many years, this country's medical schools mirrored the discriminations of our society; they were primarily the preserve of White men" (p. 663). Although the number of women and ethnic minority physicians in clinical care and entry-level academic positions may have increased substantially over the past 20 years, their promotion to higher-level academic posts and administrative positions remains incongruently slow. For both women and ethnic minority physicians, the higher the academic rank, the fewer their numbers; moreover, promotion to those positions takes longer to achieve than for their white male counterparts (Petersdorf et al. 1990). Women and ethnic minority physicians are less likely to envision academic careers for themselves as compared with white male colleagues and are also more likely to leave academic career paths than their white male colleagues (Levinson et al. 1991; Osborn et al, 1992). Underrepresentation of ethnic minority academic faculty is due to multiple factors, including an inadequate number of minority medical school graduates, indebtedness of minority postgraduate trainees, lack of awareness of opportunities in academic medical centers, lack of mentors, a shortage of role models, and environmental factors. Over recent years, the government, private industry, and some universities and medical schools have made efforts to remedy this situation. The problems, however, are complex and difficult to solve. There is a need to increase the pool of underrepresented minority students interested in careers in medicine; to promote medical student, graduate student, and house staff awareness of career opportunities in academics; to provide resources that enable students, house staff, and fellows to develop the skills necessary to succeed and survive in the academic arena; and to offer ongoing support for career development of junior faculty (Cregler et al. 1994; Rogers et al, 1990). These trends point to the need to address change strategies at the institutional/ organizational level rather than solely at the individual development level.

Institutional Change Strategies

Cultural diversity has become an increasing concern for American workplaces and business (Jackson and Associates 1992; Thomas and Ely 1996) as well as by the AAMC and the American Psychological Association (Bernal et al. 1996). Even though no published material exists about change strategies for departments of psychiatry, change strategies that can be applied may be seen from the perspectives of the American Psychological Association, the Federal Glass Ceiling Commission, and a diversity management consultant working with business.

The Bernal et al. report (1996) evolved from the activities of the Work Group on Faculty Recruitment and Retention of the American Psychological Association Commission on Ethnic Minority Recruitment, Retention, and Training in Psychology. This guide addressed many issues that academic psychiatry faces and had these specific goals:

1. Present the advantages of cultural diversity for the greater society and for the academic workplace
2. Describe various individual differences in cultural characteristics and identity among ethnic minority faculty and suggest some implications of these characteristics for faculty recruitment
3. Identify key elements of a supportive academic environment that enhance recruitment and retention
4. Emphasize the importance of plans one should consider for creating an

academic climate that values cultural diversity as a prerequisite to the
recruitment and retention of ethnic minority faculty

5. Provide guidelines for assessing the commitment of an institutional
    administration to promoting cultural diversity
6. Identify issues, pitfalls, and problems relating to affirmative action and
    faculty diversification and suggest solutions
7. Suggest concrete actions that one can take to increase the responsive-
    ness of a training program to cultural diversity

The Federal Glass Ceiling Commission, a 21-member bipartisan body
appointed by President Bush and congressional leaders and chaired by the
secretary of labor, was created by the Civil Rights Act of 1991. Its mandate
was to identify the glass ceiling barriers that have blocked the advancement
of minorities and women as well as the successful practices and policies
that have led to the advancement of minority men and all women into
decision-making positions in the private sector. Its 1995 report described
successful program characteristics common to all successful glass ceiling
initiatives:

1. They have CEO support. Strategic business plans include strategies for
    advancing minorities and women.
2. They are specific to the organization and tailored to meet specific needs.
3. They are inclusive. The entire organization benefits from accountability,
    leadership training, career development, mentoring and diversity
    training.
4. They address preconceptions and stereotypes through diversity train-
    ing required for all employees involving all levels of the organization.
5. They emphasize accountability for progress toward inclusiveness and
    track progress.
6. They are comprehensive involving outreach and recruitment as well as
    leadership training, mentoring, and career development.

Finally, a recent book by Arredondo (1996), based on her organizational
work in diversity management with business, elaborates on the actual process of creating and implementing a diversity management initiative. These
domains are elaborated upon as follows:

1. Identifying motivating factors
2. Developing the diversity vision
3. Conducting needs assessment process
4. Writing the diversity strategic plan
5. Implementing diversity-related strategies
6. Involving education and training
7. Evaluating progress and change
8. Identifying enablers and pitfalls to diversity initiatives
9. Recognizing and rewarding progress

At the University of California, San Francisco (UCSF) Department of Psychiatry, a Diversity Committee has existed since 1990 to promote faculty diversity. Practical strategies have included the following: a biennial survey report of faculty by gender and ethnicity to assess the extent of diversity, a faculty cultural competence and diversity directory based on faculty self-reports, resident recruitment and development efforts focused on ethnic minorities and women to increase the potential pool of future junior faculty, active mentoring of ethnic minority junior faculty, and the establishment of various task forces and programs on specific patient groups (Asian, black, Latino, women, HIV/AIDS, gay/lesbian) at San Francisco General Hospital. At this site in 1996, 38.2% of the UCSF faculty were from ethnic minority backgrounds. Further research needs to be done to ascertain the success of such programs in academic psychiatry.

Gays and Lesbians in Academic Psychiatry

The gay, lesbian, or bisexual psychiatrist in academia faces many of the same challenges as ethnic minorities and women, though data on the experience of sexual minorities in academic psychiatry is limited, largely because of the historical stigma of homosexuality within the field and in U.S. society. Until 1973 homosexuality was classified as a mental illness in the DSM (1968); to disclose one's sexual orientation as anything but heterosexual, therefore, posed tremendous risk for the psychiatric faculty member. Since then, with the growth of the political movement for gay rights, the visibility of gays, lesbians, and bisexuals in all aspects of society has increased, and this is true as well in academic psychiatry. Only recently have data on issues facing sexual minorities in academia become available, and the literature focuses primarily on gays and lesbians; unfortunately, very little is written about the experience of the bisexual psychiatrist, which will need to be explored in the future.

An issue that faces all gays and lesbians is whether to disclose one's sexual orientation, and if so, in what setting. Unlike women and many ethnic minorities, lesbians and gays may successfully hide their minority status without being identified on the basis of appearance. This fact represents a limitation on research among gays and lesbians, introducing a selection bias among the sample, as those more concerned about confidentiality will be less likely to respond to surveys and interviews. Disclosing one's homosexual orientation, commonly known as coming out, is an individual process that progresses over time in a manner that is neither uniform nor standard (Cabaj 1996). The choice to come out in any setting is complicated by many factors unique to the individual, including personal acknowledgment of one's orientation, support networks, acceptance by family and friends, and internalization of society's prejudices and stereotypes regarding gays and lesbians, also known as *internalized homophobia*. Once individuals make a decision to be openly lesbian or gay in at least some aspects of their life, they then also face decisions about who to tell in the workplace, if anyone, and how large a role sexual orientation should play in career choices.

In the academic psychiatric setting, choosing to be openly lesbian or gay has several possible benefits. For example, in some parts of the United States, particularly urban areas, being out may lead to a niche in working with sexual minorities and may increase referrals to a private practice or opportunities for employment in a position working with such a population. Openly gay and lesbian faculty may develop a specialization in mental health issues among gays and lesbians and offer both instruction and consultation in the academic setting. In addition, the openly lesbian or gay academic psychiatrist can serve as a role model for other professionals or trainees. As mentioned, mentorship can provide a powerful positive influence on the development of minority trainees, including gays and lesbians who may be struggling with their own coming out process and who may have had extremely few contacts with gay and lesbian professionals. Such mentorship is often informal within the academic department, but it may also be provided through national professional organizations, including the Association of Gay and Lesbian Psychiatrists and the Gay and Lesbian Medical Association. Being out as a faculty member may also provide opportunities to confront prejudice and bias and to participate in efforts toward increasing diversity and the visibility of lesbians and gays in the workplace.

Finally, being out in the workplace offers gay or lesbian individuals an integration of their personal and professional experience that may be extremely rewarding.

Certainly, there is great variability in the extent to which such benefits are possible; urban areas often provide more community support for being out publicly, as well as a larger presence of gays and lesbians. At the San Francisco General Hospital at University of California San Francisco (UCSF), there is a Gay and Lesbian Focus Psychiatric Inpatient Unit staffed by professionals trained in caring for sexual minorities; such a unit could not exist in a rural setting with few openly gay men or lesbians. Larger academic departments will have increased likelihood of contact with other lesbian and gay professionals; such numbers afford the opportunity to develop networks, committees, and seminars devoted to issues among sexual minorities.

The risks of coming out in the academic setting can be significant; among medical professionals homophobia, or prejudice against lesbians and gays, is a reality, based on surveys in the literature. In a 1986 study of physician members of the San Diego County Medical Society, 30% stated that they would not admit a highly qualified gay or lesbian applicant to medical school, and almost 40% said that they would discourage gay or lesbian physicians from seeking training in pediatrics or psychiatry (Mathews 1986). In addition, 40% of respondents stated that they would cease referrals to a colleague in these specialties upon learning that the colleague was lesbian or gay, and 40% reported being uncomfortable caring for a lesbian or gay patient. In a 1990 survey of New York medical students, respondents estimated that more than 25% of their peers and 50% of their faculty had negative attitudes about gay men and lesbians (McGrory et al. 1990). A 1991 study of homophobia at a medium-sized Canadian medical school found that 33% of psychiatric residents and 26% of psychiatric faculty scored in the homophobic range on an attitudinal instrument called the Index of Homophobia Scale (Chaimowitz 1991). In 1995, Townsend et al. (1995) surveyed U.S. psychiatry residency training directors; almost 40% reported the presence of faculty who considered homosexuality pathological. In a similar study of lesbian and gay psychiatric residents performed by the same authors, 21% of respondents reported that their program had a "pathological" stance toward homosexuality (Townsend et al. 1993), though none of the training directors did so. The authors did find a geographic variability in directors' awareness of lesbian or gay faculty at their programs; such awareness was significantly greater in the West and North-east than in the South and North Central region. Herek (1984) has found that those having little contact with gay men and lesbians are more likely to have negative attitudes toward them, and indeed, directors in the South were significantly less likely to endorse homosexuality as a normal condition, as were directors of smaller programs. Surveys of medical students also suggest a geographic variability in the extent of homophobia. McGrory et al. (1990) found little homophobia among the New York medical student respondents themselves, but in a 1987 survey of students at the University of Mississippi Medical School, Kelly et al. (1987) found that the students held both negative and prejudiced attitudes toward gay patients and people with AIDS.

How homophobia gets translated into adverse consequences for the gay or lesbian academic psychiatrist has not been adequately studied, but the results of the Mathews study suggest that the individual may face a decrease in referrals as well as barriers to advancement, secondary to prejudice among colleagues, especially in smaller towns, rural areas, and the South. There is little in the literature on the "glass ceiling" phenomenon among sexual minorities, but currently there are few openly gay or lesbian chairs of major academic psychiatric departments in the United States, and the phenomenon may become more apparent as increasing numbers of trainees and junior faculty come out. Even in urban centers with large numbers of lesbians and gays, the psychiatric department that recruits and publicly values women and ethnic minorities may not do the same with sexual minorities, who are often not seen as adding to the diversity of the workplace. Colleagues' attitudes may not be outwardly homophobic in these situations, but the gay or lesbian individual may not be regarded as an asset, either.

The unique experience of the lesbian academic psychiatrist, being both a gender and sexual minority, has been little explored in the literature. Townsend et al. (1993) in their survey of psychiatric residents did find that gay men responded in a more clearly positive way than lesbians on inquiries dealing with issues of disclosure, availability of peer and group support, and perceptions concerning their sexual orientation. Gay men were more likely to view their program as affirming of their sexuality, whereas more women felt stigmatized; gay men were also more likely to report having faculty with whom to discuss issues of homosexuality. The authors hypothesized that gay men may more easily establish mentoring relationships in a male-dominated field; lesbians have few female and even fewer openly lesbian role models. The issues faced by a gay man or lesbian are compounded when the individual is a woman and /ethnic minority, as he or she must also contend with the challenges described earlier in this chapter.

Townsend et al.'s (1995) survey of training directors had a response rate of over two-thirds, with 70% of directors reporting an awareness of lesbian or gay faculty at their programs and 70% an awareness of lesbian or gay residents. These results suggest a definite presence of gays, lesbians, and bisexuals in academic psychiatry, pointing to the need for a closer examination of their experience than currently exists in the literature. It is hoped that the growing numbers of openly gay or lesbian residents will lead to increased mentorship, recruitment, and advancement of sexual minorities, and decreased homophobia in the academic setting, such that a faculty member choosing to come out in the workplace will find that it enhances his or her career.

Summary

This chapter has highlighted the profound changes in the cultural diversity of our population, medical school enrollment, and resident census for which academic psychiatry must be prepared. Although this chapter has focused on only two aspects of cultural diversity—ethnic minorities and sexual orientation—further studies are needed to analyze the impact of other aspects of cultural diversity, such as gender, that intersect.

References

American Psychiatric Association: Diagnostic and Statistical Manual: Mental Disorders. 2nd Edition. Washington, DC, American Psychiatric Association, 1968

Arredondo P: Successful Diversity Management Initiatives. Thousand Oaks, CA, Sage, 1996

Association of American Medical Colleges: U.S. Medical School Faculty 1995. Washington, DC, Author, 1995

Association of American Medical Colleges: Minority Students in Medical Education: Facts and Figures IX. Washington, DC, Author, 1996a

Association of American Medical Colleges: Project 3000 by 2000: Year Four Progress Report. Washington, DC, Author, 1996b

Baker FM: The black woman academic psychiatrist. Academic Psychiatry 17:194–201, 1993

Bernal ME, Caldwell-Colker AT, Dela Cancela V, et al: Valuing Diversity in Faculty: A Guide. Washington, DC, American Psychological Association, July 1996

Cabaj RP: Gay, lesbian, and bisexual mental health professionals and their colleagues, in Textbook of Homosexuality and Mental Health. Edited by Cabaj RP, Stein TS. Washington, DC, American Psychiatric Press, 1996, pp 36–38

Cantor JC, Miles EL, Baker LC: Physician service to the underserved: implications for affirmative action in medical education. Inquiry 33:167–180, 1996

Chaimowitz GA: Homophobia among psychiatric residents, family practice residents and psychiatric faculty. Can J Psychiatry 36:206–209, 1991

Cregler LL, Clark LT, Jackson EB Jr.: Careers in academic medicine and clinical practice for minorities: opportunities and barriers. Journal of the Association for Academic Minority Physicians 5:68–73, 1994

Federal Glass Ceiling Commission: Good For Business: Making Full Use of the Nation's Human Capital. Washington, DC, U.S. Government Printing Office, 1995

Gruber N, Cherry LM: Grassroots, "bottom-up" strategies for a successful academic career. Acad Med 71(3):218–219, 1996

Herek GM: Beyond "homophobia": a social psychological perspective on attitudes towards lesbians and gay men. J Homosex 10:1–21, 1984

Jackson SE and Associates: Diversity in the Workplace. New York, Guilford Press, 1992

Kelly JA, St. Lawrence JS, Smith S, et al: Medical students' attitudes towards AIDS and homosexual patients. J Med Educ 2:549–556, 1987

Komaromy M, Grumbach K, Drake M, et al: The role of black and Hispanic physicians in providing health care for underserved populations. N Engl J Med 334:1305–1310, 1996

Levinson W, Kaufman K, Clark B, Tolle SW. Mentors and role models for women in academic medicine. West J Med 154(4):423–426, 1991

Mathews WC, Booth MW, Turner JD, et al: Physicians' attitudes toward homosexuality—survey of a California county medical society. West J Med 144:106–110, 1986

McGrory BJ, McDowell DM, Muskin PR: Medical students' attitudes toward AIDS, homosexual, and intravenous drug-abusing patients: a re-evaluation in New York City. Psychosomatics 31:426–433, 1990

Moy E, Bartman B: Physician race and care of minority and medically indigent patients. JAMA 273:1515–1520, 1995

Murray B: Minority faculty are still low in numbers. Monitor, (June) 40, 1996

Osborn E, Ernster V, Martin J: Women's attitudes toward careers in academic medicine at UCSF. Academic Medicine 67 (1):59–62, 1992

Petersdorf RG, Turner KS, Nickens HW, Ready T: Minorities in medicine: past, present, and future. Academic Medicine 65(11):663, 1990

Rogers JC, Holloway RL, Miller SM: Academic mentoring and family medicine's research productivity. Family Medicine 22(3):183–185, 1990

Scully J, Jones J: 1995–1996 Census of Residents Statistics. Washington, DC, American Psychiatric Association, 1996

Thomas D, Ely R: Making differences matter: a new paradigm for managing diversity. Harvard Business Review (September–October):79–90, 1996

Townsend MH, Wallick MM, Cambre KM: Gay and lesbian issues in residency training at U.S. psychiatric programs. Academic Psychiatry 17:67–72, 1993

Townsend MH, Wallick MM, Cambre KM: Gay and lesbian issues in U.S. psychiatric training as reported by residency training directors. Academic Psychiatry 19:213–218, 1995

6

International Medical Graduates

Nyapati R. Rao, M.D.

A commotion, and some shouts, told us that the emigrants had arrived.—V. S. Naipaul, *The Middle Passage*

International medical graduates (IMGs), physicians trained in medical schools in countries other than the United States, are a major presence in American psychiatry. Currently, 25% of the general members of the American Psychiatric Association are IMGs. Similarly, 41.2% of all psychiatry residents in 1996–97 were IMGs (APA 1996–97, Census of Residents, 1998). They are a heterogeneous group coming from various linguistic, cultural, and medical education backgrounds and from more than 140 countries. In this chapter, important milestones in the history of IMGs in the United States are presented. That discussion is followed by an examination of issues that IMGs face at various stages of their careers—as applicants to residency programs, as residents, and as fully trained psychiatrists. The focus in this discussion is exclusively on foreign IMGs, and it is expected that this information, along with some specific recommendations, will help both IMGs and training directors to address issues unique to IMGs and thus enhance IMGs' performance as residents and as psychiatrists.

History of IMGs

The immigration of IMGs to the United States started just prior to World War II. From the beginning, IMGs have received an ambivalent welcome from their hosts. Questions have been raised about the quality of their medical education background and their competence as physicians (Fuller Torrey and Taylor 1973). It is claimed that they exacerbate the physician surplus, resulting in the escalation of health care costs (Iglehart 1996). On the other hand, they are seen as providing an essential safety net function to the underserved population (Mick 1997). It is relevant to point out that in spite of the creation of several obstacles in the form of tighter immigration policies and tougher qualifying exams, the number of IMGs in American medicine continues to grow (S. Mick, unpublished report to the Bureau of Health Professions, July 1995). Although discussion of various aspects of this complex issue is beyond the scope of this chapter, in Table 6–1, important milestones in the history of IMGs in the United States are presented to create a context for the ensuing discussion of career issues.

Issues Confronting IMGs Seeking Residency Positions

IMGs considering psychiatric training in the United States may be at quite varied career and life stages. They may be medical graduates in a foreign country considering migration to the United States, or they may be already in the United States looking for residency positions and have a greater familiarity with U.S. medicine. They may be practicing physicians, even psychiatrists, in their own or another foreign country, or they may be practicing in the United States and contemplating a change of specialty. In any of the preceding situations, married and unmarried IMGs may have family in the United States or only in their home country. Because of this variation, the issues confronting individual IMGs are diverse, and the recommendations made next should be tailored to the individual's unique circumstances.

It is recommended that IMGs seeking residency training in psychiatry approach the task in a methodical fashion and learn about the vast differences that exist between the medical education systems abroad and those in the United States (see Table 6–2). They should familiarize themselves with various academic, economic, legal, regulatory, and interpersonal issues involved in undergoing residency training in the United States. They should also learn about how the practice of psychiatry in the United States differs from that with which they are familiar. In the following, the general differences between U.S. and foreign medical education are outlined with the caveat that particular schools may have different policies and practices. For

Table 6–1. Milestones in the history of international medical graduates (IMGs) in the United States

pre–WW II	Physicians fleeing political persecution in Europe began seeking refuge in the United States.
1949	Exchange Visitor Act passed permitting foreign professionals to seek advanced training in the United States.
1955	Requirement added to Exchange Visitor visa (J-1) that physicians return to their country of origin for 2 years upon completion of training in the United States before they are eligible to seek permanent resident status.
1956	Creation of Educational Commission for Foreign Medical Graduates (ECFMG).
1958	First ECFMG exam given.
1965	Immigration Act amended to give occupations in short supply, such as medicine, preference in granting permanent resident status.
	Quotas based on national origin abolished, resulting in Asia and Latin America becoming major sources of physicians from this point on. Previously, Europe was the major source.
1970s on	Concerns expressed regarding the presence of large numbers of IMGs in American medicine.
1976	Congress imposes immigration restrictions.
1977	Visa Qualifying Exam (VQE). Replaces one-day ECFMG Exam.
1984	Foreign Medical Graduate Examination in the Medical Sciences (FMGEMS). Replaces VQE.
1992	United States Medical Licensing Examination (USMLE).
1997	Controversies around physician surplus vs. safety net function (Mick 1997).
	Greater New York Demonstration Project launched to reduce residency positions.
	IMGs make up 23% of U.S. physician population and 24% of resident physicians in all specialties. The heaviest concentrations of IMGs are in New Jersey (44%), New York (41%), West Virginia (34.8%), and Illinois (34.3%) (AMA 1997).
1998	Clinical Skills Assessment Exam is added to ECFMG certification.

Table 6–2. Differences between U.S. and foreign graduate medical education, psychiatric training, and psychiatric practice

	United States	Foreign
Medical school	Organized experience (rotation) in psychiatry.	In developing countries, psychiatry rotation may be lacking or poorly organized.
Method of instruction	Seminars, one-to-one supervision, experiential groups, clinical rounds, and grand rounds instead of large lectures are the venues of education and have a more egalitarian atmosphere. Clinical care learned through a hands-on approach; students encouraged to demonstrate initiative and a questioning attitude; current journals form the major source of information.	Relies almost exclusively on lectures; clinical training occurs in small-group bedside rounds; the students' unquestioned acceptance of knowledge from the teacher is encouraged, and questioning in a public setting is frowned upon as showing a lack of respect to an elder.
Examination formats	Multiple-choice exams heavily used.	Oral, bedside clinical exams, and written essay exams used.
Hospital culture	Physician is member of an integrated patient care team.	Physician is sometimes the only professional making decisions regarding patient care.
Doctor/patient relationship	Egalitarian; patient has the right to question the physician's recommendation and to seek a second opinion. Legal rights of patients zealously protected by the state and legal system.	Paternalistic; some IMGs are not used to being questioned or being subjected to scrutiny in the same fashion as in the United States.
Status of psychiatry	In spite of being viewed ambivalently by other specialties, psychiatry has a long history and rich traditions.	Psychiatry does not have an established presence in many countries. Severe shortage of psychiatrists.

Care of the mentally ill	Often cared for by trained professionals and facilities.	Traditionally, family, priests, and friends care for the mentally ill.
Therapies	Talk therapies still prevalent, psychoanalytic thought and practice have a solid presence in the intellectual and cultural life of the nation.	Emphasis on biological therapies and social interventions; different models of psychological mindedness.
Service responsibilities	Postgraduate student (resident) learns the craft through a total immersion in the work of the hospital. The resident has dual education and service obligations.	Postgraduate student still considered a student with few or negligible service responsibilities.
Health care financing	Health care is not a right for citizens; insurance-based payment for health services.	In many countries, health care is a right; free health care through state-run hospitals.
Accreditation of training	Graduate medical education (GME) can be offered by any hospital with the facilities to offer such training as long as it meets both general and special requirements and is approved by the Accreditation Council of Graduate Medical Education (ACGME).	GME is usually under the aegis of universities or medical schools.
Board certification	Candidate examined by an autonomous body, the American Board of Psychiatry and Neurology (ABPN) for certification.	Diplomas are awarded by the same medical school that originally trained the candidate.

example, Philippine schools may be closer to the U.S. model of medical education than those with a British colonial history, such as India or Pakistan.

Applying and Interviewing for a Psychiatry Residency Position

Applicants should seek information about likely programs through the informal network of their IMG acquaintances, through literature on the subject, as well as through organized job fairs for IMGs such as that conducted by the Medical Society of the State of New York. In addition, the following are some issues that are unique to psychiatry that an IMG applicant may find useful to consider:

- The choice of a program in which to train is very individualized. One should consider such factors as the size of the program and contiguity of the sites, its U.S. regional location, its educational orientation, its experience in training IMGs, its reputation, the Board pass rate of its graduates, and the availability of the applicant's ethnic community and religious resources. One should interview in as many programs as possible and decide on the program only when satisfied with the information that is available.

- Many IMGs, being new to psychiatry, may be perplexed as to how to conduct themselves in an interview. They may be more adept at talking about medical or surgical cases or answering factual questions in medicine rather than talking about themselves. The psychiatric training director wants to assess the applicant's background, educational accomplishments, cross-cultural adaptation, proficiency in English, personality, genuineness of interest in psychiatry, and the candidate's fit within the program. The applicant must understand the training director's predicament: He or she may not know foreign medical educational systems, may not know what the medical school scores mean, may be put off by reading recommendation letters that do not give a picture of the uniqueness of the individual applicant, and may be confronted by communication and cultural difficulties in the interview. The training director and the faculty usually have only this one opportunity to learn more about the candidate.

- Applicants should try to present themselves in an honest manner. They must be prepared to talk about themselves openly and candidly: This includes their family background, formative experiences, scholastic performance in college as well as in medical school, and how they became interested in psychiatry. If candidates have had prior training in psychiatry, they should be prepared to discuss a case. Some IMGs may not have had prior exposure to psychiatry in medical school and, wanting to ensure that they secure a residency position, may apply to several specialties in addition to psychiatry. This may appear to the training director as a lack of genuine interest in psychiatry and that the candidate is applying to psychiatry only to get a foothold in U.S. graduate medical education. Candidates should be aware of this impression and be able to demonstrate their enthusiasm for the field in the interview. The careful consideration of these simple points can make the difference in securing a desirable residency training position.

- The National Resident Match Program (NRMP) and its importance in the residency selection process may be unfamiliar to many IMGs. The NRMP is a centralized mechanism to help candidates as well as training programs choose each other in a fair and noncoercive manner. A program's participation in the Match generally has no bearing on the quality of training it offers. All graduating U.S. medical students must participate in the Match. However, an IMG is free to obtain a residency position either through the Match or outside the Match. Historically, many IMGs, daunted by the complexity of the system or not trusting that this impersonal process will actually get them a residency position, have bypassed or unintentionally misused the system. Some may join the Match only to drop out to seize the first residency contract offered outside of the Match. This behavior may be viewed by some as unethical. The candidate who is a participant in the Match must take the same chances as any USMG candidate in being matched with the candidate's preferred program. An IMG seeking a position should either apply outside the Match from the beginning, or start and stay in the Match. In the latter strategy, candidates may rest assured that even if they should not get a position within the Match, there will be other positions open.

Issues in Residency Training

Stereotypes and Their Effect on IMG Education

IMG residents, as any minority, are subject to stereotypes that may view them as passive, poorly trained, unenthusiastic about psychiatry, and having significant difficulties with psychodynamic theory. The IMG resident may be viewed as an inferior physician who has difficulties in relating to other disciplines, has unsatisfactory clinical and communication skills, and who does not generally perform satisfactorily on certification examinations. The presence of an IMG resident may be seen as lowering the prestige of a program, and it is assumed that once an IMG is accepted into a program, USMGs will bypass that program.

Similarly, IMGs may see the host culture as a dangerous place where violence is endemic, people are self-absorbed, interpersonal relationships are superficial, and where the elderly, children, the poor, and the needy are mercilessly abandoned. Regarding their careers, they may feel that the education system uses them primarily as cheap labor and has no interest in their successful integration into the mainstream of U.S. medicine.

Stereotypes can and do create a cycle of misunderstandings between faculty and IMG residents that may result in withdrawal, rejection, and poor performance by both. Training directors must guard against this insidious and malignant process. Stereotypes frequently involve significant overgeneralization of occasional and partial truths. Each IMG is an individual and brings unique assets and liabilities much like any USMG would.

Acculturation and Adaptation

Yager and Borus (1987) defined the tasks facing IMGs in learning psychiatry as to "master psychiatry, a new culture, and often a new language, all within the same 3- or 4-year period" (p. 1045). An encounter between an immigrant and a new culture often results in culture shock syndrome (Garza-Guerrero 1974), which, briefly, is a protean psychodynamic manifestation including mourning of the lost culture, severe anxiety in adapting to the new and consequent identity disturbances. For some, the resolution of these conflicts results in either a total rejection of or a chameleon-like imitation of the new culture, both resulting in the immigrant's poor adaptation to the host culture and, for the immigrant IMG, inadequate performance as a psychiatry resident.

IMG residents must adapt simultaneously to psychiatry, which is unlike any other specialty in medicine, and to the culture at large, which is so unlike what they have left behind. Psychiatry's ambiguities, and uncertainties as a field, and the diversity of its clinical populations can be very stressful. When the IMG is feeling most deprived and anxious as a newcomer to this society, to treat very sick, demanding, and regressed inpatients very early in training can create severe existential crises. In addition, the absence of the familiar rituals and signposts of clinical medicine such as physical exams, bedside rounds, and stethoscopes all contribute to identity crises. The need to prove oneself in the midst of unfamiliar surroundings and personalities may engender performance anxieties. The training director should keep in mind that the challenges described here are part of the normal expectable development of the IMG as an immigrant and should not be viewed as pathological (Akhtar 1996).

Performance of IMG Residents

In a 1973 study of residents in the Menninger clinic, Fried et al. (1973) found that USMGs scored significantly higher than IMGs in the area of social psychiatry, even though they did not find any significant difference in overall performance. Chen (1978) surveyed 169 training programs in 1978. IMGs were rated as having a greater level of competence in clinical gerontology, organic illness, and psychopharmacological treatment. USMGs were found to be superior in their understanding and management of social and group process, efficacy in clinical leadership, nonclinical administrative skills, consultative functions, treatment of behavioral disorders, and assessment and treatment of psychological problems. In an unpublished study of training directors' assessments of the typical strengths and weaknesses of USMGs versus IMGs, Rao et al. (N. Rao, A. Meinzer, and Z. Taintor, unpublished data, October 1993) found that the greatest differences between IMG and USMG knowledge ratings were in areas that are most culture-specific, and in the descriptive and nosological areas in which culture can be seen as impacting social perception and definitions of normalcy. In addition, IMGs were seen as less competent in teaching medical students, dealing effectively with other disciplines, managing countertransference, and being comfortable with psychodynamic theory and practice.

Training Implications

Based on the preceding discussion, the following suggestions are offered to training directors to maximize their IMG trainees' potential:

1. Assess needs and focus training: The differences between foreign medical school educational methods and student role expectations and those of U.S. residency programs should be proactively addressed. Chen's findings and recommendations in 1978 are still applicable now, despite

the many changes in psychiatry since then: "Factors facilitating acculturation and professional growth *(of IMGs)* included objective and candid interactions and the clarification of learning objectives. In those
cases where faculty supervisors encouraged a task oriented approach
to learning coupled with the establishment of an understanding and
empathic relationship, trainees were perceived as having made consistent and accountable progress" (Chen 1978, p. 452).

2. Acculturation training: Acculturation programs described in the liter-
    ature have been used to help the IMG resident understand new cultures.
    These include formal instruction on various local subcultures that the
    IMG resident is exposed to, experiential group programs, socialization
    programs where faculty and residents interact, discussion groups using
    movies that depict cultural struggles of various ethnic groups, and
    focus on American colloquial language with emphasis on local subcul-
    ture syntax (Forrest et al. 1978). Helping the spouses of IMGs in over-
    coming their own social isolation will benefit the cultural integration
    of IMGs.

    Cultural learning is an ongoing process and is not completed when
    the resident finishes the first postgraduate year. Hence, the training
    director must ensure that cultural instruction occurs in all phases of
    training and is not confined to a few courses in the beginning of train-
    ing. Instruction in cross-cultural interviewing and cross-cultural thera-
    pies should be emphasized throughout training for both IMGs and
    USMGs.

3. Language proficiency: A related important area that needs the attention
    of the resident as well as the teaching staff is that of communication
    and linguistic proficiency. Psychiatry, more than any other branch of
    medicine, depends on communication for both diagnosis and therapy.
    Also, language as one of the most powerful symbols of the old culture
    may be invested with tremendous loyalty and can be quite resistant to
    change. Conflicts about letting go of the old culture may be expressed
    in difficulties in learning the new language.

    Programs should develop methods of helping their IMG residents
    with communication difficulties. English departments of local colleges
    and universities are often well equipped and eager to provide training
    in English as a second language to residents and to make the time and
    place of training readily accessible to residents.

4. Supervisory issues: Much of psychiatric learning takes place within the

context of a close relationship between the resident and the supervisor. In Indian culture, for example, the teacher is seen as a friend, philosopher, and guide who has a parental stake in the well-being of the student. Within the context of this relationship one can be deferential, dependent, reveal one's ignorance, and thus grow. South and East Asian IMGs may be more forthcoming in recognizing the supervisory situation as one in which an engaged dependence leads to invaluable growth and express their appreciation of the supervisor's help. Supervisors may be unfamiliar with this relational paradigm and be more familiar with typical USMG issues, such as independence and autonomy. Such supervisors may see IMGs as excessively needy and dependent, and misunderstandings and conflict may develop. Feelings of disappointment and rejection may result in the resident withdrawing.

5. Mentorship: Successful resolution of an identity crisis often is facilitated by a successful relationship with a mentor. Programs can promote this process by offering a well-organized mentorship experience starting at the beginning of training. Such programs would be especially useful for IMGs, many of whom come from cultures where mentorship is a basic educational paradigm. In the context of a trusting, nonevaluative, and empathic relationship, IMGs can learn to communicate better and seek solutions to educational and cultural conflicts. The IMG resident may use an identification with the mentor as a vehicle for acculturation, developing a role model, and learning psychiatry.

Finding a mentor is a difficult task for anybody but especially so for an IMG. In addition to an individual program's own mentorship resources, the resident may find a receptive mentor in researchers and teachers in the field in whose work the resident is interested. Professional literature and professional meetings are vehicles for finding such a mentor. Training directors and residents should investigate the American Association of Directors of Psychiatric Residency Training (AADPRT)/Wyeth-Ayerst IMG Mentoring Program in Psychiatry, which is designed to match selected IMGs with appropriate mentors.

6. Psychotherapy training: The Group for the Advancement of Psychiatry Committee on Therapy has described the function of psychotherapy training for all residents in terms of the acquisition of a set of attitudes: readiness to attend to all aspects of communication; adoption of a nonjudgmental attitude of attentive, active, empathic listening and observation; employment of one's own evoked emotional responses as diag-

nostic tools; consideration of multiple and hidden motivations to account for behavior; consideration and integration of patients' transference attitudes and responses into a total therapeutic plan regardless of the therapeutic modality employed; and finally, consideration of a patient as a whole person within a biopsychosocial context, whose suffering is to be alleviated without undue compromise of autonomy (Group for the Advancement of Psychiatry 1987).

These attitudes are useful to the practice of psychiatry even outside the domain of psychotherapy. Non-Western IMGs may come to their residency with culturally based attitudes quite in conflict with those just stated (e.g., professional authoritarianism that may put them in conflict with their teachers, patients, and colleagues; loyalty to group and family before the individual; and paying exclusive attention to the manifest content of both the patient's and one's own experience).

Increasing the non-Western IMG's awareness of these attitudes may have a positive impact on remediation of the difficulties identified in the psychosocial area of psychiatry. Training in psychotherapy may also help the IMG in adapting to the new culture, for example, by familiarizing the IMG with concepts of individual autonomy and with alternative modes of affect regulation and interpersonal conflict resolution. It is recommended that programs emphasize psychotherapy training as an acculturating experience for their IMG residents. An opportunity to observe an ongoing psychotherapy in a one-way mirror setting, individual supervision, experiential groups, and personal psychotherapy when indicated are some of the methods that have been found to be effective.

Career Paths After Residency

Prior to 1976 in Maryland, Weintraub and Book (1986) found that 75% of the physicians in public hospitals in Maryland were IMGs. A recent analysis done by Balon and Munoz (1996) of 27,843 responses to the APA membership survey revealed that IMGs are overrepresented in city, county, and state hospitals (10.68% of staff) when compared with USMGs (5.22% of staff). However, IMGs are underrepresented in solo office practice (22.03%) compared with USMGs (29.58%), in group office practice (4.35% versus 6.31%), and in medical schools and universities (4.25% versus 6.45%). These differences were statistically significant at the 0.01 level. Balon and Munoz concluded that IMGs practice more frequently in the area of public psychiatry, in which they serve seriously ill patients.

These data illuminate another important phenomenon that requires discussion in relation to IMGs' career issues in American psychiatry: the two-tier system of medical care. As described by Weintraub and Book (1996), the upper tier includes USMGs trained in universities who have a variety of careers open to them after completion of training. They treat more affluent and acutely ill patients and are able to work in more desirable locales with satisfactory remuneration for their work. Conversely, the lower tier includes mostly IMGs trained in nonuniversity settings, who have fewer career opportunities other than working in public institutions, and who generally treat the chronically mentally ill patients in more demanding inner city and rural areas for less remuneration.

There are multiple reasons for this two-tier system. As stated earlier, most of the IMGs are trained in nonuniversity public sector settings, and they tend to stay on as staff psychiatrists in these familiar locations. Many IMGs come from medical systems where the government is the largest employer of health care providers and so may have little conflict in continuing employment in the public sector, which provides secure jobs with generous fringe benefits and opportunities for advancement. IMGs may also be deterred by the complexity of the private health care system, especially that of managed care.

In addition, chronic patients may be more accepting of IMGs. The IMG physician is on the periphery of the American health care system and their patients, by virtue of having severe mental illnesses are deeply alienated from everyday life. They both, patient and IMG physician, may find support and succor in the other. Also, physicians in other specialties in public sector hospitals are more likely to be IMGs who will support one another across disciplines.

In private practice, IMGs are underrepresented in both solo and group settings. IMGs' private practices tend to be in inner city and rural areas. The reasons are once again their familiarity with the patient populations gained during their training in these locations, patients' acceptance, and presence of referral opportunities from IMGs in other disciplines of medicine. Many IMGs may be deterred from entering private practice by not having as role models successful private practitioners among their teachers, the seemingly complicated and unfamiliar business and legal aspects of private practice, and the insecurities inherent in self-employment. The ones who succeed in the more affluent settings still may complain of lack of acceptance by the establishment.

Although it is unfortunate that the two-tier system continues to exist, there may be exceptions based on the IMG's point of entry into the medical profession. Talented IMGs who are deeply interested in psychiatry, perhaps have had psychiatric training abroad, have entered university-based programs, and have had sufficient mentoring in their training and careers have entered positions of leadership in research and academia. These individuals must now serve as active role models.

In academic psychiatry, some IMGs have made notable contributions and occupy positions of high visibility and responsibility in prestigious institutions. However, behind the few well-known academicians, there are many IMGs who struggle at entry-level positions with minimal reward and recognition.

Many IMGs may not enter a research career due to lack of prior experience with basic clinical research in their medical schools, absence of role models, and a need to settle down and provide for their families through quicker entry into the more familiar and lucrative career of clinical psychiatry. They may lack a network from which to draw mentors interested in IMGs and have difficulty obtaining grants for research. Little research substantiates the preceding impressions, and more is needed of the sort that has been productive in race and gender opportunity.

Factors Affecting Careers

1. Licensing: Obtaining an unrestricted license to practice medicine is the first important professional hurdle that IMGs face after finding a residency position. To receive a license the IMG must have completed one to several years of graduate medical training, have passed either the now discontinued Federation Licensing Examination (FLEX) or the United States Medical Licensing Examination (USMLE), and have demonstrated proficiency in English. In addition to these general requirements, each state has its own special requirements. For example, the states of Texas and New Jersey ask for details about college education before medical school. This will create problems for an IMG coming from foreign education systems where students are admitted directly to medical schools after completion of 12 years of high school education.

Some states require quantification of the time spent in basic sciences and clinical sciences. Other states such as New York require that an IMG should be either a permanent resident or a citizen in order to obtain a license. The discriminatory nature of such requirements are quite clear: It is acceptable for an IMG to work in the state as a trainee with a temporary visa but not to be employed as a fully trained physician without a permanent resident status, which is more difficult to obtain. As a result, several hundred trainees on J-1 visas will have to leave the state once they have completed their training. Some may be able to find employment through a system of waivers in underserved areas in the country; others may be forced to return to their countries of origin.

Even if the IMG is fully licensed in one state, he or she does not automatically qualify for a full license in another state by reciprocity. Many states do not accept the ECFMG's validation of the IMG's credentials but require their own cumbersome procedures. For example, one state inquires as to how many books the foreign medical school's library had at the time the candidate was a student. Since many foreign schools are in the process of implementing computerized record keeping, these letters of validation are often endlessly delayed.

Unlike their USMG counterparts who have taken their licensing exam while still immersed in medical school, IMGs take the exam later. Those who do not pass the licensing exam on their first attempt must spend time during their residency training years studying for the exam. In some states, if they are not licensed by the end of the PGY-2, they must leave their program and seek training in another state. Additionally, not having an unrestricted license to practice medicine in the state where they are employed or planning to work will deprive them of the opportunity to take the ABPN. These obstacles to licensure will remain particular hurdles for IMGs until the credential verification process is streamlined and centralized.

2. Board certification: The pass rate of IMGs on the Board examination continues to be low (Rao et al. 1993). Many factors seem to contribute to this low pass rate. Lack of adequate preparation, performance anxiety, cultural differences, poor training, and communication difficulties are all suspect. In addition, prior to the advent of managed care, there were fewer incentives to take yet another anxiety-provoking examination. Some IMGs are trained in service-intense and academically poor programs that do not emphasize passing the Boards as a priority. Train-

ing programs that conduct mock-Board examinations will facilitate IMG residents becoming familiar with the examination process as well as learning to master the performance anxiety. This is not, however, a substitute for a comprehensive and thorough training in psychiatry.

3. Impact of managed care: The managed care of psychiatric practice has become ubiquitous. Increasingly, psychiatrists are finding that they must join managed care systems by contracting with independent practice associations, by becoming employees of staff model health maintenance organizations, or by becoming members of provider panels. IMGs, due to their low pass rates on the ABPN, may have difficulty in being accepted on panels of managed care organizations. Even if they are board certified, IMGs may find it hard to be accepted into managed care systems due to bias in these organizations in favoring USMGs. Some IMGs, even after being accepted on the panels, may find themselves without patient referrals. There has been no systematic study of this issue, but several reports claiming discrimination have reached the APA office of minority and IMG affairs.

In summary, professional life for IMGs in the United States is fraught with difficulties and complexities. IMGs continue to provide service to U.S. populations that are underserved by our medical care system. They are no longer a passing phenomenon of higher medical education, yet our policies and procedures are discouraging to IMGs and are inconsistent with those of higher education in other applied scientific and professional fields. Perhaps in the process of finding solutions to our health care crisis, a more creative and equitable approach will be found to integrate our IMG colleagues. IMGs have found greater opportunities and welcome in the United States than in any other nation, and the United States has and will continue to benefit greatly from their presence.

I would like to express my thanks to Dr. Sheldon Berman, Dr. Arthur Meinzer and Ms. Adria Keitel for their helpful suggestions in the preparation of this manuscript.

References

Akhtar S: A third individuation: immigration, identity, and the psychoanalytic process. J Am Psychoanal Assoc 43:1051–1084, 1996

American Medical Association: The demographics of IMGs. www.ama-assn.org/mem-data/special/img/demograf.htm, 1997

American Psychiatric Association: 1996–97 Census of Residents (Table 7: Source of Medical Training), 18 March 1998

Balon R, Munoz RA: International Medical Graduates in psychiatric manpower calculations (letter). Am J Psychiatry 153:296, 1996

Chen R: The education and training of Asian foreign medical graduates in the United States. Am J Psychiatry 135:451–453, 1978

Forrest DV, Ryan JH, Lazar V: American familiar language and the IMG psychiatric resident. J Psychiatr Education 2:68–82, 1978

Fried FE, Doherty EG, Coyne L: A survey of training needs, satisfactions, and social attitudes. Am J Psychiatry 130:1342–1345, 1973

Fuller Torrey E, Taylor RI: Cheap labor from poor nations. Am J Psychiatry 130:428–434, 1973

Garza-Guerrero A: Culture shock: its mourning and the vicissitudes of identity. J Am Psychoanal Assoc 22:408–429, 1974

Group for the Advancement of Psychiatry, Committee on Therapy: Teaching Psychotherapy in Contemporary Psychiatric Residency Training. New York, GAP, 1987

Iglehart JK: The quandary over graduates of foreign medical schools in the United States. N Engl J Med 334:1679–1683, 1996

Lohr KN, Vanselow NA, Detmer DE (eds): The nation's physician workforce: options for balancing supply and requirements. Washington DC, National Academic Press, 1996

Mick SS: Foreign medical graduates and the U.S. physician supply: old issues and new questions. Health Policy 24:213–225, 1993

Mick SS: The safety-net role of IMGs. Health Affairs 16:141–150, 1997

Weintraub E, Book J: Recruitment of public psychiatrists: the impact of university and state collaboration on IMGs in Maryland. Hosp Community Psychiatry 37:1017–1021, 1986

Yager J, Borus J: Are we training too many psychiatrists? Am J Psychiatry 144:1042–1048, 1987

7

Psychiatric Organizations and Professional Development

Troy L. Thompson II, M.D.

There are about 300 organizations focusing on various medical areas of interest, which have about 200,000 physician members. Membership criteria cover the spectrum from groups that are open to virtually any physician who wishes to join, to honorific, elite, exclusive groups that are limited in membership numbers and seek to select the "best and brightest" in some area. Almost all these groups have as one of their goals the continuing medical education (CME) of their members, usually through annual meetings, audiotapes, and various newsletters and journals. Some require attendance at a certain percentage of their meetings, thus assuring CME credits and active ongoing involvement of their members (Rosenow 1979). Many of these groups also attempt to develop a voice for their discipline to represent what they feel is in the best interests of their specialty and patients. If the preceding goals and objectives are successfully reached, such groups can influence the professional growth and development of their members. Some also provide self-assessment tools, recertification, peer review, and audits of performance for their members (Rosenow 1979) and otherwise try to protect their members, for example, by developing guidelines that can guard against malpractice.

The role of such organizations begins for medical students and, at some colleges, even premedical students. Medical student organizations, such as the Student American Medical Association and Student National Medical

Association, foster professional growth and development and hope to channel the energies they generate into other medical groups with similar goals and interests after the students are graduated (Johnson 1994).

Professional organizations often provide a way to meet colleagues from other institutions and locations who are in similar positions and practices. This can provide an opportunity for the exchange and development of ideas and joint projects and a source of mutual support.

Many professional organizations may play a major role in the career growth and development of psychiatrists, whether they are in private practice, academics, or some other setting. This may range from the local psychiatric hospital staff, to regional medical and psychiatric societies, to national and international organizations. Organizations exist for virtually any interest group within psychiatry and can provide support, collegiality, continuing education, and the opportunity to serve and to develop leadership skills in specific areas (Grant 1985). A list with brief descriptions of some of these groups appears in Appendix 7–A at the end of this chapter.

American Psychiatric Association— The Largest Psychiatry Organization

Founded in 1844, and currently comprised of approximately 40,000 members, the American Psychiatric Association (APA) is the oldest and largest psychiatric organization (Barton 1987). The APA conducts many educational programs and publishes the *American Journal of Psychiatry, Psychiatric Services, Psychiatric News,* and the *Psychiatric Research Report.* The American Psychiatric Press, Inc. (APPI) is a wholly owned subsidiary of APA and is a major publisher of psychiatric and mental health books. The APA also provides several other member services, including job placement, professional liability, disability, life and personal liability insurance coverage, and legal consultation. The APA Library provides special rates for photocopies and literature searches for members. A Managed Care Help Line provides assistance with managed care problems. The APA Consultation Service can provide expertise in virtually any psychiatric administrative, clinical, educational, and many other programmatic areas. A large government relations office lobbies on behalf of psychiatric interests, and a media relations office deals with public relations and media issues.

The APA has committees and task forces on every major aspect of psychiatry and service to the psychiatric community. Of particular relevance to psychiatric educators are the Committee on Medical Student Education, the Committee on Graduate Medical Education, the Committee on Research Training, and the Council on Medical Education and Career Development. The APA also maintains an Office of Research and an Office of Education.

The Office of Research is concerned with science policy, scientific assessment, and conduct of research activities. It disseminates to the psychiatric research community information about public policy that may affect financing of research of various types. It also develops programs to interest and assist young psychiatrists in pursuing research careers. Scientific assessment activities have included development of the standard (DSM) diagnostic systems in psychiatry and of scientifically based practice guidelines. The office develops and coordinates some scientific studies and provides consultation to academic departments contemplating research projects.

Since its establishment the Office of Education has been a major liaison between the APA, governmental agencies, and psychiatric educators in a number of other organizations. Its director disseminates information relevant to conducting and financing psychiatric education programs and regularly attends national educational meetings. The Office produces a number of publications dealing with education, such as the *Directory of Psychiatric Residency Training,* sponsors fellowships for residents and awards for psychiatric educators and administrators, and produces a variety of CME self-study materials.

Young psychiatrists and those new to academics in particular will probably want to regularly attend the APA annual meeting held each spring. It is a good place to get together with people you already know, but it generally is not as good a place as smaller meetings to make new contacts in your areas of interest. Psychiatrists from virtually every subspecialty area and with every type of interest will be at the APA annual meeting, but it's not likely that you will be able to have those with similar interests in one setting, at least not for very long. Some smaller organizations, and many academic departments, have receptions at the APA annual meeting, where it may be easier to make or reestablish contacts with colleagues.

The other major APA annual meeting is the Institute on Psychiatric Services, held each fall. It used to focus more on hospital and community psychiatry topics but has broadened in recent years to cover a wider range of psychiatry topics. Although it has traditionally involved many nonpsychiatrist mental health professionals, it now focuses more around the roles that psychiatrists play in the health care system and tries to appeal to a general psychiatrist audience. It is a much smaller meeting than the spring APA annual meeting, so much more networking is possible.

Smaller Organizations

There are national psychiatric organizations of a small to moderate size (i.e., several hundred to a thousand or so members) in virtually every specialty and subspecialty of psychiatry. The leaders in an academic department in the area of interest can inform a psychiatrist of one or two key small organizations in that discipline. As an example, the Academy of Psychosomatic Medicine (APM) has become the national organization for consultation-liaison (C-L) psychiatrists. This organization has grown in recent years to about 1,000 psychiatrists; almost half are young academic C-L psychiatrists. The organization provides an effective way to meet C-L colleagues who may be developing new solutions to common problems and struggling with similar career issues. Those attending often exchange ideas and strategies and initiate joint projects. The size, format, and casual tone of the meetings are such that new members also have an opportunity to meet and talk with a number of more senior members and leaders of the organization. Several receptions and other social activities are structured such that the senior members of the organization are encouraged to meet and talk with younger members and to offer mentorship.

Another similar organization is the Association for Academic Psychiatry (AAP). This is a national organization of about 1,000 members that primarily focuses on education of medical students, residents, and other medical disciplines. The AAP has sections on multiple topic areas, such as C-L, child and adolescent psychiatry, medical student education, residency education, and geriatrics. Section meetings, which typically consist of 10 to 30 members, center on discussion of projects and opportunities for collaboration and are very welcoming of new colleagues. Lectures and panel discussions of general and focused interest also occur. This is another organization in which young faculty and other psychiatrists have an opportunity to get to know and to talk with national educational leaders in psychiatry and develop a strong and supportive network.

The structures of the AAP and similar organizations foster the development of collaborative research projects. For example, the section on C-L psychiatry meets twice during the annual meeting and often discusses collaborative projects. The section developed a core reading list that was recommended for students and residents during C-L rotations. The C-L section of AAP also has been instrumental in developing guidelines of the core goals and objectives for C-L rotations and proposed to national accrediting bodies the type of C-L experience that would be considered optimal. In addition to these broader projects, a large number of smaller projects have been initiated by individual C-L psychiatrists meeting and talking during the AAP C-L section meetings. Often, papers are jointly authored based on discussions initiated during these sections. In addition, several members of the C-L section have edited books, and, based in part on discussions during those C-L sections, individuals have been asked to write chapters for those books and make other scholarly contributions.

Benefits of Activity in Professional Organizations

National Networks and Mentoring

An initial task of young academic psychiatrists in particular, but other psychiatrists with focused interests as well, should be to select one or two relatively small national psychiatric organizations focused in their areas of interest. The psychiatrist should attend these organizations' annual meetings regularly and attempt to get to know as many other active participants as possible. After attending such a meeting for 1 or 2 years and having made a number of contacts with colleagues in the group, it would be appropriate to ask those colleagues for support in playing a more active role in the organization. Young psychiatrists should also seek out and talk with the current leaders of the organization. The leaders of national psychiatric organizations are usually quite eager to get to know and to be supportive of energetic and dedicated younger colleagues (Erikson 1963). A psychiatrist should not be shy in speaking with the president, president-elect, and other officers and volunteering to serve on committees and task forces and do projects of mutual interest. The president and president-elect usually make committee assignments. If a psychiatrist has a specific idea for a project, he or she might mention this to one of those leaders and ask their advice. There is almost certainly someone in the organization in the same field of interest who either has some experience or would be interested in further discussing such an idea with them. A leader in such an organization is almost always pleased to help colleagues link up in such ways.

Psychiatrists should plan to go to at least two or three national meetings per year if they wish to develop a national network of colleagues. Many departments cannot pay for such travel in these times of fiscal constraint, but it is probably a wise investment for future professional growth and development for younger faculty to pay for such trips personally if necessary. (The costs can be deducted from income tax as a business expense.) Also, after attending a meeting, the psychiatrist may see opportunities to present at the next year's meeting, and departments are usually more prone to support a trip if a formal role, such as presenting a poster or paper, is being played at the meeting.

Young psychiatrists should try to develop mentor relationships with psychiatrists they like and respect from other departments and cities. There are obvious disadvantages to not having a mentor in your city, but there may be some advantages as well. For example, such a mentor may be able to advise you about the internal policies of your department more frankly than a local colleague, who might hesitate to speak as openly. In addition, collaborative research with mentors at distant institutions might provide access to resources not available locally.

Building Organizational and Managerial Skills

Residency education often does not involve a great deal of didactics and experience in administration and management. Administration of a mini-organization, such as an inpatient unit or outpatient clinic, or a chief residency, may provide some management experience, but activity in local, regional, and national organizations can be an important way to gain additional skills in these areas.

The head of a committee or task force must be able to facilitate the group in setting feasible and appropriate goals, run productive and efficient meetings, maintain focus and momentum over time, communicate the recommendations and accomplishments of the group clearly and effectively, negotiate for the needs of the group, and work in harmony with a variety of colleagues with different interests and personalities. Officers of organizations may have to deal with budgets; raise funds; plan, implement, and evaluate scientific/educational programs; recruit members for tasks and positions; and resolve conflicts within the organization. While honing these skills in organizations faculty members can put them to use in administrative positions within their own departments.

Advancing the Issues of Your Specialty

National organizations can advance the interests of a subgroup and represent that group's interests with other national organizations, legislative bodies, and so on. One example of this is the APM organizing an effort in the early 1990s to have C-L psychiatry recognized as a psychiatric added qualification subspecialty. The APM felt it would be useful to have subspecialty certification for C-L psychiatry as has been granted in recent years for several other psychiatric subspecialties. Therefore, the APM put together committees to look into and to address how such subspecialization approval might occur, including consulting with the American Board of Medical Specialists and the American Board of Psychiatry and Neurology (ABPN). The leaders of APM talked with the leaders of those organizations and learned what type of application process and what type of political processes are involved. The APM leaders then spoke with C-L leaders in other organizations, such as the APA, to try to receive their advice, input, and support in this endeavor. The APM learned that they must receive the support of their specialty society, so they presented their position to the APA, and the proposal was discussed and debated through the relevant councils and committees of that organization. The proposal ultimately was discussed by the Assembly of District Branches of the APA, and they voted to support this proposal. The APM then presented this proposal to the ABPN, and the psychiatry directors of that organization decided that they did not wish to support C-L psychiatry becoming a subspecialty at that time, so the matter ended.

In spite of formal subspecialty status not being approved by ABPN at that time, the process was useful in many regards. It clarified for APM members the important roles and functions of C-L psychiatrists by forcing them to put these in writing and to become clearer about their organizational goals and objectives in these regards, at times in response to rigorous questions by other thoughtful psychiatry leaders who did not agree with the proposal. The APM members involved in this learned a great deal about other organizations with which they interacted, and a great deal about political processes in the field of psychiatry. The APM and field of C-L psychiatry were undoubtedly strengthened by going through this process, and the C-L psychiatrists involved learned a great deal administratively that can be applied in other situations and settings.

Rising in Organizations

A wide range of positions and offices may be held in various organizations. The usual route to moving up in an organization is to be appointed initially to a committee or task force. A useful first step in facilitating being appointed is to talk to people who are members of the committee and then to the chair of the committee or task force. If you express your interest to them, they are often eager to have someone with similar interests work with them. They may advise you to talk with the president or president-elect of the organization, and they may wish to do so themselves. Usually the presidents and president-elects of organizations ask the chairs of various committees who they think would be most productive to work with them; they then make those appointments, particularly if they have met and like the individuals being recommended.

Once you have been appointed to a committee or task force within an organization, it is important to take an active part in developing and implementing the group's projects. As in your academic work, your productivity will be a major determinant of your success in organizations. After working actively on the committee for a year or two, you should directly express your interest in assuming the chair of the committee or other leadership roles in the organization.

Once you become a chair of a committee or task force, you usually become a member of the executive committee or a similar body within that organization. This provides the opportunity to get to better know the other leaders in the organization and to begin to collaborate more actively with the heads of other committees and task forces and the organization's officers. Similar types of bridge building and collaborative work will ensure that you will be in a position to then move up further in the organization, if that is your desire.

Because it is such a large, diverse organization, it may be harder and take longer to develop a network and assume leadership positions within the APA than in smaller, more homogeneous organizations. However, several approaches are available to those who wish to become active. First, it may be most feasible to begin on the level of the district branch, which is the local or regional chapter of the organization. District branch meetings will be more frequent, closer geographically, and less costly to attend than national APA meetings and will deal with issues of immediate concern to those in the region. Work in the district branch may then lead to more involvement at the national level, such as serving as a representative to the APA Assembly.

A second approach is to write to the APA president-elect, expressing one's interest in serving on a committee, briefly describing one's background relevant to the work, and enclosing a curriculum vitae. The president-elect will be eager to identify good people who are interested in working actively in the organization and will consider such requests seriously, even from people not personally known to him or her. Frequently, first committee appointments are as "corresponding members" who receive all written material relevant to the committee and are invited to attend its meetings, but at their own expense. Serving as a corresponding member may be a good way to get one's foot in the door, begin to learn how the committees function, and become known to other APA leaders nationally.

Finally, much of the APA's leadership is chosen by competitive election and therefore may fluctuate more than that of a smaller, more homogeneous organization. One's continued activity in the APA may depend on the election of those leaders whom one knows and whose positions one supports, so that one may wish to campaign actively to help such people attain leadership positions.

Fellowships in Organizations

Many psychiatry organizations now provide fellowship programs for residents. Residency education directors may maintain a list of organizations that provide these fellowships and speak with their residents on an annual basis about which residents might be interested in which fellowship. These fellowships often include paying for the resident to attend one or two of the organization's national meetings. When the residents attend the national meetings as a fellow, they typically receive an orientation to the organization and are often assigned a mentor. These mentors talk with the residents about their interests in the subspecialty area and sometimes will collaborate with them on various projects.

These types of fellowships are wonderful ways to begin to develop networks in areas of interest. The fellows are typically invited to receptions at the annual meetings and are often involved in the programs as participants in discussions or presenters. The fellows' opinions are valued by these organizations especially in areas of residency and medical student education. A list of fellowships in national organizations appears in Appendix 23–A in Chapter 23.

References

Barton WE: The History and Influence of the American Psychiatric Association. Washington, DC, American Psychiatric Press, 1987.

Erikson EH: Eight ages of man, in Childhood and Society, 2nd Edition. New York, WW Norton, 1963, pp 247–274.

Grant AE: Academy presidential address. What does the academy do for me? Arch Phys Med Rehab 68:277–278, 1985

Johnson AR: Student National Medical Association: its need within the forum of medical education. J National Med Assoc 86:335–336, 1994

Rosenow EC Jr: Medical specialty societies, in Medical Education: Past, Present, Future. Edited by Templeton B, Samph T. Cambridge, MA, Ballinger, 1979, pp 201–224

Psychiatric Organizations

Described here are some representative organizations psychiatrists may find useful to generate ideas and projects and develop networks and collegial support to foster career growth and development. Due to space constraints, many excellent groups have not been listed.

Academy of Psychosomatic Medicine (APM)
5824 North Magnolia Street
Chicago, IL 60660
(312) 784-2025

The APM serves as the national organization for consultation-liaison (C-L) psychiatry. It provides opportunities at its annual meeting to network with approximately 1,000 senior and junior C-L clinicians and researchers from around the world. It publishes *Psychosomatics,* sponsors educational C-L programs, develops educational standards for C-L fellowship training, and recognizes C-L psychiatry achievements through competitive awards.

American Academy of Child and Adolescent Psychiatry (AACAP)
3615 Wisconsin Avenue, NW
Washington, DC 20016-3007
(202) 966-7300

The AACAP addresses the needs and interests of child and adolescent psychiatrists in academics, private practice, and community (public) psychiatry. It is the main annual meeting in child psychiatry. The AACAP extends itself to general residents and child residents with special programs emphasizing research and mentoring. The meetings are well organized and offer a variety of programs. It is easy to meet with colleagues as this group is relatively compact as compared with the APA.

American Academy of Clinical Psychiatrists
P.O. Box 3212
San Diego, CA 92163
(619) 298-0538

This is a national organization with special interests in promoting the role of clinical psychiatrists.

American Academy of Psychiatrists in Alcoholism and Addictions (aaPaa)
P.O. Box 376
Greenbelt, MD 20768
(301) 220-0951

This is a national body of psychiatrists with interests in addiction psychiatry. It promotes the role of psychiatrists in the addiction field.

American Academy of Psychiatry and the Law (AAPL)
One Regency Drive
P.O. Box 30
Bloomfield, CT 06002
(203) 286-0787

AAPL is the leading professional society for forensic psychiatrists. It holds an annual meeting that is well attended and informative. It also publishes a quarterly bulletin that is a must for forensic psychiatrists. The membership includes most of the academic forensic psychiatrists in the nation and many abroad.

American Association of Directors of Psychiatric Residency Training (AADPRT)
c/o Department of Psychiatry University of Connecticut Health Center
10 Talcott Notch Road East Wing
Farmington, CT 06030-6410
(203) 679-6766

This group is mainly composed of residency directors and associate directors, but others interested in residency education attend. Workshops deal with curricular, administrative, and experiential aspects of residency. A major asset is the opportunity to form networks and get peer support for those in education. It also provides an opportunity to form liaisons with other groups, including the APA.

American Association for Geriatric Psychiatry (AAGP)
791 Woodmont Avenue
Bethesda, MD 20814-3004
(301) 654-7850

This group is excellent for psychiatrists interested in new research findings in geriatric psychiatry, opportunities to contact other geriatric psychiatrists through establishing networks, attending national meetings, reviewing current clinical practices, advocating geriatric patients with governmental and other agencies, and learning about approaches to the practice for geriatrics in private and other settings.

American Association for Marriage and Family Therapy
1100 17th Street, N.W.—10th Floor
Washington, DC 20036
(202) 452-0109

This group is composed of psychiatrists and other mental health professionals whose main interests are marriage and family therapy.

American Board of Adolescent Psychiatry
4330 East-West Highway, Suite 1117
Bethesda, MD 20814
(301) 718-6520

This organization provides certification in adolescent psychiatry to those who meet their criteria and pass a certifying examination.

American College of Forensic Psychiatry
P.O. Box 5870
Balboa Island, CA 92662
(714) 831-0236

The American College of Forensic Psychiatry members are practicing forensic and clinical psychiatrists. There is less of an academic membership in this college than the American Academy of Psychiatry and the Law (AAPL). The annual meeting is worthwhile as is the *American Journal of Forensic Psychiatry,* which is published by the College.

American College of Mental Health Administration
225 West Swissvale Avenue
Pittsburgh, PA 15218-1632
(412) 244-0670

This organization is open to all mental health clinicians who are administrators of programs or interested in administration. Its meetings provide a forum to advance the knowledge of attendees in this area and for networking and collegial support.

American College of Neuropsychopharmacology
320 Centre Building
2014 Broadway
Nashville, TN 37203
(615) 322-2075

This is one of the leading organizations for those interested in neurobiological investigations of behavioral disorders and the drugs used to treat those disorders. Membership is honorary, based on nomination by members and a rigorous selection process.

American College of Psychiatrists
732 Addison Street, Suite B
Berkeley, CA 94710
(510) 704-8020

This is an honorary organization for psychiatrists who have excelled in various areas of psychiatry and made significant contributions to the field. New members must be nominated and supported by several current members and are selected by a rigorous membership committee.

American College of Psychoanalysts
520 Breck Court
Benicia, CA 94510
(707) 746-7674

This is an honorary organization for physicians-psychoanalysts who have excelled in various areas of psychiatry and psychoanalysis and made significant contributions to psychoanalysis. New members must be nominated and supported by several current members and are selected by a rigorous membership committee.

American Group Psychotherapy Association, Inc.
25 East 21st Street—6th Floor
New York, NY 10010
(212) 477-2677

This organization is for psychiatrists and other mental health professionals who have a strong interest in group psychotherapy.

American Psychiatric Association (APA)
1400 K Street, N.W.
Washington, DC 20005
(202) 682-6000

APA was discussed at length in the chapter. It is the largest (about 40,000 members) psychiatry organization and encompasses almost all interest groups in psychiatry. Its publications and annual meetings provide the broadest overview of advances in the field each year.

American Psychoanalytic Association
309 East 49th Street
New York, NY 10017
(212) 752-0450

A psychiatrist who is interested in psychodynamic psychotherapeutic processes that underlie psychiatric symptomatology and are involved in the intensive psychotherapeutic treatment of these disorders will find the various meetings sponsored by the American Psychoanalytic Association useful. Each year there are two meetings, one that occurs in association with the APA spring meeting and the other in December in New York City. A large variety of topics are usually addressed in varying formats (e.g., papers, panel discussions, discussion groups, etc.).

American Sleep Disorder Association
1610 14th Street, N.W., Suite 300
Rochester, MN 55901-2200
(507) 287-6006

This is a group for those with interests in sleep circadian rhythms, dreaming, and so on. Usually in addition to psychiatrists, many biological psychologists, some psychoanalysts, and some in other disciplines are members.

American Society of Addiction Medicine (ASAM)
12 West 21st Street
New York, NY 10010
(212) 206-6770

This is a national multidisciplinary organization with about half of its members being psychiatrists. It promotes addiction medicine as a specialty and sets standards and gives an examination for certification in addiction medicine.

Association for Academic Psychiatry (AAP)
AAP Executive Office, Department of Psychiatry
Mt. Auburn Hospital
Cambridge, MA 02238
(617) 499-5198

The AAP strives to promote excellent psychiatric education through its programs, opportunities for collaboration, professional career development workshops for young psychiatric educators, and its publication of *Academic Psychiatry.* Its members not only include department chairs and journal editors, but also junior and midlevel faculty educators, who come together in a collegial spirit to share educational dilemmas and to seek common solutions. This is an excellent group for developing strong networks in these areas.

Association for the Advancement of Philosophy and Psychiatry (AAPP)
UT Southwestern Medical Center—Dept. of Psychiatry
5323 Harry Hines Boulevard
Dallas, TX 75235-9070
(214) 688-3390

This group is of interest for psychiatrists studying philosophical questions in general, but especially questions of psychiatric neurology, the relationship between mind and brain, and cognitive functions. The AAPP meets annually just before the APA and plans to launch a journal.

Association for Medical Education and Research in Substance Abuse (AMERSA)

Brown University Center for Alcohol and Addictions Studies
Box G
Providence, RI 02912
(401) 863-3173

This is a national multidisciplinary group that includes psychiatrists who are interested in teaching and research in the field of substance abuse.

Association of Directors of Medical Student Education in Psychiatry

The Chicago Medical School—Dept. of Psychiatry
3333 Green Bay Road
North Chicago, IL 60064
(708) 578-3330

This organization is for the directors of medical student education in Departments of Psychiatry and others who have a strong interest in psychiatric education of students.

Association of Women Psychiatrists

P.O. Box 61316
Durham, NC 27715-1316

Women in psychiatry would benefit, especially new practitioners, since this organization provides a large, supportive network. Male practitioners may be interested if they're interested in issues more often affecting female patients, like eating disorders, or would like to mentor and collaborate more effectively with female colleagues.

College on Problems of Drug Dependence (CPDD)

Executive Officer
Department of Pharmacy
3420 North Broad Street
Philadelphia, PA 19140
(215) 221-3242

This is a multidisciplinary group of elected members with demonstrated experience in the field of addictions. It tends to attract accomplished researchers. Its annual meeting showcases cutting-edge research.

Group for the Advancement of Psychiatry (GAP)

P.O. Box 28218
Dallas, TX 75228
(214) 613-3044

GAP is a prestigious organization. Membership ranges between 300 and 400, and one can only become a member upon invitation and subsequent election within the group.

The group is a "think-tank" that meets twice a year at the same location. Members are assigned to one of its nearly 30 committees with specific academic tasks and goals. Each committee works toward producing a written report, published as a monograph, on a given topic. Although it is not readily accessible for membership, the GAP serves the general psychiatric audience by producing these monographs, which brings together the existing knowledge on a topic and heralds future directions in that area.

International Society of Political Psychology

Professor George Marcus
Executive Director-ISPP
Department of Political Science
Williams College
Williamstown, MA 01267
(413) 597-2538

This is an eclectic group of psychologists, psychiatrists, political scientists, and others interested in the psychology of political behavior and ethnic and international relations. It provides a different perspective than what usually is involved in a psychiatric education meeting.

International Society of Psychiatric Genetics

Dr. Lynn DeLisi
T-10 HSC-Psychiatry SUNY
Stony Brook, NY 11794
(516) 444-1612

This is a good group for those interested in the genetics of behavioral disorders.

Society of Biological Psychiatry

Elliot Richelson, M.D., Treasurer
Department of Psychiatry
Mayo Clinic Jacksonville
Research Building # 1
4500 San Pablo Road
Jacksonville, FL 32224
(904) 953-2439

This is a group focusing on biological psychiatry research advances including etiology and treatment. It holds annual meetings, usually just before the APA meeting, which center on scientific presentations. New members must be nominated by current members.

Society for Light Treatment & Biological Rhythms
P.O. Box 478
Wilsonville, OR 97070

This is a group for professionals interested in the mental health effects of light and biologic rhythms.

Society for Professors of Child and Adolescent Psychiatry
Jean DeJarnette, Administrative Assistant
3615 Wisconsin Avenue, N.W.
Washington, DC 20016
(201) 966-7300

This group would especially appeal to division heads or residency directors of child programs. The meetings primarily discuss educational concerns and economic impacts affecting child and adolescent training. Membership is open to present or past residency directors.

Society for the Scientific Study of Sex (S.S.S.S.)
P.O. Box 208
Mt. Vernon, IA 52314
(319) 895-8407

This is a group for medical educators and is an excellent forum for staying current with educational efforts and advances about the teaching on human sexuality to medical students and residents. It is also an excellent resource for teaching aides (e.g., videotapes) in this area.

II

Psychiatric Research

8

Development as a Researcher

Soo Borson, M.D., Dorcas Dobie, M.D., and
Gary J. Tucker, M.D.

Advancement of knowledge is the *summum bonum* of the scientific enterprise. Medical schools and departments of psychiatry, judged in earlier eras on the quantity of their publications and the quality of their teaching and clinical work, now command respect largely on the basis of the research dollars they draw. This seeming paradox—in which the criterion of success has become increasingly monetary—is ironic, and perhaps more in the American entrepreneurial spirit than in the European tradition of scholarship. Although creating an ethos of excellence in training and patient care is a critical function of academic clinical departments, research activity creates its external reputation. This tension between the search for new knowledge and its application in the practice of medicine often divides departments internally and can disturb the collegial environment and detract from the quality of training and service. The manner in which these three elements are balanced within a department is a critical aspect of how well, and in what domains, it is prepared to foster the development of junior faculty. This chapter focuses on dimensions of faculty development that are specifically related to preparing junior faculty for careers in scientific research.

Major research universities in this country identify themselves by their primary commitment to investigative activity, giving teaching and patient care important, but secondary, billing within their overall mission. Perhaps 20 institutions today see themselves as "research universities," and in these, the atmosphere of research pervades nearly all departments from undergraduate to graduate programs. A relative handful of departments of psychiatry are recognized as major research sites today; half of all psychiatric researchers are concentrated in 15 of the 116 departments nationwide (Pincus 1995; Pincus et al. 1993, 1995). In these research-intensive settings, rules for advancement are clear. Faculty promotion comes only with the achievement of investigative independence, evidenced by scientific publication and peer-reviewed funding, and full professorship follows only after national or international recognition of one's work. The rules for advancement are less clear and exacting in departments where research activity is less plentiful and high priority is placed on the preparation of clinicians to meet a community or regional need. As departments grow and meet this identified need, research often tends to assume new prominence.

The implicit conflict that has grown up between research, clinical care, and teaching has led, in many departments, to the formation of two academic tracks, that of the clinician-teacher, and that of the researcher. *Clinician-teachers* often participate in clinical studies and clinical trials, write illustrative case reports, develop innovative programs, and receive teaching awards from medical students and residents, frequently becoming local legends. On the other hand, *full-time researchers* vigorously pursue a focused investigative program, supported by competitive grant funding (and are in some jeopardy if this is not obtained); set a life pace separate from the needs of patients, students, and residents; and help to create the image of the department to the world through national attention to their research accomplishments. Both groups work equally hard in the pursuit of these divergent scholarly aims, but their daily lives may appear quite different.

The Academic Culture of a Department

Considering the relatively small number of major research departments of psychiatry, what does this mean for the remaining 100? Although each may have one or two partial to full-time researchers, the majority of the faculty are mainly clinician-teachers who may do some clinical investigation. The approximately 10% of residents who wish to pursue academic work must understand the type of effort expected (Yager and Burt 1994). They must grasp the culture of a department and its unstated, as well as explicit, rules for advancement. Departments can vary, from those that pursue their mission with close attention to the highest academic standards, expecting knowledgeable and scientifically informed practice and significant research, to simply large group practices whose faculty members enjoy clinical care, teaching, and salaried positions. The academic culture of a department is judged primarily on two relatively objective criteria. One is the number of peer-reviewed funded grants its faculty holds. The greater the number, the greater the likelihood that research is the predominant culture and that the department's resources will include research mentors and an infrastructure for supporting new investigators. A second criterion is the number of faculty publications and the reputation of the journals in which these appear, as an indication of scholarly quality. Although the number of publications is frequently a reflection of the number and size of funded grants, some departments without extensive research funding are strongly oriented to research, and their faculties are extremely well represented in the literature. In past years, the theoretical orientation of a department was a defining criterion of its mission, but the easy distinctions of the past, between departments with strict psychoanalytic or equally strict biologic orientation, have now become blurred by diversification within the field itself. The quality and nature of a faculty's publications are better indicators of department's orientation than what it says about itself, and, in some cases, the appearance of important research may reflect an isolated segment of departmental activity not available to the aspiring junior faculty member.

The current demands for fiscal viability have made successful competition with the private sector for patients necessary and brought new emphasis on community service and clinical care to academic psychiatry. These pressures result in the expansion of the clinician-teacher track and the number of faculty doing only clinical work and can further divide the bulk of the department from those doing research. As funds to support both clinical care and research become tighter, local support for developing new researchers has become more difficult to secure. Specifically, newly hired junior faculty must generally seek outside funding to ensure "protected" time for establishing a research program and plan. Departmental priorities in the mid-1990s are being refocused to meet the challenge of new organizational structures for delivering health care. Research funding has simultaneously become more competitive, forcing new attention on strategies for providing appropriate mentorship for developing researchers and funding their work. However, both clinical medicine and scientific inquiry have always depended mainly on the curiosity and passion of their practitioners for new and deeper knowledge. It is likely that the sea-change now taking place within academic psychiatry will stabilize over the next decade in new, but still easily recognizable forms. Those who feel the "call" to investigative work may take comfort in their fundamental commitment and in the emergence of new mechanisms for supporting their chosen direction. It is more often the drive of the individual, coupled with the support of a competent and caring mentor, that makes the successful researcher, rather than the availability of funds, fellowships, or splendid laboratories (however, these certainly facilitate the process). In the following sections, we review the nature of contemporary psychiatric research, the importance of mentorship in developing new researchers, and some of the mechanisms by which early career support may be financed.

Types of Research: "There Is Research, and There Is Research"

Many different types of research contribute to the development of psychiatry as a specialty (Table 8–1). Perhaps the most resource-intensive is *laboratory* or *bench research*. The infrastructure needed for basic laboratory research is extensive and expensive. In this fast-moving field, the mentors must be actively engaged, almost full-time, in research and have collaborators and colleagues available to them for cooperation and cross-fertilization.

Psychiatry in the 1950s, 1960s, and 1970s used much of its federal support for training clinicians and teachers. Few institutions foresaw the dramatic developments that have taken place in psychiatric neurobiology and developed the research infrastructure (departmental laboratories or basic research equipment) necessary for success. Consequently, the bulk of laboratory space is occupied, in most medical schools, by departments of

Table 8–1. Types of psychiatric research

	Technical skill needed	Creative potential	Mentoring requirements
Basic neuroscience (including imaging)	High	High	High
Health services	High	High	High
Clinical phenomenology	Moderate	Moderate to High	Moderate
Treatment outcomes	Moderate	Moderate	Moderate
Clinical drug trials	Low	Low	Low

basic science, medicine, and a few surgical subspecialties. Most of these specialties put their training moneys into the development of researchers and of an infrastructure of laboratories, equipment, and mentors that provided a firm base for laboratory investigation, which continues to grow today. Psychiatry has come relatively late to this enterprise as a result of the recent explosion of methodologies in the behavioral neurosciences. Consequently, aspiring researchers who choose a career in laboratory investigation must find a department already so engaged, or spend time outside the home department. Few others will have the resources to develop substantial basic research divisions de novo in the near future.

Clinical research involving patients and patient care has also become more structured and specialized than in the past. A relatively new example is *health services research,* in which large populations are examined with structured instruments for detecting prevalent psychiatric disorders and outcomes of current treatments, and for testing alternative practice patterns. The rigorous methodology required for meaningful results frequently involves collaboration with epidemiologists, statisticians, and other clinician specialists committed to the research topic. Some departments have the resources to support these highly trained personnel, whereas in others, the necessary collaboration must be supported by a series of interrelated grants awarded to investigators in different departments or schools.

The systematization of psychiatric diagnosis based on the empiricism of DSM-III (American Psychiatric Press 1980), and successive generations of its approach, has stimulated much interest in research on diagnostic criteria and methodologies. This kind of research often requires fewer resources, and many small but informative studies of specific diagnostic groupings and *clinical phenomenology* are still within the scope of investigation by the clinically trained individual investigator, whose primary commitment is to improving patient care.

Many departments provide the clinical infrastructure for *clinical treatment trials,* most often designed and supported by the pharmaceutical industry, which requires busy clinical practice sites to establish the safety and effectiveness of new treatments. Although these studies may offer little in the way of intellectual, creative, or academic interest to investigators, they can provide seed money for the development of other research endeavors. However, the indirect costs demanded by academic institutions have made the private practice sector more attractive as sites for such trials, and industry support has diminished in many academic centers.

The last type of investigation in psychiatry is *clinical synthetic research*. This traditional form of scholarship provided the early foundation of psychiatry in Europe and continues to flourish in a few centers both in America and abroad. Experienced physicians offer a synthesis of their own clinical experience within a historical context, integrating it, often in the form of a topical monograph, with contemporary perspectives on diagnosis and treatment, that can be the culmination of a life's work. These are usually most successful when written by a senior professor who has already established prominence in the field; books such as *Delirium* by Lipowski (1990), and *Organic Psychiatry* by Lishman (1980), are examples of exquisitely documented clinical texts that have contributed to the evolution of an entire field. Such works charge a new generation of researchers with the tasks of validating and explicating the fundamental mechanisms underlying the phenomena observed in patients.

Where to Start

Faced with these disparate forms of scholarly activity, aspiring faculty members must begin by identifying the type of research best suited to their temperament and interests, and by searching out potential resources available within the department they wish to join. Chief among these resources are *mentors* who are able and willing to help develop the careers of others and can assist them in acquiring the essential *technical expertise*. Although diagnostic and phenomenological research, clinical trials, and synthetic research may superficially appear simpler for beginning faculty to undertake, these areas may be poorly funded and the work must be left to one's ever-diminishing spare time. Progress in these areas is correspondingly more difficult and may rapidly reach a ceiling beyond which no significant further development can take place. For launching a viable research program in today's funding climate, formal research training is almost—if not certainly—mandatory. Table 8–2 provides a set of questions for prospective junior faculty that may be useful in deciding whether a department of interest is ready to meet his or her needs.

Technical Training

While individuals vary enormously in energy levels and maturity, the acquisition of technical expertise requires formal methodologic training at

Table 8–2. Checklist for prospective junior faculty

---

1. Are my specific interests welcomed in the department?
2. Is there a senior research mentor available within the department? If not, can I identify external mentoring support?
3. What options are available for research training? Will these help me achieve my goals?
4. What choices do I have for allocating my time?
5. How committed is the department to advancing new knowledge?
6. Does the contract offered to me support or hinder my research development? Can I negotiate alternatives?
7. Are my overall career development needs recognized in sufficient detail (including possible interruption for starting a family)?

---

some stage in career development. Some new investigators will develop research skills without assurance of funding, protected time, or the support of their families, whereas others will only do so when these assets are readily available. These divergent temperaments and facts of experience are both compatible with eventual success, but a high level of preparedness undeniably eases the transition into faculty life. Some residents come to psychiatry with intensive background for investigation. Increasingly, these are dual-degreed M.D./Ph.D.s with specific expertise in, for example, basic pharmacology, molecular biology, quantitative neuroimaging, experimental psychology, or genetics, and a desire to use their skills to advance knowledge of the basic causes of mental illness. Others may become committed to research through participation in a mentor's project during residency training. The person with sophisticated research training prior to becoming a faculty member often needs little more than time and minimal support (depending on the type of research) to develop a project and become competitive for outside funding. However, mentorship is still important for guidance in assuming faculty responsibilities and advocacy with senior members of the department. Frequently, a well-prepared junior investigator will negotiate protected time as part of an initial contract, but the person must have a clear understanding, preferably in writing, of how much time is to be allocated to research, the resources to be provided, opportunities for further training, and the potential for collaboration. Most such contracts are time-limited, allowing 2 to 3 years for development that is expected to culminate in extramural funding.

For prospective faculty without prior research training, a period of formal postresidency fellowship is becoming an increasingly important requisite. The National Institutes of Health offer on-site fellowships in specialized lines of research, but some academic departments at major research universities hold institutional training grants that provide substantial support for developing technical research skills. It is difficult, if not impossible—in most settings today—for young investigators to gain effective research training only after joining a faculty and assuming the necessary clinical obligations this entails. As research becomes more complex and collaborative, departments seek junior faculty who come with a foundation that will not only continue to grow but also complement existing expertise and enrich the total research enterprise. Unfortunately, general residency programs cannot be expected to provide sufficient research training experience to enable a graduate to successfully pursue an academic career. Hence, fellowship training may be an essential developmental step. For those intending to do laboratory research, this requires 2 to 4 years of nearly full-time apprenticeship to a senior scientist. For those expecting to do clinical research in either health services or diagnostic, phenomenological, or therapeutic aspects of psychiatry, several years may be devoted to a course of study ending in a master's degree in public health or another health-related discipline, usually as part of a funded fellowship program. Not surprisingly, though, demands for increased clinical productivity have affected fellowships as well as faculty positions. The aspiring academician should evaluate fellowship programs carefully, with an eye toward the amount of actual research training and protected time available in the curriculum. An inquiry as to funding sources and levels provided within the fellowship structure is one way to assess whether research training is a priority. In most instances, candidates must be prepared to sacrifice, temporarily, the faculty-level income expected by their peers who accept positions primarily dedicated to clinical service.

Mentoring

A decisive factor in successful entry into an investigative career is the availability of role models and mentors who are willing to invest their own time in the development of junior faculty. In large departments of psychiatry, it is easy for junior members to get lost in the diverse demands of academic life and to fail criteria for promotion, coming up short with regard to evidence of research productivity after being swamped with clinical work or stuck at some stage of their research because of insufficient senior faculty guidance. Like medical practice, research training is an apprenticeship and requires a significant investment of time to reach maturity.

Some large departments have developed formal mentoring programs to facilitate faculty career development (Fried et al. 1996). At the University of Washington (with 155 faculty members and considerable funded research), it became apparent that junior faculty were being hired but not promoted, a problem due largely to insufficient research productivity and particularly affecting women physicians. As a result, a formal structure for mentoring was developed and modified by faculty input provided during a departmental retreat. The proposal adopted (presented in Table 8–3) requires each junior faculty member hired to be supported by a three-person mentoring committee to look after the individual's academic development, attending specifically to research, teaching, and clinical skills. Faculty meet with their committees twice a year, after which a written progress report is sent to the chair and the individual's service chief. The chair and service chief then meet with each faculty member to discuss accomplishments and future needs. After 4 years of implementation, a departmental review of this mentoring program was undertaken. Most faculty reported that this new program contributed significantly to the research development of junior investigators, by providing a forum for systematic monitoring and advising to help maintain focus and overcome obstacles. The participation of the service chief on the mentoring committee was cited as a potential concern, allowing a vehicle for exploitation of faculty on busy clinical services. Nevertheless, the committee mechanism has received wide acceptance by both junior and senior faculty and promises to help protect young faculty from overly burdensome demands on their time while they establish research credentials. It keeps promotion time lines and criteria visible to mentees and makes established faculty accountable in the development of their junior colleagues. The following is a composite example of a mentorship committee report and gives the sense of how the process works. Dr. M. is a late-blooming but promising physician-investigator whose promotion is in jeopardy.

> Dr. Mentee's committee met with him last week to discuss his progress over the last six months. His clinical work and teaching are acknowledged as excellent. He encountered difficulties with promotion last year because he had not yet defined a productive research direction. He has

Table 8–3. A mentoring plan

---

1. On acceptance of a new junior faculty appointment (assistant professor and below), an individual mentorship committee is assigned to assist in defining an appropriate career path. Members include:
   - some or all members of the search committee active in his/her recruitment, or
   - persons appointed by the chair, vice-chair for research development, and clinical service chief, if no search committee was convened.

   This initial committee serves for the first 6 months, counseling the mentee on early career development and identifying the appropriate composition of a permanent mentoring group best suited to his/her needs and interests.

2. After 6 months, the mentee, together with the chair, vice-chair, and service chief, meet to select and appoint the permanent committee.

3. The permanent committee will consist of three individuals, usually senior in rank, and generally includes the research mentor (to whom the mentee relates in day-to-day research interactions) and the service chief.

4. The functions of the mentorship committee are two:
   - to foster and oversee career development in each of the major areas of faculty life: research, teaching and supervision, and clinical care/administration where relevant.
   - to advise the chair on progress.

5. Its activities include *supporting the faculty,* by
   - helping to identify a research focus (if needed) and/or a research mentor (or collaborators, if classical mentorship is not needed).
   - facilitating access to appropriate individuals for research and clinical development.
   - identifying specific needs for research and teaching support services
   - observing and critiquing teaching and clinical care
   - meeting with mentees at least twice a year, and ad hoc if problems arise

   and *assisting the chair,* through

   - advising on solutions to structural tensions (e.g., heavy clinical loads, special needs such as family leave) that impede scholarly progress
   - preparing an annual written progress report to be used in yearly meetings with each faculty member

6. The mechanism for troubleshooting: Changes in the composition of the mentorship committee may be requested by the mentors or by the mentee. Requests are handled at the committee level, with input as needed from the service chief, chair, or vice-chair.

7. Mentorship committee appointments will be publicized, to give recognition to mentees and their mentors throughout the department and to serve as an ongoing mechanism for highlighting faculty activities.

---

made substantial progress but more is required, and, to that end, the committee supported his decision to relinquish his time-consuming administrative job and strongly encouraged his continued work with the established depression research group he joined three years ago. He has taken the lead on a very promising project investigating plasma ragase levels after plagyminol challenge in recovered patients with major depression, and he plans to test the results in a model for predicting relapse. The plagyminol studies will be resubmitted this spring as a considerably stronger RO-1; two members of the committee have worked closely with him on structuring appropriate revisions in response to reviewers' comments, which should improve its chances for funding. We have also advised him on revisions of three research manuscripts that should promote publication in good journals. His work is interesting and nicely complements the direction of his collaborative group; he is a quick study and has been very responsive to suggestions. Committee members were in agreement that his promotion will hinge on whether his outstanding teaching record and signs of increasing research productivity will be enough.

Two groups of junior faculty are especially vulnerable to delayed or inhibited success as researchers: women and M.D.s without prior research training. The development of women faculty members has been historically very difficult in clinical departments and requires specific efforts toward remediation (Fried et al. 1996; Kaplan et al. 1996). The interruption of a career for the bearing and rearing of children is a watershed in the lives of most women, coming for most at an extremely vulnerable time in their academic evolution, and this has particularly powerful effects on talented women without prior research training. Creating appropriate structures and mechanisms for supporting women—who are more often pulled "off track" by competing needs to nurture children while their career clocks keep ticking—has only just begun in academic medicine generally. Ample data indicate that women tend to cluster in the lower ranks and salary ranges and in more demanding clinical jobs, may be less academically productive, and often find less institutional support for their research than their male counterparts (Kaplan et al. 1996). They tend to progress through the ranks more slowly even when academic indicators are comparable (Tesch et al. 1995), and they are more likely to suffer from perceived gender bias, inappropriately lowered career expectations, and limited access to information critical to their development (Fried et al. 1996). The roots of these problems are complex but surmountable with concentrated departmental efforts (Fried et al. 1996). Career path modifications (e.g., part-time assignments; delaying the tenure clock during this phase; intensive, mentored efforts to find research support while temporarily delaying full entry into clinical and administrative duties without prejudice) are one institutional mechanism for acknowledging the particular requirements of women during the years of necessary preoccupation with childbearing and childrearing. Even when such attempts are made, however, women must still navigate the changing sense of self that comes with motherhood and struggle with concerns about diminished competitiveness by virtue of adding a new identity to their carefully nurtured professional selves. Furthermore, the academic ethos has historically demanded a devotion to the research enterprise that is difficult for a new mother to sustain. Attending national meetings to meet colleagues and gain the national visibility necessary for promotion is unrealistic for many women caring for young children, and research productivity may plateau for an extended period. Current academic structures do not recognize this normative phase for women with significant family responsibilities, or that productivity may rise steeply once children become more autonomous. Whether the academic mission can sustain an interest in doing what is necessary to recruit and keep gifted women faculty, during a time of relative economic tumult and competitive pressure, remains to be seen. The emerging research literature in this area provides an essential tool for supporting new developments in this direction.

It is evident that in many departments of psychiatry, faculty of both sexes who enter with Ph.D.s and structured research training are much more likely to achieve senior ranks than those who begin with M.D.s and little research training, who are hired into positions requiring large clinical time investments. Unlike the full-time researcher, who has the resources to shift schedules to participate in the logistics of child care or the demands of the family, the young clinician must be present, at specific hours, for any and all problems that arise; energies are easily exhausted by these demands. It is for this group that postresidency research fellowships are most urgently needed.

Life Cycle of a Researcher

The lifestyle of the full-time researcher is at least as demanding as that of the clinician. His or her activities and funding depend on a high level of personal investment, long work hours, and sufficient autonomy and freedom to follow where the science leads. Certainly, the existence of the researcher is more precarious than that of the clinician (as one can always find patients who need care). The increasing competition for research dollars demands much of the investigator but also much of academic administration. In this section, we describe the three phases in the life cycle of an investigator and some elements of administrative foresight that foster successful transitions from one phase to the next.

Early Career: Building the Foundation

The first step is the development of research skills and knowledge, usually through a project under the direction of a senior investigator. This period of apprenticeship prepares junior faculty members to move to the next stage as independent investigators, capable of generating and sustaining their own research support. Mentorship programs provide specific support during this period.

Midcareer: Establishing and Maintaining Scientific Creativity

During this stage, which ideally lasts throughout the life of an investigator, the primary products are new knowledge, publications, expanded mastery of a chosen field, and development of a flexible network of scientific colleagues. It is typical at this stage for investigators to be involved collaboratively in projects developed by others, in addition to deepening their investment in their own particular area. They take on responsibility for training students and sometimes residents in research, and they must maintain a reasonably stable stream of funding for themselves and their trainees. They may join research review panels that decide on the merit of their colleagues' proposals. The skills required for successful traverse of this stage of development are stamina and hardiness, broad intellectual curiosity without sacrifice of focus, the ability to communicate effectively with other members of the scientific community, and interpersonal talents that foster productive working relationships. Hazards include inimical changes in departmental administration that lower the priority of one's work, the emergence of personality flaws that inhibit collaboration and scientific growth, and unpredictable personal hardships that divert attention from professional activity. Effective navigation of this stage evolves naturally into the next, that of generativity.

Late Career: Building the Next Generation of Researchers

Generativity, the manifestation of mature investment in both scientific work and the welfare of departmental and organizational structures that support it, has received very little formal attention outside the social sciences, and, within academic medicine, the scientist much past 60 continues to be held in some suspicion as possibly incapable of innovation (Johnson 1996). However, solid and creative mentoring and programmatic contributions, on both a local and a national scale, are the hallmarks of this stage and are compatible with continued scientific growth and with new discovery. One's own success established, that of junior scientists becomes a personal priority and a source of intense satisfaction. Generative mentors find pathways to national recognition for their younger colleagues, through helping them consolidate their research directions and critiquing their papers and proposals to enhance their chances of success. They develop training programs, become editors or members of editorial boards of specialty journals, and participate in policy-setting bodies of professional organizations. There is some reason to think that skills for generativity are partially learned during the early phases of career development, through identification with valued mentors who gave generously of their time and talents. They are also learned through the mistakes and failures of one's mentors. Hazards to achieving real generativity, given success—and sometimes great creativity—as an investigator, fall primarily in the domain of personality. Inability to master competitive drives can lead senior scientists to stifle the development of their juniors, by failing to credit their work or appreciate their growing autonomy, neglecting key areas in which their support is vital, or behaving in other ways that are overtly or covertly undermining. An aspect of working generativity is teaching one's mentees to move to independence when the time is right. The low esteem in which traditional (but fast-disappearing) academic tenure in medical schools has been held is owed, in large part, to failures of senior faculty to take the mantle of responsibility conferred upon them by their own past contributions. Studies of predictors of third-stage career success are an important step toward building robust faculties of the future.

The elements of this three-stage pattern of career development have changed little since Osler's time, but the mechanisms for achieving it have changed dramatically. At the turn of the century, good observational skills, an experimental turn of mind that could be applied to any type of clinical or investigative problem, and a scholarly attitude were all that were required, provided a department chair was willing to commit resources to the support of promising young faculty. At least one recent Nobelist has noted that his ideas never would have found a home within today's environment for research support by centralized peer review. The broadening, differentiation, and formalization of the scientific methodologies required for different forms of scholarship have made apprenticeship in medicine a lengthier and more rigorous process than it was in Osler's day. A specialized set of skills in mentors and departmental administrators are needed that make complex entrepreneurial talents a more prominent feature of administrative life than in former times.

These skills depend on the cultivation of an attitude oriented toward the continuous updating of knowledge of funding mechanisms appropriate for faculty at differing stages of career development. The National Institutes of Health, the Department of Veterans' Affairs, and, increasingly, private foundations that support research have created pathways for supporting career growth that partially pay salaries to enable junior faculty to enhance their research skills. Residents seeking research careers as faculty members should inquire about how a prospective academic "home" department has made use of these opportunities in their own fields of interest. Table 8–4 presents a sampling of options. Departments wishing to support these important mechanisms may benefit from creating offices of research development, to provide the necessary infrastructure for the preparation of grants, keep abreast of developments, facilitate the research process, and complement the more personalized mentorship activities offered individually to junior faculty. Finally, administrative promotion of opportunities for collaborative research among investigators within a department or school should be welcomed by senior faculty as extensions of their mentorship roles. An example is the creation of interdisciplinary training programs, such as those in behavioral neuroscience that have begun to emerge in several major universities. As yet, these rarely include psychiatry faculty as leaders in their development, but the interdisciplinary relationships fostered within them help to buffer the unpredictability of research funding for individual investigators, and more importantly, they create a climate of mutual assistance and excitement on which the academic enterprise ultimately depends.

Table 8–4. Some mechanisms for supporting early research career development[*]

National Institutes of Health

- Postdoctoral fellowships in Bethesda
- Small grants
- Coinvestigator roles on senior faculty research grants
- Institutional National Research Service fellowships
- Individual postdoctoral fellowships (at the home site)
- Mentored Research and Clinical Scientist development awards
- FIRST awards
- Academic career awards

A Few Foundations (examples of types of research supported)

- Alzheimer's Disease and Related Disorders Association (biological, clinical, and social/behavioral aspects of neurodegenerative diseases)
- American Suicide Foundation (suicide and its prevention)
- Bristol-Myers Squibb Foundation (neuroscience)
- Burroughs Wellcome Fund (neuroscience, psychopharmacology)
- Carnegie Corporation (social research, child and adolescent)
- Commonwealth Fund (health services, child/adolescent, aging)
- Robert Wood Johnson Foundation (health services, alcohol/substance abuse)
- Henry J. Kaiser Foundation (health services, child/adolescent, aging, substance abuse, minority and women's issues)
- McArthur Foundation (diagnosis, mood disorders, health services, consultation-liaison, child/adolescent, aging, violence)
- National Alliance for Research on Schizophrenia and Depression (neuroscience, clinical psychobiology, psychopharmacology, affective disorders, psychosis)
- Pew Charitable Trusts (cognitive neuroscience, health services, child/adolescent, poverty)
- Sandoz Foundation for Gerontological Research (geriatric psychiatry, aging issues)
- Scottish Rite (clinical psychobiology, psychopharmacology, psychosis)

---

[*]*Many other resources exist. For a more comprehensive treatment, see Pincus HA (Ed), 1995.*

References

American Psychiatric Association: Diagnostic and Statistical Manual of Mental Disorders, 3rd Edition. Washington, DC, American Psychiatric Association, 1980

Fried LP, Francomano CA, MacDonald SM, et al: Career development for women in academic medicine: multiple interventions in a department of medicine. JAMA 276:898–905, 1996

Johnson HA: "Osler recommends chloroform at sixty." Pharos 59(1):24–26, 1996

Kaplan SH, Sullivan LM, Dukes KA, et al: Sex differences in academic advancement: results of a national study of pediatricians. N Engl J Med 335:1282–1289, 1996

Lipowski ZJ: Delirium. New York, NY, Oxford University Press, 1990

Lishman WA: Organic Psychiatry, 3rd Edition. Oxford, England, Blackwell Science, 1997

Pincus HA (ed): Research Funding and Resource Manual: Mental Health and Addictive Disorders. Washington, DC, American Psychiatric Association, 1995

Pincus HA, Dial TH, Haviland MG: Research activities of full-time faculty in academic departments of psychiatry. Arch Gen Psychiatry 50:657–664, 1993

Pincus HA, Haviland MG, Dial TH, et al: The relationship of postdoctoral research training to current research activities of faculty in academic departments of psychiatry. Am J Psychiatry 152:596–601, 1995

Tesch BJ, Wood HM, Helwig AL, et al: Promotion of women physicians in academic medicine: glass ceiling or sticky floor? JAMA 273:1022–1025, 1995

Yager J, Burt VK: A survival guide for aspiring academic psychiatrists: personality attributes and opportunities for academic success. Academic Psychiatry 18:197–210, 1994

9

Generating and Implementing Research Ideas

Michele T. Pato, M.D.

Research can be simply described as systematically posing a question and attempting to answer it. This definition is not meant to belittle the effort that goes into pursuing research endeavors, but to make the point that research is within the reach of any good clinician. At the core of pursuing the care of any patient is the generation of a hypothesis (diagnosis), or question, and the generation of an experiment (treatment) to test whether the hypothesis (diagnosis) was correct (Rutter 1990).

The problem then is finding a way to form a question so one can answer it with the resources available. The resources for answering these questions come in many forms, but the most important resource is a personal one, enthusiasm for what you want to study. Without enthusiasm, it will be hard to sustain interest through the inevitable frustrations and setbacks in pursuing the answer to the questions.

This issue of enthusiasm begs the questions, "Why do research?" The answer can be found on both a professional and personal level. Professionally, research advances the field, contributes to the better care of patients (directly or indirectly), advances your own career, and gains you the respect of colleagues and peers. Perhaps more important, the care one gives patients, the treatments we offer, should be based on proven effective interventions and not on tradition or anecdote. There are also the personal rewards that come from satisfying your own curiosity, from seeing something through to completion, from furthering your own thinking as you get feedback and critique from colleagues, and from finding new ways to enjoy what you do as a clinician (Burke et al. 1986; Garfinkel et al. 1989).

Although enthusiasm may be the critical component in sustaining the research effort, obviously other skills and attributes are needed as well. Burke et al. (1986) noted five such attributes: (1) values and motives, (2) clinical care of patients, (3) creativity and disciplined thinking, (4) management skills for the organization and maintenance of the research effort, and (5) technical skills. Although there may be a tendency to think of the technical skills as the ones most needed for the clinician to make the transition to research, they are, in fact, noted Burke et al., the easiest and quickest to acquire. The values, motives, and management skills are slower to acquire and require a more developmental learning curve. In fact, the technical skills often do not have to be a barrier at all to doing research. As long as the question is posed in an answerable form, one can seek out those with the expertise and collaborate with them to get the answers.

Where Do Ideas Come From?

If research is within the reach of all those who wish to pursue it, then the issue becomes, "How do you do it?" The first order of business is having an idea. For most clinicians, the most ready sources of ideas come from their patients, or more broadly their clinical experience (Hulley and Cummings 1988; Leibenluft et al. 1989). Ideas can arise from things as simple as a side effect, a treatment response, or a diagnostic dilemma. Rutter (1990) writes: "We need to train ourselves to recognize when something unexpected occurs, and to be able to appreciate when there is an important generalizable lesson in that surprise" (p. 446). Other sources of research ideas may come from administrative experience, supervisory experiences, or philosophical exploration. Hulley and Cummings (1988) extend the notion of research a bit further, defining research as "the process of drawing inferences about the truth in the universe from events observed in the study sample" (p. vi).

Perhaps most critical to forming a researchable question is recognizing a question as important and being creative in your approach to it. Hulley and Cummings (1988) suggest the "so what" approach; namely, that the answer to the question should contribute usefully to the state of knowledge about the subject. They define a hypothesis simply as a researchable question: "A hypothesis is a version of a research question that has the purpose of providing the basis for testing the statistical significance of the findings" (Hulley and Cummings 1988, p. 4).

Thus, early in the process of formulating a researchable question, a hypothesis, statistical considerations become important. The concept of biostatistics often seems to loom as a major stumbling block for clinicians trying to pursue research because they often do not have formal training in this area. But, at its core, biostatistics is a simple process. Glantz (1988) gives a definition of biostatistics that should be comforting to anyone, even the neophyte. He says: "Biostatistics provides the tools for turning clinical and laboratory experience into quantitative statements about whether, and by how much, a treatment or procedure affected a group of patients" (Glantz 1988, p. 3). Thus, two of the most critical aspects of turning a notion into research are picking a question and describing your results in a quantitative way (statistics).

Steps in the Formulation of a Research Project

The first order of business is asking a question that can be answered. Once a topic or item of interest has been identified, you have to pose a question (hypothesis) you wish to answer. Usually, it is helpful to read some literature related to the topic. Find out what has already been written. Not only does this tell you what questions have already been asked and answered, but it will also give you hints about what methods have been used to answer questions in your area of choice. It is often best to start with a current review article or a short chapter, because these will give a broad overview and will usually include the most relevant and recent references to further direct one's reading. However, one should shy away from books or lengthy chapters, which will often take you too far afield from focusing on the question and finding a way to ask it so it can be answered. Along with a short review, it is important to look at any recent articles that have asked and answered the same or similar questions. December issues of most journals include an author and subject index for the entire year and can provide a quick way to get some recent articles before you head to the library or your own home computer to do a Medline search. Further reference searching can most easily be done through on-line computer searches. There are several software packages such as Grateful Med that can give you access to the MEDLARS database of the National Library of Medicine (NLM). This database is frequently updated though there can be at least a 2-week gap in entries appearing in it. More current citations can be accessed also through Current Contents, which is updated weekly by The Institute for Scientific Information, but it contains mostly titles and is not always indexed in an easily accessible way. An alternative for very recent citations might be SDI (Selective Dissemination of Information). This service, for a price, will do a periodic search (usually monthly) of citations and abstracts in specific topics of your choosing and send them to you. The selections are made from the more than 3,000 titles on file at the NLM. (The interested reader is referred to Sackett et al. 1991 for details and further references.)

Once you've read a few (three to five) articles, you should begin to ask yourself questions such as, Can I formulate my question or hypothesis just a little differently to both replicate and then extend the previous work? This is often a good way to get a project off the ground. It is also important to remember that the way the question is posed will also affect the design of the study. Ideally, the question posed should lead to a study that is feasible, interesting, novel, ethical, and relevant (Hulley and Cummings 1988). This leads naturally to a consideration of resources that are available to do the study. The first question is who, or what, will be the subject of the study.

When one mentions the word *subject* what initially comes to mind is a whole living patient, but this is too narrow a definition of a subject for research purposes. A subject can take many forms, from a live patient to the patient's chart to some of the patient's cells or blood or to an animal who exhibits behavior similar in some way to that seen in humans so that it can be used as a model for human behavior. Even past literature, written by others, can be seen as the subject of a research project where you might reanalyze that data to answer your own research question.

One of the key issues in choosing your subject pool is to remember that in answering the question, you want your results to be as generalizable as possible to the larger population of similar subjects that you were not able to study. One is usually not in the position to study the entire subject pool, either because it is too big, too expensive, or in some other way not feasible. Thus, the study population must be selected from the whole target population sample in such a way that is still representative. Once the "subject" type has been chosen, there are two questions that must be answered: (1) Who are the subjects? (subject selection), and (2) How will they be selected? (sampling design). Subject selection involves establishing inclusion and exclusion criteria that will allow you to choose a sample of subjects that is representative of the target population you want to study. Sampling design involves decisions about how subjects meeting the inclusion and exclusion criteria will be chosen to enter the study. (See Hulley and Cummings 1988, pp. 18–30, for further details.)

The next decision involves what measurements to use to get your results. Again, the choice of measurements must be related to the question being asked. It is often helpful to think of the data being collected in two categories. The outcome variables, the things you want to find out, and the predictor variables, those things that may affect the outcome. In statistical terms, the outcome variables are often referred to as the dependent variables and the predictor variables as the independent variables. Although there are exceptions to the rule, it is probably easiest to think of these variables in terms of the researcher manipulating the predictor variables (independent variables) and then measuring the outcome variables (dependent variables) as the results.

In choosing ways to measure variables, the researcher should keep several things in mind. First, the ideal measurement is one that is appropriate, objective, and sensitive yet specific. In addition, the measurement instrument must be able to detect differences over a wide range of values. Measurements come in many varieties, including rating scales, diagnostic interviews, laboratory results, demographic data, and neuroimaging results just to name a few. But in every case, three factors must be considered because they affect the precision of a measurement. These factors are the observer, the subject, and the instrument itself. When designing the research study, one should remember the primary question (hypothesis) and make sure that, in collecting the data to answer this primary question, the measurements are as accurate as possible. For example, if you are doing a study of side effect differences between two medications, a rater-administered side effect scale would be advisable over a self-report scale, since the latter may be inaccurate because of subject bias. However, if the main question in the study is one of treatment efficacy, a subject self-report rating scale of side effects is fine, because it is not the primary research question.

The final step in developing a research project is often a statistical one. Some of the more clinically based and descriptive pilot studies described in the following section, "Types of Projects and Publications," might not always require statistical analyses. But as one moves from more anecdotal and descriptive research to analytic and experimental studies, the following two questions must be addressed: (1) How large must my study sample be? (i.e., issues of power), and (2) How will the data be analyzed? A detailed answer to these questions is beyond the scope of this chapter, but Table 9–1 provides some basic definitions of statistical factors that may be involved in answering these two questions. It is important to ask these two questions *before* one begins to collect data, because answering these questions could be critical to the amount and type of data collected. More specifically, one can tailor the type of data collected to statistical methods that one is familiar with or in which one's collaborators have expertise. It is also wise to avoid study designs and collection of data types that will be beyond the scope of the investigator to later analyze and interpret. The interested reader is referred to Hulley and Cummings (1988, pp. 139–150) for a concise and understandable explanation of estimating sample size and to Glantz (1988) for the basics on biostatistics. In addition, it is often helpful to collaborate with a statistician early on so that he or she can contribute to the design of the study.

Types of Projects and Publications

Although the most critical aspect of pursuing any research project is to first pose a single answerable primary question (hypothesis), it is not always easy to figure out what form the question and ultimately the project should take. One thing that might help is to think hierarchically and to ask oneself a series of questions. The first question is, Do I want to stand apart from the study or intervene in the events of the study? The former will dictate a more observational study, the latter will require experimental manipulation of some sort. The second question is, If the study is observational, will it be a single occasion, a cross-sectional study, or over a period of time, a longitudinal study? And the final question is, Will the study involve past and present events, retrospective, or future events, prospective? (Hulley and Cummings 1988).

As researchers answer these questions, the type of study to be done begins to take shape. The simplest type of study is a descriptive study, in which one simply describes the phenomena. This type of study usually leads to publications such as letters to the editor, case reports, and systematic case series and, in a more abstract sense, may be simply a review of the literature. The next stage in the hierarchy is the analytic study. Analytic studies look at cause-and-effect relationships. Studies like this can appear in the literature as retrospective and prospective chart reviews, literature reviews, commentary or editorial pieces, and reports on questionnaire find-

Table 9–1. Basic definition of statistical factors

Statistical test or principle	Reason to compute or assess	What it can contribute to developing the research project
Power	To make sure the sample you are studying is large enough for your conclusions to be valid.	Helps you decide how many "subjects" to study.
Reliability	To assess a measurement can be made consistently, over repeated administration or different raters.	Helps ensure adequate measures of symptoms are being used.
Validity	To assess if the variables chosen actually measure the phenomena they intend to measure.	Helps ensure adequate measures of symptoms are being used.
Kappa (or Interclass Correlation Coefficient, ICC)	To demonstrate agreement between two raters taking into account that some agreement may occur by chance.	Assesses whether measurements are reliable when more than one "rater" is being used.
Analysis of variance (ANOVA)	Answers the question: Is the difference seen between the means of the groups being studied just due to chance or due to the experimental manipulation?	Allows for testing of significance of results. Tests whether the groups studied (usually more than two groups) showed a true difference in results.
T-Test	A simplified ANOVA that only involved two groups.	Allows for testing of significance of results. Tests differences *only* between two groups.
Correlations	To measure how one variable changes in relation to another variable.	Gives information on the relationship between two or more variables but does *not* necessarily imply causation.

(*continued*)

187

Table 9–1. Continued

Statistical test or principle	Reason to compute or assess	What it can contribute to developing the research project
Nonparametric tests	To test for differences in variables that are nonarithmetic, or not normally distributed. These tests usually measure categorical differences rather than numeric ones.	Allows for significance testing of qualitative data or of data from skewed distributions.
Chi squared	A nonparametric test that compares expected and observed results of a "treatment."	Allows for significance testing of categorical results, e.g. response vs. nonresponse to a treatment in two different groups.
Relative risk and odds ratio	To measure the association between a predictor and an outcome variable.	Allows for epidemiologic study of populations rather than individual subjects. Allows for comment on associations between variables as a correlation might do.

Adapted mostly from Glantz 1988.

ings. The most complex studies are experimental studies. In these studies, one tries to establish the effect of an intervention. Such studies often appear in the literature as small clinical trials, prospective blinded clinical trials, or basic science hypothesis-driven trials. Often in the course of pursuing a particular line of research, one will engage in all three aspects of study design—starting first with observation reports such as letters to the editor or a small case series, then moving to retrospective studies of a group of patients who one predicts might have a similar reaction, and finally designing and executing a blinded clinical trial. (See Table 9–2 for some examples.)

Many think of research with a capital "R," implying that it requires formal grants and research proposals and usually a great deal of money. Although many research projects that are pursued in a systematic way will ultimately require some, even considerable, funding, in reality most research projects start small. Many projects go through stages, moving in a natural progression from single patient experience to a complicated research endeavor. Your own contribution to the field, even if it doesn't lead you to a large research grant, may contribute along the way to others doing research. Thus, in terms of getting from a notion to a research project, it is helpful to examine how small projects can move to bigger projects and what your options are in contributing to the research literature.

Teaching How to Do Research

The focus of this chapter has been on going from a notion, or a question, to designing and implementing a research project. Obviously, reading this chapter will not suddenly make one a researcher, but it may begin to let one think and formulate ideas to begin a project. Initial projects are best done in collaboration with others, ideally someone who has already done research. However, not everyone has such acquaintances. In addition, it has been my experience that just because someone can do research does not mean they can teach how to do research.

To try to deal with the difficulties in finding good mentors and learning to do research, I developed a seminar series called "The Scientific Approach in Psychiatry." The seminar systematically presents how to do research. It takes the student of research through thinking about how to ask questions, as this chapter does. Then, it goes through the different types of study designs from case reports to chart review studies to blinded clinical trials to laboratory experiments and large sample prospective and retrospective

Table 9–2. Examples of types of studies

Types of study or publication	Strengths	Weaknesses
Letters to the editor	Descriptive. May generate hypothesis. May inform others of important issues.	No control of variables.
Case series	Descriptive. May generate hypothesis. May inform others of important issues. Can begin to point toward associations.	No control of variables.
Literature review	May allow for reanalysis of data in new light; may generate new hypothesis. Descriptive. May inform others of important issues.	Can draw erroneous conclusion since not based on primary data but just interpretations of interpretations being published.
Open clinical trial	May allow for some inference about relationships between variables. Can do more cheaply than randomized clinical trial (RCT) so often used as a pilot study to decide whether to pursue an RCT.	Allows for minimal control of some variables. Run the risk Type II error especially because sample size typically too small from a power point of view.

Study type	Advantages	Disadvantages
Case-control study	Allows for *some* inference about relationships and causation. Allows some control of variables.	Requires large sample so can be expensive. Usually retrospective so don't have control over as many variables.
Cohort study	Allows for *more* inference about relationships and causation. Often prospective so easier to control variables.	Requires large sample. Even more expensive than case-control study because is prospective and potential dropouts cause more problems.
Randomized clinical (controlled) trial (RCT)	Most powerful results. Allows for *most* inference about relationships and causation because allows for most control over independent variables.	Often expensive because power mandates adequate size. Often difficult to complete because stricter inclusion and exclusion criteria mean fewer subjects eligible to participate.

epidemiologic studies (see Table 9–2). Finally, as is described in Chapter 3, the seminar explains how to write up and publish one's findings.

This seminar often seems a daunting task to set up at a given institution, especially one that is not particularly strong in research. However, invariably, some topics related to research design and methodology are already being taught. If one organizes the existing lectures in sequence, it can often be easy to see what is missing, be it lectures on how to write and critique, how to do a chart review study, or how to structure a case-control study. It is important to draw upon the expertise of your own faculty to make the experience of doing research seem real and doable to the trainee. Thus, less attention should be paid to the specific topic of the research and more to the form or design of the research project. One can often find faculty in other departments to fill in the gaps in types of research that may exist in the curriculum of the seminar.

A writing and publishing experience is also part of this seminar. The format for writing up one's "findings" in this seminar is to have every participant write a Letter to the Editor reporting on some specific finding on a patient. Some participants have written about side effects and others about a novel treatment that did or didn't work. The focus of the letter is to think of it as a small anecdotal research paper. Much like a report of a more systematic investigation, a Letter to the Editor should contain an introduction where one cites the existing literature. Next, the methods section contains two parts, the subjects and the procedure. In the case of the Letter to the Editor, the subject is usually one patient and the procedure is usually no more complicated than a specific treatment, for example, the administration of a particular medication. One may strengthen the conclusions of the report by building in a rechallenge phase in the methods section, in which one attempts to reproduce the side effect or therapeutic effect by giving the medication a second time, assuming that ethical considerations allow for this. The results section, also brief, simply reports what happened to the patient. The conclusion or discussion section should offer some explanation, hypothesis, of why the result occurred and then, if possible, cite the current literature to support one's hypothesis. The Letter to the Editor format has the added benefit of a word limit. This requires writers to be precise and concise in their report of findings. This is good practice for producing larger manuscripts and grants in the future, where rambling and verbosity will often distract from the results or diminish the likelihood of publication.

The Letter to the Editor not only acts as a good exercise in writing up findings but also serves as a stepping-stone for discussing issues of the risks and benefit of anecdotal findings. For instance, "What are the pitfalls of an n of 1 study?" More specifically, "What is the potential for random error, chance, and systematic errors and bias that one might encounter in reporting findings with one patient?" The same question should be applied when considering studies with a few patients, and even with a larger sample. It also affords the opportunity to discuss issues of generalizability. How can the findings with one patient be applied to others? Why is it important to describe patients in enough detail so that they can be compared with other similar patients? All these questions, generated by this simple writing experience, will often begin for any clinician what can be a lifelong pursuit of doing research and contributing to the literature, for patients, for colleagues, and for oneself.

References

Burke JD, Pincus HA, Pardes H: The clinician-researcher in psychiatry. Am J Psychiatry 143:968–975, 1986

Garfinkel PF, Goldbloom DS, Kaplan AS, et al: The clinician-investigator interface in psychiatry: I—Values and problems. Can J Psychiatry 34:361–363, 1989

Glantz S: A Primer of Biostatistics, 2nd Edition. New York, McGraw-Hill, 1988

Hulley SB, Cummings SR: Designing Clinical Research. Baltimore, MD, Williams & Wilkins, 1988

Leibenluft E, Summergrad P, Tasman A: The academic dilemma of the inpatient unit director. Am J Psychiatry 146(1):73–76, 1989

Rutter W: Interface between research and clinical practice in child psychiatry some personal reflections. Paper presented at the Royal Society of Medicine, May 1989

Sackett DL, Haynes RB, Guyett GH, et al: Keeping up to date, in Clinical Epidemiology: A Basic Science for Clinical Medicine. Edited by Sackett DL, Haynes RB, Tugwell P. Boston, MA, Little, Brown, 1991, pp 335–378

A special thanks to Carlos Pato, M.D., for his editorial assistance on this chapter.

10

Getting Funding for Research

Natalie Walders, M.A., Terri Tanielian, M.A., and Harold Alan Pincus, M.D.

Psychiatric researchers face unique challenges when seeking research grant funding. Despite the high prevalence and severe consequences of mental illnesses and substance abuse, support for psychiatric research is proportionately and significantly less than that for biomedical research in other areas. For example, whereas the economic consequences of mental illnesses and substance abuse totaled $313 million in 1990—more than the costs of cancer ($104 billion in 1987), respiratory disease ($99 billion in 1990), AIDS ($66 billion in 1991) and coronary artery disease ($43 billion in 1987)—research funding support for mental health and addictive disorders represented less than 5% of all health research dollars (American Psychiatric Association 1996). On the strength of the science and the skills of the investigators—as well as through increased lobbying efforts and public awareness campaigns launched by professional and scientific organizations (such as the American Psychiatric Association) and consumer-based advocacy organizations (such as the National Alliance for the Mentally Ill, the National Mental Health Association, and the National Depressive and Manic Depressive Association)—federal research funding to departments of psychiatry has increased significantly in recent years (see Table 10–1). Nonetheless, overall resources remain quite limited, and competition for federal, foundation, and industry grants is increasing. Due to the competitive funding climate, it remains vital that mental health researchers seek support from diverse sources, ranging from federal agencies to philanthropic orga-

Table 10–1. NIH extramural support to institutions of higher education by department (*dollars in millions*)

	FY 1993		FY 1984*	
	Dollars awarded	% of H.E.	Dollars awarded	% of H.E.
Higher Education	**6,263.0**	**100.0**	**2,912.1**	**100.0**
Medical Schools	*4,285.8*	*68.4*	*2,002.3*	*68.8*
Medicine	1,218.1	19.4	603.2	20.7
Psychiatry	**300.9**	**4.8**	**82.5**	**2.8**
Pediatrics	260.0	4.2	94.3	3.2
Biochemistry	247.1	3.9	157.3	5.4
Pathology	231.2	3.7	109.5	3.8
Physiology	231.1	3.7	130.0	4.5
Microbiology	229.3	3.7	108.5	3.7
Pharmacology	200.9	3.2	104.1	3.6
Surgery	174.1	2.8	84.9	2.9
Anatomy	172.8	2.8	88.1	3.0
Other	1,020.3	16.3	439.9	15.1

Other than Medical Schools	1,977.2	31.6	909.8	31.2
Biology	277.6	4.4	132.6	4.6
Chemistry	204.1	3.3	110.3	3.8
Psychology	183.9	2.9	63.3	2.2
Public Health & Preventive Med.	129.3	2.1	36.3	1.2
Biochemistry	128.9	2.1	77.8	2.7
Other	1,053.4	16.8	489.5	16.8

Note: Includes NIAAA, NIDA, and NIMH. *NIAAA, NIDA, and NIMH contracts in 1984 not included; they are not available to type of institution or by department within institutions of higher education. However, contracts made up less than 2% of NIMH extramural funding in 1984.

The data indicate that within medical school departments, psychiatry has moved from being tenth in 1984 to being second in 1993 in terms of overall NIH funding. That is, funding to psychiatry department has gone from 2.8% of the total higher education funding to 4.8%, representing a 71.4% increase. In dollars, psychiatry department funding has gone from $82.5 million to $300.9 million, a 265% increase; in terms of actual buying power, they have gone from $82.5 million to $195.6 million (adjusted 1984 dollars), a 137% increase in constant dollar funding.

Source: NIH, DRG, ISB, SAES.

nizations. To succeed, researchers must be equipped with the knowledge and skills required to successfully compete for grant support, and they must understand the structure of mental illnesses and substance abuse research funding and the process of gaining support.

The purpose of this chapter is to provide psychiatric faculty with assistance in preparing high-quality grant proposals and with tools for securing grant support. This chapter will serve as a resource to (1) provide basic information on the different types of funding agencies, (2) highlight steps for identifying funding options, (3) identify strategies for preparing polished grant proposals, (4) describe the review process for proposals, and (5) outline additional sources of information on federal and private funding sources.

Identifying Funding Options and Targeting Where to Seek Support

The federal government, specifically the National Institutes of Health (NIH), remains the primary source of support for biomedical research. Although the National Institute of Mental Health (NIMH), National Institute on Drug Abuse (NIDA), and National Institute of Alcohol Abuse and Alcoholism (NIAAA) have traditionally been the principal sources of funding for psychiatric research (see Figure 10–1), many other NIH institutes, federal agencies, foundations, and state mental health authorities, as well as industry, are important components of the anatomy of psychiatric research support. Psychiatric researchers need to be prepared to target those federal agencies with a specific mental health focus, but they must also be alert to funding opportunities from agencies that one would not intuitively consider as a source for psychiatric research funding.

Federal Funding Sources

It can be challenging for researchers to maneuver within the complex structure of the federal government. The first step to follow when soliciting support from a government source is to review the federal funding options across a wide range of mental health and related areas. Appendix 10–A lists agencies that have some past or potential funding for areas related to mental health and substance abuse. The American Psychiatric Association's *Research Funding and Resource Manual: Mental Health and Addictive Disorders* contains a detailed profile on each federal agency with a concentra-

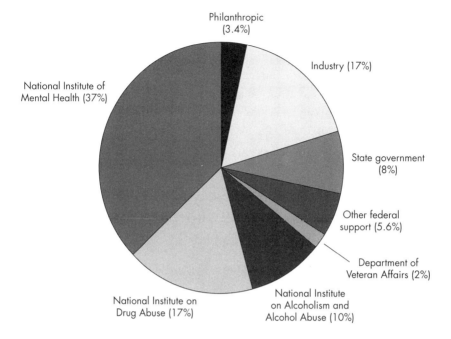

Figure 10–1. Sources of financial support for mental illness and substance abuse research in 1988.

tion in this area and serves as an excellent reference for researchers during this initial phase (Pincus 1995).

   The following section describes the NIH and the Department of Veterans Affairs (VA), the major institutions and agencies involved in federal grant support for psychiatric research. The NIH is the research arm of the Public Health Service and the Department of Health and Human Services. It serves as primary liaison on health-related research and is composed of 17 institutes with specific health missions, such as the NIMH, NIAAA, and NIDA, as well as four centers, and main administrative divisions. The NIH fund research uses three major mechanisms. These are described briefly in the following.

National Institutes of Health

1. Research Grants: This mechanism encompasses the largest category of NIH research funding and supports research projects, research centers, career development awards, and other research grants (e.g., cooperative

agreements, and other research-related programs) (National Institutes of Health 1994). The category of research projects includes traditional research projects (RO1 grants) and program projects (PO1 grants), First Independent Research Support and Transition (FIRST awards), and other research project mechanisms (e.g., Small Business Innovation Research, Outstanding Investigator awards, etc). Traditional research projects are awarded to domestic or foreign institutions to support work on a discrete project in the principal investigator's area of competence. Program projects support broadly based, long-term research programs involving a group of investigators (often multidisciplinary) working on research that contributes to the overall objective of the program. FIRST awards are granted to new investigators to develop their research capabilities and competence and enable them to demonstrate the merit of their research ideas. Potential applicants should consider which mechanism best fits their research proposal.

Research centers (P50 awards) support multidisciplinary, long-term research development programs at research centers. These awards are made to an institution on behalf of a program director and a group of collaborating investigators. Research center awards usually have a clinical orientation and respond to a specific need announced by the awarding NIH institute/center.

Career development awards support the development of outstanding scientists, enabling them to expand their research potential. These include the Mentored Clinical Scientist Development Award (K08) and the Mentored Research Scientist Award (K01). Career development awards typically provide salary support for investigators and funding for the conduct of their research.

It should be noted that not all institutes support all of these individual mechanisms.

2. Research and Development Contracts: This mechanism is utilized to support basic, applied, or developmental research or to test or evaluate products, materials, and devices for use in research communities. The research initiatives usually originate within NIH and are announced through request for proposals. Contracts are then negotiated with qualified organizations.

3. Training Awards: This mechanism provides funding to support the research training of scientists for research careers in both the behavioral and biomedical sciences under the authority of the National Re-

search Services Awards Program (NRSA). Training awards include institutional training grants (T awards, i.e., T32, T35) and individual fellowships (F awards, i.e., F32) (National Institutes of Health 1994). In addition, there are fellowship programs aimed specifically at increasing the number of research-trained minority investigators (e.g., the APA's Program for Minority Research Training in Psychiatry (PMRTP)—which provides funding for short- and long-term training opportunities in psychiatry at three levels: medical school, residency, and post-residency).

The Department of Veterans Affairs (VA)

The Department of Veterans Affairs (VA) is another major source for mental health and addictive disorders research. The VA provides funding for mental health research through the Department's Medical Research Services, Health Services Research and Development Service, and the Rehabilitation Research and Development Services (Pincus 1995). These programs support a wide range of research conducted in VA facilities or by VA personnel. For example, the VA has provided support for psychopharmacotherapy studies, clinical trials, multisite research initiatives, and Alzheimer's research.

State-Level Funding

State support for mental illness and addictive disorders research varies considerably from jurisdiction to jurisdiction. Recent evaluation of state-sponsored research showed that approximately 57% of states directly fund mental health research, and 29% support substance abuse research. Research-directed funding, however, totaled only approximately 0.3% of total state expenditures for mental health (Pincus 1995). The factors influencing state-level funding practices have been identified as differences in state mental health authorities, differences in the level of consumer-based advocacy, and the presence or absence of a strong academic community.

Industry-Sponsored Research

Industry provides considerable support for mental illnesses and substance abuse research. However, in comparison to industry support for overall biomedical research and development, industry involvement in mental health research is comparatively limited. Several factors have created barriers that have limited the role of industry in supporting psychiatric research. Reluctance to seek mental health care due to the continued stigma attached to mental illness restricts the market for psychopharmacological interventions. Furthermore, the limited access to and restraints placed on psychiatric interventions by insurance companies and managed care organizations also contribute to limiting the market. One additional factor that may restrict industry sponsorship of mental health research is the extensive drug approval process implemented for psychoactive substances (Pincus 1995). Despite these barriers, the recent success of several major central nervous system (CNS) drugs has increased industry interest in this area, and opportunities for securing industry support are expanding.

Foundation Support

Although the majority of researchers focus on securing funding from government agencies, private foundations are also an important resource. (Refer to Appendix 10–B for a listing of foundations that support mental health and addictive disorders research.) The American Psychiatric Association's *Research Funding and Resource Manual* (Pincus 1995) defines five different types of foundations. The most common type of foundation is the "independent foundation," which includes nonprofit organizations that direct the distribution of support from a single endowment source. "Company-sponsored foundations" are defined as entities supported by for-profit corporations that are usually established as a public service outreach effort. "Community foundations" constitute a relatively small amount of overall foundation giving. They are supported by a diverse pool of donors and tend to offer community-based grant programs. "Operating foundations" are organizations that maintain some central purpose or focus (e.g., the United Way) and seek foundation status for tax purposes. The final type of foundations are "medical research organizations," which are connected to a hospital and support research within that particular setting. These foundations will vary in their organization, eligibility requirements, areas of interest, and procedures for grant review.

Choosing a Source of Funding

In targeting either a private or public entity for support, it is important to gather "intelligence" data to identify the areas of focus that may relate to your proposal. During this stage, it is important to confirm that your research fits into the organization's larger mandate/agenda. This background investigation is not only key to identifying an organization that may fund your project, but also provides insight for how best to frame your proposal so that it receives full consideration. An effective first step for either foundation or federal proposals is to compose a short summary statement of your project prior to any contact, enabling you to streamline your thoughts and refine your proposal. Second, it can be productive to network with colleagues to help identify which agencies' agendas intersect with your project's objectives.

A critical step when approaching a foundation (but often true for other sources) is establishing "warm contact" with the organization. It is important to remember that no matter how strong a foundation grant proposal may be, it must fit in the organization's scope of interest or it will be a wasted effort to submit. If possible, speak directly to the program director or executive director of the organization to find out if your proposal is in their interest and purview. Request a copy of relevant foundation's annual reports and mission statements if they are available. In your investigation of a foundation, try to obtain the following information: How many grants are awarded annually? What is the average grant award amount? What is the length of the average grant? Is overhead funded?, and so on. Answers to these types of questions will guide you in the development of your proposal. The cornerstone of most successful foundation proposals is demonstrating how your work will make a difference for populations of interest to the agency.

Preparing a Strong Grant Proposal

An essential component of any successful grant proposal is strict adherence to the detailed application instructions of the funding agency. Make certain that you are eligible for the award for which you are competing and that you honor all restrictions placed on length, nature of information, and necessary documentation and forms. For example, the NIH has specific guidelines on the number of publications allowed in the appendices that accompany a grant application (no more than 10) (National Institutes of Health 1990). If you should have any questions concerning the proposal, call the agency program personnel for advice and direction.

Foundations often have specific guidelines, but the organization and structure of a proposal are usually left up to the grant seeker. In some cases, foundations require an initial letter of intent before allowing the submission of a full proposal from the grant seeker so that the foundation may review the investigator's funding idea. Generally, foundations request thorough, succinct proposals between 5 and 10 pages in length (Reif-Lehrer 1991).

Foundations are generally more open to innovative projects and pilot work than federal grants, and they are often interested in providing seed money to start an innovative investigation. At the same time, foundations usually do not want to "adopt" a grantee and provide ongoing, continuous funds. Once initial support has been provided, foundations hope that other funding will be received to make a worthwhile project continue. Therefore, your plans for obtaining future funding should be emphasized. In addition, most foundations limit or do not provide support for indirect costs (although some administrative expenses may be included in direct costs).

Overall, for both federal and foundation proposals, it is essential that you present a clearly organized and persuasive research outline on a topic that you find meaningful and timely. To achieve a well-executed proposal, as noted already, gather data to ensure that you are targeting the correct audience with a "marketable research focus." As part of that data collection process, investigate the techniques used by successful researchers, and, when possible, obtain copies of previously funded proposals.

An attractive proposal succinctly presents an innovative and workable research question and actively states how and why you are capable of addressing the issue effectively. Although formats may vary, the following elements must be articulated: (1) significance—show that the question you are analyzing is in an important area where your project will fill a critical gap; (2) methods—describe how the study will be conducted in a scientifically rigorous manner with design, sampling procedures, measures, analysis, and so on aimed at ensuring reliable and valid results; (3) feasibility—demonstrate how you will complete the project successfully in a timely and efficient manner; and (4) special features—emphasize those attributes of you and your institution that make it particularly appropriate for you to be conducting this research (Steinberg and Kennedy 1995).

Dedicate an extensive amount of time to the development and fine-tuning of your proposal to ensure that the finished product is as "user-friendly," strong, and specific as possible. Also, the importance of a realistic and accurate budget and budget narrative should not be underestimated. The best proposals are polished, professional, and succinct. First impressions are important and appearance is critical. Regardless of the specific format of a proposal, reviewers often consider preparation and presentation of an application to be a reflection of the management and administrative skills of the applicant (Ogden 1991). Achieving a flawless application calls for careful revision, attention to detail, and a well-edited manuscript.

One of the most important ways to strengthen your proposal is to use the technical assistance provided by the agency or foundation to which you are applying. Program officers are generally available to discuss your proposal and suggest ways to improve its presentation. Prior to submission to a funding organization, it is also advantageous to ask professional colleagues within your organization and within your field of expertise to review and critique your draft, identifying weaknesses and possible improvements. A similar way to critique your proposal is to submit it to a "mock" internal review group (IRG), a group of professionals within your organization who will grade your draft as if they were participating in the peer review process and provide you with valuable input. It is important to check on the possibility of receiving input from the agency prior to submission —some federal or foundation officials are willing to review and comment on draft proposals.

Review Process for Federal and Foundation Grant Proposals

Depending on the nature of the funding organization, the review and funding process may be as simple as submission of a proposal, staff review and recommendation, and eventual approval by the board of directors at a foundation. In other cases, the applicant will be expected to understand complex peer review structures, such as those employed by the NIH.

The NIH review system begins with an evaluation of the scientific merit of submitted proposals by an IRG, a study section of 12 to 15 people, that often contains several ad hoc members. It provides applicants with formal summary statements containing priority scores, percentiles, and from one to five pages of critique about the proposals. Following IRG review, the proposal usually goes to an Institute's advisory council and then to Institute staff for ultimate funding decisions. The entire NIH review process takes about 9 months. It is unusual for someone other than the assigned reviewers to read an entire proposal carefully, so it is important to find out who is on the standing advisory panels or review committees to see if the appointed reviewers have sufficient expertise in your area of research. Discuss any concerns with the individual organizing the review so that an ad hoc reviewer may be added, if needed, to a standing committee. It is also important to make certain that any issue regarding conflict of interest is addressed.

Foundations often differ from government agencies in the amount of personal influence foundation personnel or the executive director have in awarding funds. Because of this influence, developing a personal communication with foundation staff is important for improving the odds of getting your research funded. In some foundations, a proposal may even be developed collaboratively by the grantee and the staff at the foundation.

Foundations vary widely in their proposal review as well. Some use a peer review system with reviewers meeting periodically. Others will have a much less formal review, with an ad hoc review board or a single foundation staff member overseeing the technical review of a proposal. Mail/telephone critiques and reviews may supplement or substitute for a typical advisory panel meeting. In other cases, foundations may rely on outside reviewers. Regardless of the review process, final approval for funding a proposal is decided by the board of directors of the foundation. Approvals for grants usually occur during board meetings, which may take place only one or two times a year. Knowledge of this approval schedule is essential in knowing when to submit a proposal. Reviews usually take between 3 and 6 months or may be less if personal relationships with the foundation exist.

The Reality of Competition: Steps to Follow If Your Proposal Is Not Funded

The reality of grant seeking is that competition for grant funding is intense. In 1994, the success rate for competing research projects at the NIH was 25.4%. Success rates for competing research projects at NIMH, NIDA, and NIAAA were 20.7%, 32.9%, and 29.3%, respectively (National Institutes of Health 1994). Researchers should be prepared to face the possibility that their research will not be funded. There are steps to take if your proposal does not receive funding support. First, try to meet with your contact person or discuss the results with a member of the review team in a professional manner. Accept comments as constructive criticism and revise your proposal accordingly. Try to identify concrete weaknesses in your submission or other reasons why your proposal was not funded.

It is vital to not get discouraged if at first you do not receive funding. After receiving feedback, you will have an increased chance of securing funding during a future submission. A revised proposal is generally more successful than one which has not yet been reviewed. Data from the NIH document indicate that grant applications are more likely to be paid after they have been revised and resubmitted, and second revisions are even more likely to be paid than first revisions. Most successful proposals have gone through multiple resubmissions, although also be aware that the NIH has limited submissions to three times within 2 years (National Institute of Mental Health 1994).

Recommendations for Additional Resources

There are a wide variety of publications advising how to write grant proposals and providing other resources to assist investigators in isolating funding sources. Many of these technical resources are available on-line, through the Internet, or on CD-ROM. The Foundation Center, a nonprofit organization headquartered in New York City (with regional offices around the United States) serves as an information clearinghouse on foundations and publishes the *Foundation Directory,* a collection of abstracts on foundations in the United States. Federal resources can be tracked in the *Catalogue of Federal Domestic Assistance,* the *NIH Guide,* the *Federal Register,* and *Commerce Business Daily.* Other publishing houses offer many publications and resources on grants and grant funding, such as the *Directory of Research Grants* and *Directory of Biomedical and Health Care Grants,* published by Oryx Press. Other research funding resources for psychiatry include *Psychiatric Research Report,* a newsletter published by the APA Office of Research, and the APA's Psychiatric Research Resource Center (also maintained by the APA Office of Research), which serves as a clearinghouse on funding information. The APA has recently published the *Research Funding and Resource Manual: Mental Health and Addictive Disorders* (Pincus 1995), a compendium of information on where and how to get funding for mental health and addictive disorders research along with other important information on science policy issues, scientific journals, and so on.

References

American Psychiatric Association: Opening Windows Into the Future, Psychiatric Research in the 21st Century. Washington, DC, American Psychiatric Association, 1996

National Institute of Mental Health: Research Information Source Book, Fiscal Year 1994. Rockville, MD, National Institute of Mental Health, 1994

National Institutes of Health: Helpful Hints on Preparing a Research Grant Application to the National Institutes of Health. Bethesda, MD, National Institutes of Health, 1990

National Institutes of Health: NIH extramural trends; fiscal years 1984–1993 (NIH Publ No 94-3506). Bethesda, MD, National Institutes of Health, 1994

Ogden TE: Research Proposals: A Guide to Success. New York, Raven, 1991

Pincus HA (ed): Research Funding and Resource Manual: Mental Health and Addictive Disorders. Washington, DC, American Psychiatric Association, 1995

Reif-Lehrer L: Tips for applying to private foundations for grant money. The Scientist 5:20–25, 1991

Steinberg J, Kennedy C: Successful research grant applications, in Research Funding and Resource Manual: Mental Health and Addictive Disorders. Edited by Pincus HA. Washington, DC, American Psychiatric Association, 1995

This appendix, which provides a listing of the names and acronyms for federal institutions involved in supporting mental illness and substance abuse research, is a useful reference that identifies the key federal agencies to target when seeking psychiatric research funding. Complete federal funding agency profiles (including such information as contact names, agency addresses, agency descriptions, and sample program announcements) are available in Pincus 1995.

Department of Health and Human Services (HHS)
Public Health Service (PHS)
  National Institutes of Health (NIH)
    National Institute of Mental Health (NIMH)
    National Institute on Drug Abuse (NIDA)
    National Institute of Alcohol Abuse and Alcoholism (NIAAA)
    National Institute on Aging (NIA)
    National Institute of Child Health and Human Development (NICHD)
    National Institute of Neurological Disorders and Stroke (NINDS)
    National Cancer Institute (NCI)
    National Heart, Lung, and Blood Institute (NHLBI)
    National Institute on Deafness and Other Communication Disorders (NIDCD)
    National Institute for Nursing Research (NINR)
    National Institute of Allergy and Infectious Diseases (NIAID)
    National Institute of Arthritis and Musculoskeletal and Skin Diseases (NIAMSD)
    National Institute of Dental Research (NIDR)
    National Institute of Diabetes and Digestive and Kidney Diseases (NIDDK)
    National Institute of Environmental Health Sciences (NIEHS)
    National Eye Institute (NEI)
    National Institute of General Medical Sciences (NIGMS)
    National Library of Medicine (NLM)
    National Center for Human Genome Research (NCHGR)
    National Center for Research Resources (NCRR)
    Fogarty International Center (FIC) for the Advanced Study in the Health Sciences

Substance Abuse and Mental Health Services Administration (SAMHSA)
  Center for Mental Health Services (CMHS)
  Center for Substance Abuse Prevention (CSAP)
  Center for Substance Abuse Treatment (CSAT)
Other Public Health Service Programs
  Agency for Health Care Policy and Research (AHCPR)
  Center for Disease Control and Prevention (CDC)
  Food and Drug Administration (FDA)
  Health Resources and Services and Administration (HRSA)
Other Health and Human Services Programs
  Administration for Children and Families (ACF)
  Administration on Aging (AOA)
  Health Care Financing Administration (HCFA)
  Social Security Administration (SSA)

Department of Veterans Affairs (VA)
Medical Research Service (MRS)
Health Services Research and Development Service (HSR&D)
Rehabilitation Research and Development Service (Rehab R&D)

Department of Education (ED)
National Institute on Disability and Rehabilitation Research (NIDRR)

National Science Foundation (NSF)
Directorate for Social, Behavioral, and Economic Sciences (SBE)
Directorate for Biological Sciences (BIO)

Department of Justice (DOJ)
Office for Victims of Crime
National Institute of Justice
Office of Juvenile Justice and Delinquency Prevention

Department of Defense (DOD) and Related Organizations
Air Force Office of Scientific Research (AFOSR)
Army Research Office (ARO)
  Army Research Institute for the Behavioral and Social Sciences (ARI)
Office of Naval Research (ONR)
  Life Sciences Programs Directorate
  Navy Personnel Research and Development Center
  Naval Medical Research and Development Command
North Atlantic Treaty Organization (NATO)

National Aeronautics and Space Administration (NASA)
Department of Agriculture (AG)
Department of Energy (DOE)
Department of Transportation (DOT)

The following resource lists the major foundations and nonprofit institutions that provide or have provided support for research related to mental health/substance abuse. This listing is not all-inclusive; it should be considered as an initial reference source. Foundations and nonprofit organizations are subject to shifting concentrations and priorities. Consequently, it is always recommended that investigators do their own background research on a potential funding source. Complete federal funding agency profiles are available in Pincus 1995.

AARP Andrus Foundation (AARP)
Alcoholic Beverage Medical Research Foundation
Allied-Signal Foundation
Alzheimer's Disease and Related Disorders Association, Inc. (ADRDA)
American Health Assistance Foundation (AHAF)
American Medical Association Education and Research Foundation
  (AMAERF)
American Paralysis Association
American Suicide Foundation (ASF)
Arca Foundation, The
Bristol-Myers Squibb Foundation, Inc., The
Burden Foundation, Florence V.
Burroughs Wellcome Fund, The
Carnegie Corporation of New York
Clark Foundation, The Edna McConnell
Commonwealth Fund, The
Culpeper Foundation, Charles E.
Cummings Foundation, The Nathan
Dana Foundation, The Charles A.
Diamond Foundation, The Aaron
Ford Foundation, The
Foundation for Child Development
French Foundation for Alzheimer Research, The
Fulbright Scholar Program
Glenn Foundation for Medical Research
Grant Foundation, William T.
Grass Foundation, The
Guggenheim Foundation, The Harry Frank

Harris Foundation, The
Hartford Foundation, The John A.
Hood Foundation, The Charles H.
Howard Hughes Medical Institute (HHMI)
Huntington's Disease Society of America
Ittleson Foundation, Inc.
JM Foundation, The
Jacobs Foundation, Johann
Johnson Foundation, The Robert Wood (RWJ)
Kaiser Foundation, The Henry J.
Keck Foundation, W. M.
Kenworthy-Sarah H. Swift Foundation, Inc., Marion E.
Klingenstein Fund, Inc., The Esther A. and Joseph
Life and Health Insurance Medical Research Fund
Lilly Endowment Inc.
MacArthur Foundation, The John D. and Catherine T.
Mailman Family Foundation, Inc., A.L.
McDonnell Foundation, James S.
McKnight Endowment Fund for Neuroscience, The
Merck Fund, The John
Milbank Memorial Fund
Mott Fund, Ruth
National Alliance for Research on Schizophrenia and Depression (NARSAD)
National Alliance for the Mentally Ill (NAMI)
National Parkinson Foundation
New-Land Foundation, Inc., The
Packard Foundation, The David & Lucile
Pew Charitable Trusts, The
Retirement Research Foundation, The
RGK Foundation, The
Sandoz Foundation for Gerontological Research
Supreme Masonic Council, 33, Scottish Rite
USX Foundation, Inc.
van Ameringan Foundation, Inc.
Whitehall Foundation, Inc.
Wills Foundation, The

11

Doing Research Without Grant Support

Mantosh Dewan, M.D., Edward K. Silberman, M.D., and Deborah A. Snyderman, M.D.

In an age of shrinking resources, the "publish or perish" monster continues to menace junior faculty. Although research productivity traditionally has been the single most important criterion for academic promotion, a minority of psychiatry faculty ever receive external grant support for research (Burke et al. 1986). Therefore, their scientific output depends on their ability to mount studies with resources available within their own institutions.

This chapter describes strategies for conducting research despite a paucity of funds, and appeasing the monster honorably and with professional satisfaction. Our recommendations are based on our own experience and on an empirical study of published research conducted without external funding (Silberman and Snyderman 1997). In this study (itself conducted without external funding!) we identified reports of unfunded research in 14 leading psychiatric journals for the year 1992. We profiled articles for type of methodology and topic of study and surveyed first authors about their professional demographics, duties, and the resources needed to accomplish their study.

Our guide to low-budget research will deal with the following questions: What kinds of studies can be done without grants? Who does unfunded research? How are research ideas generated? What resources are required, and how are they obtained? Where are unfunded studies published? What makes a good environment for unfunded research?

What Kinds of Studies Can Be Done Without Grants?

Unfunded studies comprise a substantial portion of the psychiatric research literature; about 25% of research in our sample was accomplished without external funding (literature reviews, case reports, and conceptual articles were excluded). Among the types of small-scale studies with which the authors have experience are questionnaires, chart reviews, and clinical studies of biology, phenomenology, and medication-response.

Questionnaires are a valuable and especially cost-effective mode of scholarly activity (Dewan et al. 1988; Huszonek et al. 1995). The $200 that was almost not worth begging for a few years ago can now fund stamps for return envelopes on 600 questionnaires (a nice size study), depending on the subject under study, thereby raising the sample size and increasing the chances of being published.

Small clinical studies tend to test a simple hypothesis and could be closely aligned with a researcher's everyday duties and practice. For instance, when the dexamethasone suppression test (DST) became a rage, we tested its specificity for the diagnosis of depression by performing the DST on 20 nondepressed schizophrenic patients. Unexpectedly, 30% were DST positive. This inexpensive study (cost: we bought $100 worth of test tubes for an endocrinologist's research lab in exchange for his running the cortisol assays) resulted in a paper in the *American Journal of Psychiatry* (Dewan et al. 1982). Obviously, clinical studies do not have to be biologically driven. For instance, we were able to compare the defense mechanisms used by depressed and nondepressed inpatients (Margo et al. 1993). This study required no funds but did utilize some of the department research assistant's time.

Clinical drug trials are a rich source of funds as well as a source for contacts with other researchers in that particular area of study. Usually, drug trials enable the investigator to have some, often substantial, monies left over that can be used to fund other research projects. Another advantage of doing drug trials is that they sometimes allow an investigator's research to be added onto the prescribed protocol.

Prospective, hypothesis-driven studies tend to be more valuable, scientifically rigorous, and expensive. However, even these can be successfully completed on a shoestring budget. For instance, we attempted to characterize biologically a cohort of 23 schizophrenic patients by utilizing CT scan, EEG, WAIS, Halstead-Reitan neuropsychological battery, platelet MAO and serum DBH, and selected clinical parameters. The total cost of this complex study was only $10,000 but resulted in a significant number of published papers (Boucher et al. 1986; Dewan et al. 1983a, 1983b, 1986; Pandurangi et al. 1984, 1986). The success of this project depended on combining many of the previously described strategies. For instance, we actively collaborated with other faculty and obtained free services from neurology (25 EEGs worth $5,000), neuroradiology (25 CT scans worth $15,000), neuropsychology (WAIS and HRB analysis worth $2,500), and a researcher at The National Institute of Mental Health (NIMH) (platelet MAO and serum DBH assays worth thousands more), for a total savings of more than $22,500. We did pay for a part-time research assistant for two years and supplies for neuropsychological testing and biochemical assays.

Our survey of unfunded research suggests that our own experiences are typical of small-scale researchers. Seventy-one percent of the studies we surveyed were prospective, involving some type of direct examination or assessment of subjects, and 9% were prospective questionnaire studies; 28% of studies used retrospective methodology, either chart review (19%) or analysis of data from a previously collected database (9%). (Percentages do not add up to 100% because some studies used more than one type of methodology.) This research was typically (although not exclusively) low-tech: 67% of studies in the sample used no higher technology than interviews or paper-and-pencil examinations. Only about 10% of the studies used technology that was not routinely available clinically, such as SPECT scans or serum serotonin metabolite assays.

The most common topics of study were those compatible with low-tech methods. As seen in Table 11–1, 16 topics were represented in the study sample, but phenomenology/epidemiology, drug therapy, and systems and utilization account for almost three-quarters of the reports. (Phenomenology and epidemiology were considered as a single category because they were usually closely linked, such as a study assessing degree of comorbidity of specified disorders.)

Twelve percent of studies concerned patients with mood disorders, 10% patients with schizophrenia spectrum disorders, 9% with medical/surgical illness, 8% with anxiety disorders, and 8% with nonpatient volunteers.

Table 11–1. Research topic areas

Topic area	%
Phenomenology/epidemiology	40
Drug therapy	19
Systems and utilization	14
Neurobiology	10
Diagnosis	9
Cognitive/neuropsychological testing	5
Psychotherapy	3
Rating scales	3
Legal/regulatory issues	3
Psychosocial rehabilitation	2
Brain imaging	2
Electrophysiology	2
Educational issues	2
ECT	2
Economic issues	1
Other	2

However, the most common way of defining study population was by clinical service site or clinical setting (41%). Forty-three percent of studies were performed on inpatient units and 31% were set in outpatient clinics, but only 2% were based in hospital emergency services. Therefore, an available clinical population in a setting that allows for research appears to be an important factor in determining what type of low-budget research is undertaken.

Who Does Unfunded Research?

In our sample, the typical principal investigator of unfunded studies was a full-time, paid, junior faculty physician without a second graduate degree, and no grant support for other studies. Ten percent of studies were done by residents and 16% by full professors; 23% did have graduate degrees other than the M.D., and 32% had external funding for other current projects. Clinical duties accounted for the greatest proportion of investigators' time (44%), while teaching accounted for 15% and administrative work for 14%. Two-thirds of the investigators spent no more than 25% of their work time in research. Thus, the modal investigator was a clinician-educator or clinician-administrator, rather than someone with a primary researcher identity.

How Are Research Ideas Generated?

You do not have to be a Nobel Prize candidate to generate research ideas. Elegant ideas often come from clinical challenges (e.g., I wonder what the next step should be: After 6 to 8 weeks if an SSRI antidepressant produces an inadequate response, should you increase the dose or add another medication?) or simple clinical questions (e.g., given a therapeutic range, are higher blood levels of lithium more efficacious than lower blood levels in the prophylaxis of mania?) that occur in everyday practice. Your particular area of interest may help focus on the unanswered questions—and every area has many unanswered questions, some of which are quite basic. For instance, after 30 years of using antipsychotic agents, we still cannot agree on dose equivalencies. A review of the standard texts revealed a 500% variance in the dose of haloperidol (from 1 mg to 5 mg) that is reported to be equivalent to 100 mg of chlorpromazine (Dewan and Koss 1995).

Colleagues often raise possibilities that elicit the "that would be neat to study" response from you and could lead to a collaborative project. Similarly, residents may raise a question you do not know the answer to or talk about an area that they are excited by. Just such a discussion with one resident led to an interesting paper. He had experienced that some of our medical colleagues looked down on psychiatrists and he wondered how prevalent that was. Our survey found that, in fact, other doctors had an overall very positive view of psychiatry and psychiatrists (Dewan et al. 1988). Another resident noted the growing interest in alternative therapies among our patients and wanted to know if and how often traditional doctors integrated the two systems. Our survey of 572 primary care physicians found that two-thirds were willing to refer patients for five unconventional treatments. These were relaxation techniques (86%), biofeedback (85%), therapeutic massage (66%), hypnosis (63%), and acupuncture (56%) (Blumberg et al. 1995).

Personnel and programmatic issues that arise in the routine course of administering a training program are rich sources of investigation. A flow of excellent articles can be found in *Academic Psychiatry*, published by the American Association of Directors of Residency Training and the Association for Academic Psychiatry, and serve as useful examples. (For a discussion on how to turn ideas into formal research protocols, see Chapter 9.)

Data from our survey support the conclusion that research ideas most commonly arise out of investigators' daily work and informal discussions with colleagues. Forty-six percent of our sample of investigators reported that the idea for their project came from their own clinical experience, 46% from their own reading, 44% from prior research projects, and 40% from discussions with colleagues. By contrast, only 2% reported that a departmental research seminar was the source of the project, 1% that grand rounds was the source, and 1% that journal club was the source. (Respondents could report several sources of ideas.)

Close collaboration with colleagues was especially important for junior faculty. Forty-six percent of junior faculty versus 29% of senior faculty ($P < .04$) listed discussions with colleagues as a source of ideas, and 56% of junior faculty versus 19% of senior faculty ($P < .001$) said they had a mentor for their project. By contrast, prior research was more likely to a source of ideas for senior faculty (56% vs. 38%, $P < .04$). Thus, once initiated, research often perpetuates itself.

What Resources Are Required and How Are They Obtained?

Time

Most small-scale research projects are not done on "protected time," but on time squeezed in among the investigator's other duties. Fortunately, a great deal of time is not necessarily required. Eighty-three percent of investigators in our survey spent no more than 5 hours weekly (on average) on their project, and 77% estimated 12 hours or less spent by all study participants. The mean time from initiation of the project to submission of a manuscript was 21 months. At the same time, researchers were willing to devote time during "off hours" to work on their projects. Eighty-seven percent of our respondents reported working on their study during evenings and weekends, and they estimated that an average of 50% of the work was done during these times. This finding is especially important because it dispels the widely held belief that research and writing are completed from 8 to 5.

Money

Departments and medical schools sometimes have "seed money," which tends to be relatively noncompetitive, particularly if earmarked for new faculty. Not surprisingly, this is not always prominently advertised. Ask around, try to understand the politics, and definitely apply, no matter how small the amount or forbidding the odds of obtaining funds. If there is a cutoff that excludes you (for example, faculty must apply within their first year), use another faculty colleague as a "front" and collaborator. This could be beneficial to both of you. Similarly, some departments have monies earmarked to support resident research that can be accessed collaboratively with a resident as a front. Pharmaceutical companies can be helpful, and sums of a few hundred to a few thousand dollars can sometimes be allocated at a local level in a noncompetitive manner. Finally, faculty have done extra clinical work in exchange for keeping the fees for their research. This is to be avoided but may be a necessary evil to begin your research if the previous options listed are not viable.

In our sample, only 41% of studies were supported directly by funds from the department or medical school, and when money was given, it was usually in small amounts: 30% of studies received $500 or less, 60% received $2,000 or less, and 90% received $12,000 or less. Internal funding was most often used to pay for personnel (78%), but it was also used for equipment (38%), supplies (38%), laboratory studies (12%), pay for subjects (5%), and a variety of other uses, such as computer time, travel, and postage. Of note is that 83% of investigators used personal computers in completing their study, 78% of which were either assigned exclusively to, or owned by, the investigator. Thus, a personal computer is an indispensable tool that can support many projects and should be high on the list of capital equipment requests for those who wish to pursue research.

In closing the discussion of money, we point out that unfunded studies themselves can be a source of future grant money. Twenty-two percent of the investigators in our survey had applied for grants based on their study. Of these, 32% had received a grant, 44% were not funded, and 24% were awaiting the outcome of their application. Thus, one might estimate that about 40% of such grant applications were eventually successful, a very good batting average in today's economy.

Personnel

The first rule of recruiting personnel is to look for helpers who cost no money. Rich sources of competent help include residents (on a research rotation if your department has one, or as an elective), psychology interns, work-study students (excellent for doing your library searches and entering data), and pre-postgraduate students—these are graduates who will volunteer to do research to strengthen their application for a master's program. These (usually biology or psychology) students are often bright, motivated, and free!

Only 17% of investigators in our survey reported paying for research help. Instead, 61% had help from volunteer participants, such as just described, and 65% were able to assign research-related tasks to support staff. In fact, the most commonly reported type of helper was secretaries (59%) followed by other faculty (53%), consultants (40%), research assistants (39%), students (19%), nurses (18%), and residents (17%). Data collection was the most frequent type of contributory activity (76%), followed by clerical work (65%), design or statistical analysis (60%), and technical procedures (23%).

If you do have some money to spend on a genuine research assistant, *never* hire your own full-time person unless you are very sure that you have enough projects to fully utilize a full-time person. Given a typical faculty member's multiple responsibilities, research is often done in spurts, and there may be periods of weeks to months when you cannot even supervise an assistant. Scarce funds cannot be wasted on an assistant who has significant "down time." You must also be sure that you have enough money for at least several years. You want to spend your time doing research, not finding renewal funds each year. Another drawback is the fringe benefits cost (around 20%–30%) that must be added to a full-time salary. A recommended alternative is to hire part-time assistance without fringe benefits (perhaps on an hourly basis), preferably a person who has the flexibility to increase hours temporarily when necessary. Another suggestion is to buy assistant time from another researcher who may not be fully utilizing his or her full-time assistant and may actually welcome the additional support in an era of dwindling resources.

Collaboration

Research is no exception to the adage that there is strength in numbers. Some of the most fruitful low-cost research can be accomplished by combining forces with other faculty and taking advantage of whatever infrastructure they have put together. One-third of the unfunded studies we identified were done as part of larger ongoing projects, half of which were themselves unfunded. Such collaborations are especially valuable for studies that need highly technical procedures; 32% of "piggybacked" studies used high-tech procedures, whereas only 9% of freestanding studies did so ($P < .002$).

Multidisciplinary studies are currently looked upon with favor. These can be done in conjunction with either high-tech or low-tech departments. With high-tech departments, access can be gained to cutting-edge investigative tools such as functional MRI, SPECT, and PET scans. Low-tech departments such as Internal Medicine and Family Medicine are invaluable because of access to a high volume of patients, many of whom have psychiatric illnesses. With the advent of managed care, there is renewed interest in primary care, such as the diagnosis and treatment of depression in medical patients, or the detection and treatment of alcoholism in nonpsychiatric practices.

Basic scientists are valuable collaborators. Those who operate animal laboratories allow the testing of a hypothesis in a relatively short time. For instance, a rat study may take a month to complete as compared with a human study, which could drag through several years, especially if you are on a low budget and only able to devote time for research in sporadically. In addition, to add another study to the schedule of an already operational laboratory may cost you little, since you may be able to negotiate paying for just the animals and chemicals (perhaps a few hundred dollars). Basic scientists also tend to be dedicated full-time researchers as opposed to the average clinical faculty who has numerous clinical, educational, and administrative duties, with research being an after-hours perk.

Frequently, "barter" arrangements can be made instead of monetary payment for use of equipment, technical or research assistant time, or patient access. We found that compensation in such arrangements is most often in the form of coauthorship on publications, but teaching, clinical work, performance of technical procedures, and help on a collaborator's study may also be viable payments.

A study from our own research experience illustrates many of the principles of collaboration and resource utilization that we have described. One of us (EKS) has a long-standing interest in the relationship between seizure disorders and psychopathology. Within his institution, there was an epilepsy center whose medical director had an interest in behavioral neurology and a desire to publish. The two designed a project investigating the relationship between epileptic aura phenomena and interictal psychopathology. The study required EEG-based clinical diagnoses, demographic and historical information about the participants, MMPI testing, a self-report of social functioning, and separate structured interviews to assess aura phenomena and determine major DSM diagnoses.

The center's nurse was trained by the principal investigator to administer the aura inventory, and she scheduled patients for the study during their regular visits. As the study was being designed, the psychiatry department's psychology internship program was looking for additional training opportunities in psychiatric diagnosis. The principal investigator offered to train and supervise interns in administering and interpreting a structured diagnostic interview in return for having them perform the interview with all patients in the study. Clinical data on patients was available from the epilepsy center records. Consultation on scoring of the MMPI was provided by a member of the psychology division. Data were stored and analyzed on the principal investigator's computer, with the help of the epilepsy center's administrator, who was expert in using the available statistical package. No funds were allocated directly to the study.

The study found that the degree of complexity of epileptic auras predicted interictal anxiety and depression, but not level of social functioning. It was published in the first journal to which it was submitted, with the epilepsy center medical director, nurse, and administrator as co-authors (Silberman et al. 1994).

Where Are Unfunded Studies Published?

Many small-scale studies may be published in obscure or newly launched journals that may be less rigorous than the more widely read journals. However, our survey demonstrated that unfunded studies are publishable in many of the same places as funded studies. Table 11–2 shows the number of unfunded research reports and their percentage of the total research in each journal we reviewed. The wide range of proportions most likely represents the type of research featured by the various journals. Journals such as the *Archives of General Psychiatry* or *Biological Psychiatry,* which publish research requiring high technology, very large samples, or longitudinal study of patients, include relatively few reports of unfunded research. By contrast, *General Hospital Psychiatry,* the journal with the highest proportion of unfunded studies, specializes in consultation-liaison research, which is often based on data routinely collected as part of clinical work. High-quality small-scale research may find its way into very selective journals; in our survey, the journal publishing the greatest number of such articles

Table 11–2. Unfunded research by journal

Journal	Number	Percentage
General Hospital Psychiatry	14	63
Journal of Nervous and Mental Disease	29	57
Canadian Journal of Psychiatry	27	53
Comprehensive Psychiatry	16	47
Hospital and Community Psychology	32	38
Journal of Clinical Psychiatry	17	35
Journal of Clinical Psychopharmacology	12	32
Journal of the American Academy of Child &		
Adolescent Psychology	25	27
American Journal of Psychiatry	48	28
Psychosomatic Medicine	6	20
Community Mental Health Journal	4	18
Biological Psychiatry	20	14
Journal of Studies on Alcohol	2	4
Archives of General Psychiatry	2	3

(although not the highest percentage) was the *American Journal of Psychiatry.*

For a discussion of picking an appropriate journal for your study, writing it up, and dealing with the review process, see Chapter 3.

What Makes a Good Environment for Unfunded Research?

Some departments provide more fertile soil than others for growing small-scale research. Our own experience, supported by the results of our survey, suggests several factors that make a difference for young faculty trying to start research projects:

1. *Leadership*—Small-scale research will not flourish unless it is valued and supported by the department chair. First, the chair must recruit a critical mass of faculty who have the motivation and training to do research. Second, the chair must clearly articulate the importance of small-scale research to the departmental mission and support faculty for academic promotion based on it. Third, although monetary support may not always be necessary, it never hurts. The chair must be willing

to maintain a start-up fund for promising projects and money for faculty to travel to meetings to present their results. Finally, the chair is responsible for establishing a departmental culture and infrastructure that can sustain such projects.

2. *Collegiality*—A collaborative rather than competitive atmosphere is a great asset for generating research projects. Formal departmental activities may not be as important to faculty as having opportunities for informal discussions. Whether such opportunities exist may depend on how close faculty are to one another geographically, whether there is a convenient communal place to eat lunch, and whether faculty have the time ever to go there.

3. *Richness of the Environment*—The more academic activity taking place in a department (or an institution as a whole), the more new activity it can generate. A core of productive researchers (working in a collegial rather than highly territorial atmosphere) are an invaluable source of ideas, expertise, and research infrastructure. In our survey, all the institutions in the top 10% in publishing unfunded research were also in the top 25% of research funding from NIMH.

4. *Accessible Patient Populations*—Faculty generate research ideas out of their own clinical experiences and choose which projects to undertake based on what types of patients are available. Therefore, it is imperative that a department have control over sufficient clinical services if research is to be possible; research cannot be accomplished in clinical settings where there is indifference or hostility to research goals.

5. *Staffing*—Although formally protected time is not necessary to accomplish research, departments in which faculty have multiple jobs, requiring every minute to be spent providing service, are not likely to generate much unfunded research. The same may be said for departments with bare-bones support staff. Secretaries who are stretched among large numbers of faculty would not be available to make their vital contributions to small-scale research projects. Thus, the general infrastructure of the department must be sufficient to accommodate time spent in research.

Conclusion

We have tried to provide practical suggestions for conducting small-scale, low-budget research that may be applicable in a variety of academic settings. The data support the notion that grant funding is not necessary to do research that is a genuine contribution to our knowledge and also a substantial contribution to the academic success of the faculty member who produces it.

References

Blumberg DL, Grant WD, Hendricks SR, et al: The physician and unconventional medicine. Altern Ther Health Med 1(3):31–35, 1995

Boucher M, Dewan M, Pandurangi A, et al: Relative utility of three indices of neuropsychological impairment in a young chronic schizophrenic population. J Nerv Mental Dis 174:44 46, 1986

Burke JD, Pincus HA, Pardes H: The clinician-researcher in psychiatry. Am J Psychiatry 143:968–975, 1986

Dewan MJ, Koss M: The clinical impact of reported variance in antipsychotic potencies. Acta Psychiatr Scand 91:229–232, 1995

Dewan MJ, Pandurangi AK, Boucher ML, et al: Abnormal dexamethasone suppression tests results in chronic schizophrenic patients. Am J Psychiatry 139:1501–1503, 1982

Dewan MJ, Pandurangi AK, Lee SH, et al: Central brain morphology in chronic schizophrenic patients: a controlled CT study. Biol Psychiatry 18:1133–1140, 1983a

Dewan MJ, Pandurangi AK, Lee SH, et al: Cerebellar morphology in chronic schizophrenic patients: a controlled computed tomography study. Psychiatry Res 10:97–103, 1983b

Dewan MJ, Pandurangi AK, Lee SH, et al: A comprehensive study of chronic schizophrenic patients: quantitative computed tomography. Acta Psychiatr Scand 73:161–171, 1986

Dewan MJ, Levy B, Donnelly MP: A positive view of psychiatry and psychiatrists. Compr Psychiatry 29:523–531, 1988

Huszonek J, Dewan MJ, Donnelly MP: Factors associated with antidepressant choice. Psychosomatics 36(1):42–47, 1995

Margo G, Greenberg R, Fisher S, et al: A direct comparison of the defense mechanisms of non-depressed people and depressed psychiatric inpatients. Compr Psychiatry 34:65–69, 1993

Pandurangi AK, Dewan MJ, Lee SH, et al: The ventricular system in chronic schizophrenic patients. A controlled computed tomography study. Br J Psychiatry 144:172–176, 1984

Pandurangi AK, Dewan MJ, Boucher M, et al: A comprehensive study of chronic schizophrenic patients. II: Biological, neuropsychological, and clinical correlates of CT abnormality. Acta Psychiatr Scand 73:161–171, 1986

Silberman EK, Snyderman D: Research without external funding in North American psychiatry. Am J Psychiatry 154(8):1159–1160, 1997

Silberman EK, Sussman N, Skillings G, et al: Aura phenomena and psychopathology: a pilot investigation. Epilepsia 35:778–784, 1994

Psychiatric Education

12

Preclinical Undergraduate Curricula

Myrl R. S. Manley, M.D., and David Trachtenberg, M.D.

Course Content

Preclinical medical student courses in psychiatry have conventionally included a survey of psychopathology and something called "behavioral science." Typically behavioral science has been taught in the first year and psychopathology in the second year, although at some schools they have been combined in a single course given either first or second year. We will consider them separately here.

Behavioral Science

Describing a behavioral science curriculum is like shooting at a moving target. The scope and content of this area is in flux with considerable variation between schools, and over time, within schools. Some programs have abandoned behavioral science teaching altogether, and many have replaced courses taught exclusively by departments of psychiatry with multidisciplinary courses.

Behavioral science courses became widespread in the late 1960s when the National Institute for Mental Health (NIMH) made grants available to academic departments of psychiatry to expand their preclinical teaching. The courses became universal and fixed in medical school curricula when the National Board of Medical Examiners (NBME) added behavioral science questions to its Part I examination in 1971 and 1972, and then began reporting a behavioral science subsection the following year (Brownstein et al. 1976).

From the beginning there was widespread disagreement on what courses in behavioral science should teach. The NBME proved to be of limited help in defining course content when it designated as "behavioral science" an impossibly comprehensive list of topics ranging from sociology to medical anthropology to medical economics, including subjects such as epidemiology and biostatistics that were already taught by nonpsychiatry departments.

A 1983 survey of North American medical schools by Arnett and Hogan revealed that only a single topic was taught in more than 50% of behavioral science courses and that only five topics were included in at least a quarter of all programs. A decade later (2 decades after the courses were first required) another study found an emerging consensus in the content of behavioral science (Table 12–1). However, the consensus topics appeared heavily centered on psychoanalytic theories of development and relatively neglectful of the by then extraordinary advances in the neurosciences and molecular biology. Medical schools across the United States and Canada were increasingly teaching the same thing in behavioral science, but it was no longer clear they were teaching a balance of topics that reflected the evolving concerns of psychiatry (Manley 1994).

We would like to pose three key questions as the necessary first steps in designing a course in behavioral science:

1. *What should be taught?* Considerable time, attention, and thought should be given to defining the core topics of behavioral science. It is a mistake to cobble together a course out of existing resources. Such a

Table 12–1. Behavioral science topics taught in at least 75% of schools, 1990 survey

Child psychological development
Psychodynamic theory
Adult psychological development
Human sexuality
Doctor–patient relationship
Behavioral learning theory

Source: Manley 1994.

pastiche is likely to be perceived by students and deans as makeshift. Whether the core is defined by the individual course director or by committee of basic scientists and clinicians, the process of definition is important.

We are including three different approaches to the content of behavioral science. The outline contained in Table 12–2 was prepared by the American Psychiatric Association Committee on Medical Student Education (1994). Table 12–3 is based on the content outline of the 1996 United States Medical Licensing Examination (USMLE; Federation of State Medical Boards of the United States and the National Board of Medical Examiners [FSMB-NBME] 1995).

Our proposal is presented in Table 12–4. It is divided into primary subject areas—those of likely importance to a broad spectrum of schools—and secondary subject areas—those more likely to be of

Table 12–2. Behavioral science topics proposed by the Committee on Medical Student Education of the American Psychiatric Association, 1994

A. Medical interviewing and physical diagnosis
   1. Cultural influences on health and health-related behaviors
   2. Health and illness in relation to social identity, role, and social context
   3. Family interactions and how they contribute to developing and maintaining illness and facilitating recovery
   4. The explicit and implicit "contract" between doctor and patient
   5. The use of various forms of psychotherapies in medical treatment
B. Behavior and neuroscience
   1. Human development throughout the life cycle
   2. Neuroanatomical, biochemical, genetic, physiologic, and immunologic correlates in normal behavior and in psychiatric and medical illnesses
   3. The doctor–patient relationship
   4. The application of psychodynamic understanding to patient, physician, and family behavior
   5. Learning theory
   6. Health behavior
   7. Psychological issues related to gender
   8. Human sexuality
   9. Chronobiology
   10. Domestic violence
   11. Suicidal and homicidal behavior
   12. Alcoholism and other forms of substance abuse
   13. Psychosocial responses to acute chronic illness and disability

Table 12–3. Behavioral science topics listed in the content description of Step I of the USMLE, 1996

A. General principles: Psychosocial, cultural and environmental influences on behavior, health and disease process
   1. Progression through the life cycle
   2. Psychologic and social factors influencing patient behavior (includes psychodynamic and learning theory, doctor-patient relationship)
   3. Patient interviewing, consultation, and interactions with family
   4. Medical ethics, jurisprudence, and professional behavior
   5. Organization and delivery of health care delivery
B. (For each organ system:) Psychosocial cultural and environmental considerations
   1. Influence of emotional and behavioral factors on disease prevention, progression, and treatment
   2. Influence of disease and treatment on person, family, and society

Table 12–4. A core curriculum in behavioral science

I. Primary topics
   A. Human growth and development
      From infancy through old age and senescence, a survey of the interplay between physical maturation and cognitive, emotional, and social growth; in childhood and adolescence. (More emphasis on brain plasticity and environmental triggers, and milestones of development than on purely theoretical models of staged development)
   B. Human sexuality
      Female and male sexuality, anatomy and physiology; sexual response cycles; full range of normal sexual behaviors across the life span
   C. Behavioral medicine
      The doctor–patient relationship; compliance; acute stress syndromes; adaptation to chronic illness
   D. Neurobiology of behavior
      Memory; mood and anxiety regulation; chronobiology; psychoneuroimmunology; behavioral genetics; sleep physiology
II. Secondary topics
   A. Culture and medicine
   B. Death, dying, and bereavement
   C. Drug and alcohol-related topics (neurobiology of addictions, epidemiology, and sociology of drug/alcohol use; specific disorders may be included in psychopathology)

interest to individual programs based on available teaching hours and faculty resources. It is intended to be minimal rather than comprehensive, a foundation on which given departments and medical schools may build according to their particular strengths and orientations.

2. *What is already taught elsewhere?* Having defined a core, the course director needs to ascertain whether individual topics are being taught in other courses and if they are, whether they should remain there, be duplicated in behavioral science, or shifted to behavioral science.

3. *Who should teach?* The course director must decide which areas will be better taught in collaboration with another department. A variety of solutions are being arrived at across the country and although it is not possible to describe them all, we can give some representative examples.

Many schools now offer a first-year course called "Introduction to Clinical Medicine" (ICM) or something similar. It is often interdisciplinary, sometimes run from the department of medicine, and typically includes active involvement by the department of psychiatry. It provides supervised, small-group clinical exposure during the first year of medical school. Common to many ICM courses are medical interviewing, physical diagnosis, and a range of issues concerned with the doctor-patient relationship (e.g., medical ethics) and behavioral medicine (e.g., compliance). Where they exist, ICM courses have largely supplanted the clinical component of conventional behavioral science courses.

Some medical schools include a separate course on reproductive medicine. Nearly always multidisciplinary, it may include obstetrics-gynecology, urology, endocrinology, and physiology. Psychiatry may take responsibility for topics in normal and abnormal sexual behavior (including sexual response cycles in men and women) and a discussion of sexual dysfunctions.

A course in neurosciences may be expanded to include, in addition to the usual neuroanatomy and neurophysiology, behavioral neurobiology. This attractive solution firmly grounds psychiatry in the medical model and establishes that normal and abnormal behavior derive from biological brain processes.

Psychopathology

Compared with behavioral science, courses in psychopathology are a breeze. The subject matter is clearly defined, the clinical focus catches students' interest, and the topics are thoroughly familiar to the faculty. Nevertheless, it is helpful to think of some key questions while planning a course in psychopathology:

1. *Which psychiatry?* Most psychiatry residency programs now describe themselves as "eclectic." It is understandable that residents, over the course of 4 years of intensive full-time training and exposure to multiple schools and clinical approaches, would be expected to forge their own synthesis. This is unrealistic for medical students whose time with psychiatry is much briefer. Unless they are presented with a single, clear theoretical focus, the field will seem anarchic. We believe that the appropriate model of psychiatry for medical students is medical: phenomenologic-descriptive psychiatry, strongly grounded in biology.

2. *Which disorders?* It is unlikely that any psychopathology course will be able to present all known psychiatric disorders, and some will be very restricted indeed. Judgments will have to be made about what to include and what to omit. Here are some principles that will help in deciding.

   a) Choose common disorders over uncommon: schizophrenia instead of erotomanic delusional disorder, HIV encephalitis instead of Creutzfeldt-Jakob disease.

   b) Emphasize diagnostic categories. It may be sufficient to give a few representative examples of the broader category, to teach, for example, a few personality disorders to illustrate the general concept of a personality disorder.

   c) Play to your strength. If your department includes a world expert on multiple personality disorder, you may want to include that topic in your course.

   d) Consider including disorders that illustrate important principles. Alzheimer's disease, in addition to being common, allows us to make correlations between brain pathology and clinical symptoms (degeneration of amygdala and hippocampus associated with memory loss). HIV encephalitis helps to illustrate the difference between cortical and subcortical dementias. Narcolepsy—identified by sleep-onset REM—is the exception that helps clarify the broader generalization that there are not yet biological markers for psychiatric disorders.

   e) Make sure students understand that the list of disorders is incomplete. It may be useful to suggest additional topics for self-study or USMLE preparation.

3. *What do you do with DSM-IV?* DSM-IV (American Psychiatric Association 1994) is great in getting us to think in the same conceptional categories and speak the same language. It is pretty good at increasing diagnostic reliability. It is not meant to be a textbook of psychopathology for beginners. Trying to understand schizophrenia by reading diagnostic criteria is a bit like trying to visualize a truck by reading a parts manifest of gear ratios and axle lengths. Although DSM-IV is useful in providing the organization for diagnostic categories and common agreement about what the diagnoses mean, students should not be made to memorize diagnostic criteria. They will not be asked them on the boards, and the criteria will change in a few years.

A successful psychopathology course will emphasize the clinical. Lecturers will illustrate key phenomena with video demonstrations, readings will include case descriptions, and students will be given the chance to talk with psychiatric patients. They can meet in small groups once a week on the psychiatry services to interview patients, perform mental status examinations, take psychiatric histories, and to see in person the clinical reality of what they are hearing in lecture. Above all, psychopathology courses can help to demystify psychiatric illnesses. The majority of students will enter fields other than psychiatry. They should take with them the knowledge that these disorders can be medically understood, rationally diagnosed, and in most cases treated or controlled.

The Role of the Course Director

Course directors are like Hollywood producers. They assemble the component parts of the course—topics, reading assignments, lecturers, small-group preceptors, examinations—and oversee the production through to its completion. Successful course directors will also remain highly visible and personally identified with a course. They should attend all lectures, sit in on small-group discussions, personally proctor examinations, and be easily accessible to students. Course directors represent the course at departmental meetings and schoolwide curriculum meetings and stand accountable for a course's failures as well as its triumphs.

For a lecture-based course, it is desirable for the course director to personally give, if not all the lectures, a great proportion. A single lecturer over several weeks is able to give a course unity, cohesiveness, and direction. He or she can make the course tell a story, drawing from earlier topics and expanding on them. By personally lecturing over several weeks, course directors develop a rapport with their class, recognize faces, call on students by name, understand more quickly when a topic is clear or mysterious, and perfect their timing so the jokes don't fall flat.

Some lucky course directors face the dilemma of departmental superstars—widely published faculty with national or international reputations who travel extensively giving grand rounds and lecturing at meetings of professional associations. The course director may be tempted (or pressured) to use superstars in preclinical courses. They are, after all, part of the unique richness of an institution, and they advertise the strength of the individual department.

There is no question that students should be engaged with the most talented, productive, and creative people within a department, but required preclinical courses may not be the best forum. Superstars tend to be extraordinarily busy. Their lectures are likely to be prepackaged and delivered from a series of slide projections that may not hit the appropriate level of training and knowledge. The very depth of their knowledge may make it harder for them to appreciate which topics are conceptually difficult for beginners and which vocabulary is foreign. It is often wiser to introduce students to superstars outside the confines of a specific course: at local grand rounds or special lectures, psychiatry club meetings or discussions in informal settings.

Course directors have two constituencies: their students and their teaching faculty. Attention to the former should not result in neglect of the latter. Much of course directors' time and energy will be in faculty development. They will need to continually recruit new lecturers and group leaders, often from among the junior faculty who are eager to begin building an academic career. Becoming coach, mentor, and senior adviser to beginning teachers can be one of the most rewarding parts of a course director's work. Like students, faculty are eager for feedback. They need encouragement and supportive criticism. Course orientations, teaching workshops, and instructional packets are part of the standard armamentarium of faculty development. It has been our experience, however, that none of these devices are as helpful in the long run as frequent, informal, personal, one-to-one conversations, which serve to sustain the vision of a particular course while solidifying personal relationships.

Collaboration With Other Departments

In 1984 the American Association of Medical Colleges (AAMC) issued a report titled "Physicians for the Twenty-First Century" calling for fewer classroom hours and more interdisciplinary teaching. The trend was strengthened in 1992 when the Parts I and II of the NBME were reorganized as Steps 1 and 2 of the USMLE. Topics on the old exams were organized and reported as categories that corresponded to preclinical courses: anatomy, biochemistry, physiology, and so on. The new exams have a section on general principles and another on organ systems, each of which includes normal and abnormal processes. Among the "normal and abnormal processes" are included psychosocial, cultural, and environmental considerations. A given question may require knowledge from several disciplines. Many schools have responded to these changes by attempting to weaken departmental boundaries in order to decompartmentalize preclinical courses (and perhaps to strengthen central control over the curriculum.)

Problem-based learning (PBL), pioneered at McMaster University and Michigan State University in the early 1970s became widely popular in the mid-1980s as a way not only to increase interdisciplinary teaching but also to radically revamp preclinical medical student education and strengthen self-directed learning (Neufeld et al. 1989; Schmidt 1983; Tosteson 1990). In PBL, students meet in small groups to discuss written cases. As students work through the cases they must first identify what they need to know, then seek out the information on their own and report back to the group. The cases are constructed to draw on information from all disciplines. For example, the case of a patient with renal failure may raise questions about acid-base balance, renal anatomy and physiology, adaptation to chronic illness, patient-doctor communication, and medical economics. The groups are led by a "facilitator"—by design not an expert in a given field—whose task is more to monitor and guide discussion than to impart factual information or answer questions of content. The PBL group discussions may be supplemented by lectures and laboratories, but in its purest form these are optional resources from which students may draw to work through the written cases.

Proponents such as Kaufman et al. (1989) have argued that PBL would teach problem solving, increase motivation, promote self-directed learning skills, and impart knowledge better than traditional teaching. Above all, it would be more fun. Advocates and converts have at times seemed to have

an almost messianic zeal. Unfortunately their enthusiasm has not been supported by research data. By all available measures, the graduates of PBL
and traditional schools are indistinguishable (Berkson 1993). Moreover, there
are serious difficulties with PBL. Because all learning is confined to cases
and since only one or two cases will be prepared each week, there are limits
on the number of topics that can be taught. It is not uncommon for all of
psychopathology to be limited to discussions of schizophrenia, mood disorders, and anxiety disorders. The demands on faculty teaching time are
heavy and sustained. Since most group leaders are nonexperts, students
miss out on the valuable experience of thinking *along with* a senior colleague, to observe how a seasoned clinician reasons from the information
at hand. There may be great differences in students' abilities to use a self-
directed curriculum. (It should also be remembered that the clinical years
in traditional schools have always been "problem based.")

Less radical approaches to multidisciplinary teaching are also being
implemented by many medical schools. Course boundaries and departmental identification with a given course may be preserved while the course
director recruits lecturers, discussants, and group leaders from other departments. A pharmacology course might include lectures by clinical psychiatrists on psychopharmacology, an anatomy course lectures and prosec-
tions by surgeons. In addition, the sequence of topics in conventional
department-based courses may be coordinated so that all courses deal with
a particular organ system simultaneously (sometimes called "vertical integration").

In the past few years considerable controversy has been generated over
the issue of psychiatry collaborating with primary care or family practice.
The debates have been impassioned, fueled by uncertainty over the future
direction of psychiatry as a medical specialty and changing patterns of
reimbursement. Because there is a trend among HMOs to establish primary
care physicians as gatekeepers to specialist services, and because of concern
that the gatekeepers will refer services traditionally supplied by psychiatrist
to lower-cost nonphysician providers, some have argued that psychiatry
must establish itself as a primary care specialty (Shore 1996). Others have
argued for increasing specialization, citing the advances in criterion-based
diagnosis, growing knowledge of the neurobiology of psychiatric disorders,
and absence of empirical evidence that psychiatrists are better psychotherapists than trained psychologists, social workers, and nurses (Lieberman
and Rush 1996). Although we hope preclinical course directors will remain

involved with these issues, we also urge them to recognize that their responsibilities to their students and their responsibilities to their field are not coterminous. Medical students in the first 2 years are not being taught psychotherapy. If their introduction to the doctor-patient relationship, medical interviewing, and medical ethics can be strengthened through collaboration with primary care and family practice, we strongly support such cooperation. It will help keep those topics from becoming marginalized, and it further serves to establish psychiatry as a medical discipline, fully integrated in the work and culture of the medical center. Those areas in which psychiatrists do hold unique expertise—the assessment and treatment of psychiatric disorders—will be presented in the psychopathology course and more thoroughly in the psychiatry clerkship.

One word of caution: When curriculum hours or course ownership are relinquished, they are seldom regained. It is not realistic to think that psychiatry teaching time can be given over to interdisciplinary courses on an experimental basis. Once it is gone, it is likely gone forever.

Teaching Formats

Lectures

Lecture courses have long been the mainstay of preclinical medical school education. Although recent efforts have been undertaken to limit the number of hours students spend in lectures, they remain the predominant form of teaching at most medical schools. Lectures have been criticized by just about everyone. Students tend to see them as dull, irrelevant to clinical work, and inefficient ways to learn material for exams. Faculty often feel frustrated trying to teach complicated, rapidly evolving topics in such a short period of time. Deans and course directors worry about adding to the biotechnology information overload that risks leaving students confused, overwhelmed, and focused on memorization and exam preparation. The 1984 American Association of Medical Colleges report concluded:

> Medical faculties should examine critically the number of lecture hours they now schedule and consider major reductions in this passive form of learning. In many schools, lectures could be reduced by one third to one half. The time that is made available by reducing lectures

should not necessarily be replaced by other scheduled activities. ("Physicians for the Twenty-First Century" 1984, p. 12)

The idea that lectures are a "passive form of learning" has been repeated so frequently as to have become a truism. Too often, bad lectures obscure the potential for lectures as a teaching modality. We believe that lectures can be an exciting, dynamic, active process with strengths not shared by other teaching formats.

At its best, when not simply a recitation of facts for students to copy and memorize, a lecture is a place where students are asked to think and reason along with a senior colleague. Thinking is active. It should be cherished as one of a physician's most important activities. Good lecturers will provide the conceptual scaffolding around which knowledge is constructed. They identify what is core and what is subsidiary. They draw from their own clinical experiences and critical analysis of current issues.

Good teachers also help students develop their own capacities for self-learning and critical thinking by identifying key principles and by demonstrating how to formulate and solve problems. For example, a lecturer on the genetics of schizophrenia, rather than asking students to memorize twin concordance data, may stress the interpretation of that data and ask students to identify and critique some of the underlying assumptions of twin studies. Similarly, a lecture on personality disorders may present the problem of categorical versus dimensional diagnosis instead of outlining DSM-IV diagnostic criteria. Lectures are for ideas, not lists.

When lecturers pose problems, ideas are generated, new questions get formulated, and creative thinking is most likely to take place in students' minds. Students who attend a lecture (unlike those reading a transcript) can see the teacher thinking, outlining main ideas, clarifying points, and giving examples. The student can ask questions and challenge assumptions.

Videos, movies, slides, and other audiovisual aids can help a lecture. Used promiscuously, however, they can sink it. The power of a lecture is the personal connection between teacher and student. When the personal is repeatedly disrupted by the technological, the power weakens. We do not favor the practice of lecturing from a series of slide projections. The practice is widely used by faculty too busy to adequately prepare a lecture. It focuses students' attention on the projection screen rather than the person of the lecturer. Dimming the house lights breaks the immediacy of connection between speaker and students. Here are some tips for better lecturing:

1. Don't read the lecture. Nothing is deadlier. Use notes sparingly or not at all. Don't hide behind a lectern. Get out in front and look at your audience. Make them look at you.
2. Use the blackboard. Write while you are talking and thinking. Students will keep better pace with you as they write their own notes.
3. Use slides only for what cannot be easily written on the blackboard such as complicated diagrams or photographs of brain pathology. Students should receive printed copies of all projected diagrams.
4. If your lecture is built around a series of slides with list after list of facts, take them out and burn them.
5. Video clips should be short (e.g., no more than 3 minutes) and shown for a clearly defined purpose. The lecturer should introduce the taped segments by telling students what to look for, and at the conclusion, summarize what they have seen. It will engage students' interest to pose a problem for them to solve; for example, "The manic patient on this tape uses a clang association. See if you can identify it."

Small Groups

Small-group learning has become an increasingly popular alternative to lecture-based courses. Small teaching groups are presumed to require more active participation by students in the form of preparation and in-group discussion. They facilitate faculty-student interaction and encourage student self-education. Small-group preceptors get to know their students as individuals, appreciate their strengths and areas of need, and observe firsthand their skills and attitudes. Some modalities of small-group teaching are outlined in Table 12–5.

Careful attention to patient selection will increase the success of clinical small groups. A common difficulty among beginning students is overidentification with patients and minimization of pathology ("Of course he's depressed, I would be too if I were in his situation.") On the other hand, the life circumstances of some patients may be so alien to students that they find it difficult to summon up any compassion, empathy, or even curiosity. The ideal patient will be willing, sufficiently verbal to be interviewed, with obvious pathology but with whom empathic resonance is still possible. If a given site is relentlessly homogenous, having, for example, only deteriorated chronic schizophrenia patients, efforts should be made to rotate students among different sites.

Table 12–5. A sampling of small-group formats

Clinical Small Group—Live patient interview with a preceptor, case is then discussed. *Example*: Medical students and preceptor meet with a psychiatric inpatient, take a history and perform a mental status exam.

Case Conference—Similar to preceding, typically faculty does the interview, focus is often on the "case findings" rather than the patient. *Example*: Demonstrating memory impairment or neurological signs in a patient with dementia.

Seminar Discussions—Readings and/or topics are assigned (there is no "live" patient), discussion is usually guided by faculty, may involve formal preparation and questions. *Example*: Reviewing and critiquing a paper describing structural brain abnormalities in schizophrenia.

Problem-Based Learning—Groups are assigned a facilitator, often a "non-expert" who encourages group discussion and team interaction around investigating a written clinical case presented in several parts. *Example*: The case of a woman with heart disease raises questions of cardiac physiology, adaptation to chronic illness, complications of tricyclics, possible panic disorder, and medical economics.

Small-Group Tutorials—Groups centered on a specific topic, paper, patient, or done for exam preparation. Usually involves only a few students together with a preceptor. Allows for more student–preceptor interaction, individualization of learning. *Example*: Students who do poorly on the midterm receive tutoring in preparation for the final.

Small-group teaching inevitably means the recruitment of a large teaching faculty. Residents can be quite helpful, especially in clinical groups. Voluntary faculty may be needed as well, and department chairs can be extremely useful in reminding voluntary faculty of the teaching obligation that comes with university appointment. Wherever recruited, faculty will need guidance. An orientation allows the course director to personally welcome faculty, distribute course materials, and discuss the mechanics of the course. In our experience, the most valuable part of any orientation is providing teachers with clearly defined goals and objectives.

Grading, Promotion, and Remediation

Grading practices vary. Some schools give only pass/fail grades, some pass/fail with Honors. Some have letter grades in preclinical courses and pass/fail in clinical courses, others just the opposite. Some schools have so expanded pass/fail grades (Honors, High Pass, Pass, Low Pass, Unsatisfactory) that they are functionally equivalent to letter grades. Whatever the grading policy of an individual school, three principles should guide the course director in this area:

1. The basis for evaluation should be made explicit at the start of a course, preferably in writing, including requirements for passing, the relative weights of examinations, small-group and clinical exercises, and what remediation will be required in the case of unsatisfactory work.
2. Timely midcourse evaluations should be given so that students with deficiencies are given the chance to bring their work up to passing standards. (This is not possible, of course, when a grade is determined by a single final examination—one reason why grading by a single exam is undesirable.)
3. Evaluations should be meaningful; it must be possible for a student to fail. It is unfair to students who work hard, and a terrible disincentive to all students, to routinely pass everyone without regard to the quality of their work or whether the standards of the course have been met.

Preclinical psychiatry courses are in the advantageous position of routinely including small-group discussions and clinical sessions. It may be more possible in these than in other basic science courses to evaluate professional behavior and personal social interactions. We believe that these are important aspects of professional education and that students should be evaluated on their behavior as well as on exam scores. It should be possible for a student to fail a course because of unprofessional conduct, even though examination grades are passing. Behavioral evaluations must be purely descriptive and nondiagnostic. "John was 20 minutes late for each small-group session" is acceptable. "John was passive-aggressive (or hostile, entitled, narcissistic, depressed, etc.)" is inappropriate.

Medical schools and individual departments also vary in the work required to remediate a failing grade. Makeup exams are often given for students who score below passing on the initial exam. Students who do poorly in small groups or clinical exercises may be required to undertake a series of tutorials, or to submit a paper. In extreme cases, students may be required to repeat the course. (Course directors and lecturers usually dread having someone in class who has already heard all the jokes.) For a fuller discussion of evaluations, see Chapter 15 by Bryce Templeton in this book.

Course Evaluations

Centrally administered course evaluations are mandated by the AAMC for accreditation and are now fixtures of all medical schools. Students are asked to rate anonymously a range of items such as quality of lectures, course organization, and accessibility of faculty and to indicate a global rating of satisfaction. Rating questionnaires are commonly distributed at the time of major examinations to maximize student participation. (It is worth pausing to consider the implicit assumption in this decision, that students will not be in full attendance at lectures, laboratories, or small-group activities.) A summary of the data is returned to each course director and usually to the respective department chair. Comparisons over time within and between departments are compiled and often widely circulated.

These evaluations are almost certain to remain a fact of course directors' lives for the foreseeable future, and it is wise to consider their strengths and weaknesses, uses and misuses. They have the advantage of providing regular, detailed feedback about student satisfaction. They offer a way to monitor the impact of innovations and changing curriculum, and they provide a means for the formal recognition of superior teaching.

There are a number of potential problems, however, in overreliance on evaluations of this sort. Since the ratings are collected at examinations, they are vulnerable to the distorting effect of an unusually difficult or unpopular exam. Obviously invalid ratings on one item may call into question this validity of the whole (e.g., a course receives midrange ratings on its computer instruction when it offers none at all).

There is also the risk when course evaluations are given strong emphasis that course directors will begin to play to the numbers, subordinating their own judgment to the annual ratings, embracing the safe and familiar and becoming reluctant to innovate. For example, if a potentially exciting clinical exercise receives bad ratings its first year out, there may be the temptation to drop it rather than to work on improving it over the next several years. Moreover, evaluations are of little use to a course in progress. They cannot identify the profoundly disaffected students who will go on to give the lowest possible rating for every item. They are of no help with midcourse corrections.

Students can indicate their level of satisfaction with a course, but there is much information they cannot provide. They cannot tell if courses are teaching what they should, if the content is widely accepted, accurate, and up-to-date. This is critical for a field as rapidly changing as psychiatry. (It is sometimes argued that scores on Steps 1 and 2 of the USMLE provide a check on course content, but, of course, they may be more an indication of students' ability to supplement the formal curriculum with self-study.) Some schools are now addressing this problem by supplementing student course evaluations with external reviews. Members of other departments, representatives from other medical schools, or other outside experts are invited to meet with the director and faculty of a course, to review the curriculum, interview students, read examinations, and in some cases to serve as external examiners at students' orals. The outside reviewers then prepare individual reports offering comments and suggestions.

Above all, it is critical that course directors not rely on central evaluations to the exclusion of their own judgment. They must monitor lectures, sit in on small-group discussions, and attend clinical exercises. They must arrange to meet regularly and frequently with students to attend to early dissatisfactions, and they must be willing to respond quickly to students' comments. If a particular lecturer was incomprehensible, the material may be summarized in a handout, additional reading may be recommended, or a clarifying makeup lecture offered. If there are complaints about a group preceptor, the course director must be willing to work with that person and, in extreme circumstances, find a replacement. Boring lecturers may be (tactfully) interrupted with intriguing and provocative questions.

Course directors who take this active role and who remain at the center of a course are positioned to use intelligently the information from central evaluations within the context of their own experience. They will be able to accept and make use of criticisms with which they agree but also to reject those with which they do not.

Some departments supplement central course evaluations with internal departmental evaluations. Although they may put students at some risk of evaluation overload (resulting in more superficial, thoughtless responses), internal evaluations can be tailored to the specific needs of a course, identifying unique areas of strength and weakness. They may also be a source of information used to identify teaching excellence for departmental recognition and promotion.

Special Problems

Antipsychiatry Bias

Beginning course directors are sometimes jarred to find not only skepticism among their students, but outright hostility. Numerous surveys have found that medical students consider psychiatry soft and unscientific and psychiatrists fuzzy thinkers (Eagle and Marcos 1980; Nielson and Eaton 1981). In preclinical courses, this bias may reveal itself in nonattendance, sarcasm, and cheekiness. When combined with the heavy academic demands of gross anatomy, biochemistry, pathology, and physiology, a milieu may be established in which dismissive disregard for psychiatry courses is tolerated.

The origins of antipsychiatry bias are multiple and often beyond the reach of an individual course director: the culture and traditions of the medical school, school admissions policies, societal stereotypes. Although widespread, the negative attitudes are neither intractable nor inevitable. In many schools, psychiatry courses are highly rated and their faculty win best teaching awards. Although course directors may not be able to eradicate completely preexisting bias, they can create a climate of scientific curiosity in which the course material is taken seriously. Some suggestions include the following:

1. Be unapologetic. Course directors themselves must believe in the value of their material. Saying "I know most of you aren't interested in psychiatry" is instantly self-fulfilling. Skepticism is healthy and scientific. Uninformed antagonism is not and should not be accepted.
2. Don't try to buy respect with kindness. A kindly, indulgent, forgiving attitude reinforces stereotypes and fosters dismissive contempt. The greatest kindness a course director can show students is giving them their money's worth with a solid, well-organized, high-level academic course—a course that challenges intellect and stimulates creativity. It must be possible to fail the course; otherwise passing has no meaning.
3. Be visible. Course directors and psychiatry faculty should take active, visible roles in the medical school community, chairing committees, serving as academic advisers, participating in campuswide clinical pathology conferences, interviewing applicants, performing at talent nights, taking part in student-faculty athletic events. Psychiatry will not be seen as an integrated medical discipline if its representatives maintain disdainful isolation.
4. Be honest. Students have extraordinarily well-tuned radar for intellectual dishonesty. If you don't know something, say so. Discuss how you can find the answer. Look it up and bring it back to class.
5. Be respectful. Disparaging remarks about surgeons or other medical specialists are totally out of place. Many of your students are thinking

of becoming surgeons, and your comments will sound defensive and insulting.

6. Don't analyze students. Your position with students is as educator, not therapist. It is desirable that the teaching functions and student counseling functions of the department be kept as separate as possible. It is a conflict of interest for faculty to treat students and also judge their academic performance. Students need the reassurance that in the classroom your concern is with their learning and not with their hidden emotional conflicts or private behavior. Students who do bring personal problems to the course director can be listened to sympathetically and, if necessary, guided to independent evaluation and treatment.

Recruitment

In the last several years, a decline in the number of American medical graduates matching psychiatry residencies has stimulated national concern. Although the number of psychiatrists actually needed in the country remains unclear (at least one prominent educator has argued there is no shortage of psychiatrists; Michels 1990), psychiatry course directors may find themselves under considerable pressure from department chairs and residency training directors to increase the number of their graduates choosing psychiatry careers.

In this climate, course directors need to recognize dual obligations. They should be able to identify, nurture, and mentor the small number of students who express an intense interest in psychiatry. At the same time they must not forget or neglect their responsibilities to the entire class, the great majority of whom will be going into other fields.

If a program has no graduates choosing psychiatry it is worth asking whether the teaching is turning off potential interest, but the success of a program should not be measured by the number of students entering the field. It should be possible, however, to make students comfortable with choosing psychiatry. High-quality, demanding, and well-organized courses will help the most. Psychiatry clubs may establish a cohort of self-support. Strong, happy, productive faculty provide good role models. When psychiatry teaching is well respected and thoroughly integrated among the medical disciplines, career choice in psychiatry becomes less culturally deviant. In Chapter 14 of this book, Theodore Feldmann discusses positive ways to encourage psychiatry.

Computer Instruction and the Internet

The use of computers in medical education will increase. Most students now enter medical school with some degree of computer literacy, some with highly sophisticated expertise. Some schools require all students to own computers. All schools make computers available. The consequence of these trends is unknown but a fertile area for speculation. Some observers such as Chodorow (1996) predict an utter transformation in teaching:

> The development of new multimedia teaching materials will break apart the old molds we have used for centuries to organize teaching and learning. Our effective contact with students will not be bound by time and place; our distinction between elementary and advanced will be virtually impossible to maintain; our traditional pacing of teaching and learning will lose some of its usefulness and justification. (p. 224)

Others have urged that we not be caught in a stampede of enthusiasm and that we consider the meta-effects of supplanting the personal with the electronic.

> Perhaps our networked world isn't a universal doorway to freedom. Might it be a distraction from reality? An ostrich hole to divert our attention and resources from social problems? A misuse of technology that encourages passive rather than active participation? What's most important in school? Working with good teachers who can convey method as well as content. Except to the extent that students are involved with a caring teacher, schooling is limited to teaching facts and techniques. In this sense, network access is irrelevant to schooling— it can only prevent this type of interaction. The computer is a barrier to close teaching relationships. (Stoll 1995, p. 118)

What seems certain is that preclinical course directors will not have the option to ignore these powerful tools. They will need to educate themselves or have ready access to good computer consultants to ensure the tools are used wisely. It is useful for those of us made uneasy by the fact that we have less experience and facility with these modalities than do our students to review what interactive computer programs and the Internet do well and what they do rather more poorly. Among their greatest strengths are the following:

1. Information storage and retrieval: Information that would fill a library shelf can be efficiently sorted through and accessed. Literature searches, once requiring laborious review of volume after volume of *Index Medicus* or *Psychological Abstracts* can now be done in a few minutes with the click of a switch. Information on drug interactions, the newest available antidepressants, glossaries of terms, textbooks, and abstracts of current journal articles are all immediately at hand.

2. Visual information: The extraordinary sophistication of computer graphics offers imagery unequaled by any other medium. It is possible, for example, for a student studying Alzheimer's disease not only to move back and forth through serial sections of a head CT scan but also to move back and forth through time to study the disease progression on sequential CTs. It is possible to call up a three-dimensional model of the basal ganglia and rotate it so that it can be viewed from different perspectives.

3. Rote review: Several software programs and Internet sites such as the New York University (NYU) Department of Psychiatry home page provide series of questions on selected topics with immediate feedback and suggested references for follow-up study. They offer great flexibility in permitting students to practice in their own time and at their own pace.

A list of some useful Internet sites is provided in Table 12–6.

We believe that computers do less well in presenting new concepts and in clinical training. The most brilliant interactive program cannot approach the interactive quality of a person-to-person encounter—the teacher's ability to detect the faint shadow of doubt or uncertainty on a student's face, or the ability to grasp the misperception embedded in a poorly worded question and to rephrase the question before answering. No computer training can be a substitute for working with living patients, for touching their bodies and hearing their words, for fine-tuning our powers of perception and learning to deal with the near infinity of unexpected and idiosyncratic responses of patients.

The best education is personal. Our minds have evolved an extraordinary capacity to learn from one another, and the relationship between teacher and student can be one of the strongest motivating forces available.

Table 12–6. Selected Internet addresses of interest to preclinical course directors

Search engines	
Lycos	http://lycos.cs.cmu.edu/
Yahoo	http://www.yahoo.com/
Deja News	http://www.dejanews.com/forms /dnquery.html
Training	
New York University Department of Psychiatry	http://www.med.nyu.edu/Psych/NYUPsych .Homepage.html
University of Iowa "Virtual Hospital"	http://vh.radiology.uiowa.edu
CUSI at Northwestern	http://www.eecs.nwu.edu
Publishing	
Interpsych	http://www.shef.ac.uk/uni/projects/gpp /ip.html
Archives of General Psychiatry	http://www.ama-assn.org/sci-pubs/journals /standing/psyc/psychome.htm
American Journal of Psychiatry	http://www.appi.org/ajp
Psychiatric Service	http://www.appi.org/psjournal
Psychiatry on Line	http://www.cityscape.co.uk/users/ad88 /psych.htm

Source: Adapted from Lim 1996.

When our students begin to know us, when we become important people in their educational lives, when we are seen to embody the knowledge and discipline to which they aspire, our personal knowledge and judgment of their progress becomes extremely important. The experience of sitting face to face with a respected and admired teacher, and hearing the teacher say, "I'm disappointed in your work; I know you can do much better," is more powerful than receiving an exam grade or reviewing a transcript. When education is personal, our students will gradually internalize the judgments and expectations of valued teachers. They will learn to set and meet their own demands and be started on the difficult road of self-education.

References

American Psychiatric Association: Diagnostic and Statistical Manual of Mental Disorders, 4th Edition. Washington, DC, American Psychiatric Association, 1994

American Psychiatric Association Committee on Medical Student Education: A Guideline for a Medical Student Curriculum in Psychiatry and Behavioral Science. Washington, DC, American Psychiatric Association, 1994

Arnett JL, Hogan TP: The role of behavioral sciences in North American medical schools: an overview. J Med Educ 58:201–203, 1983

Berkson L: Problem-based learning: have the expectations been met? Acad Med 68(Oct. Supplement):579–587, 1993

Brownstein EJ, Singer P, Dornbush R, et al: Teaching behavioral science in the preclinical curriculum. J Med Educ 51:59–62, 1976

Chodorow S: Educators must take the electronic revolution seriously. Acad Med 71:221–226, 1996

Eagle PF, Marcos LF: Factors in medical students' choice of psychiatry. Am J Psychiatry 137:423–427, 1980

Federation of State Medical Boards of the United States and the National Board of Medical Examiners (FSMB-NBME): United States Medical Licensing Examination, 1996. Step 1: General Instructions, Content Description, and Sample Items. Philadelphia, PA, Federation of State Medical Boards of the United States and the National Board of Medical Examiners, 1995

Kaufman A, Mennin S, Waterman R, et al: The New Mexico experiment: educational innovation and institutional change. Acad Med 64:285–294, 1989

Lieberman JA, Rush AJ: Redefining the role of psychiatry in medicine. Am J Psychiatry 153:1388–1397, 1996

Lim RF: The internet: applications for mental health clinicians in clinical settings, training, and research. Psychiatr Serv 47(6):597–599, 1996

Manley MRS: An emerging consensus in behavioral science course content. Academic Psychiatry 18:30–37, 1994

Michels R: Address to New York County District Branch, American Psychiatric Association, New York City, 1990

Neufeld VA, Woodward CA, Macleod SM: The McMaster M.D. program: a case study of renewal in medical education. Acad Med 64:423⇒–432, 1989

Nielson AC, Eaton JS: Medical students' attitudes about psychiatry: implications for psychiatric recruitment. Arch Gen Psychiatry 38:1144–1154, 1981

Physicians for the twenty-first century: Report of the Project Panel on the General Professional Education of the Physician and College Preparation for Medicine. J Med Educ 59(11 Pt 2):1–208, 1984

Schmidt HG: Problem-based learning: rationale and description. J Med Educ 17:11–16, 1983

Shore JH: Psychiatry at a crossroads: our role in primary care. Am J Psychiatry 153:1398–1403, 1996

Stoll C: Silicon Snake Oil. New York, Anchor Books, 1995

Tosteson DC: New pathways in medical education. N Engl J Med 322:234–237, 1990

13

Psychiatric Clerkships

Amy C. Brodkey, M.D., and Frederick S. Sierles, M.D.

Characteristics of Clerkships and Directors

The average required third-year (rarely, fourth-year) psychiatry clerkship lasts 6.1 half weeks, with a range of 4 to nine 9 weeks; the majority are 6 weeks, about 25% are 8 weeks, and about 10% are 4 weeks. Anecdotally, some psychiatric educators report having to shorten their clerkships to accommodate new clerkships in primary care. Most directors perceive that 4 weeks is too brief for a meaningful clinical experience in psychiatry. Despite the current emphasis on ambulatory settings in all clerkships, the most common clinical site in psychiatry remains an inpatient service (Links et al. 1988; Sierles and Magrane 1996).

The average psychiatry clerkship director is 46 years old and has occupied the position for almost 6 years. More than 90% are board-certified psychiatrists. Their distribution in academic ranks of assistant (36%), associate (32%), and full (27%) professor does not differ significantly from residency training directors. More than 90% carry one or more additional administrative duties, most often director or codirector of medical student education in psychiatry (66%), course coordinator in psychopathology or behavioral science, or clinical service chief. Half are members of their department's executive committee.

Directors work an average of 51.7 hours per week, including 13.6 hours teaching and another 11.2 on educational administrative duties. Teaching hours are divided among clinical (5.5) and didactic (4.1) instruction of students and of residents (3.9). Other activities include clinical practice (15 hours), which most feel enhances their teaching, and conducting research (5.9 hours). Most directors do not perceive that conducting research is essential to their position (Sierles and Magrane 1996).

Diverse roles exist for faculty participating in a clerkship. In departments with multiple clinical sites, each may have a site director who implements the educational program and ensures comparability of experience and consistency with the clerkship's goals. Clinical and didactic teaching must be widely shared among faculty. Certain strongly involved faculty may serve on a clerkship or medical student education committee. Other roles include facilitating a student psychiatry club, evaluating students, and advising interested students.

Administering the Clerkship

Typical administrative duties of the clerkship director are listed in Table 13–1. Evaluating students is covered in Chapter 15.

In addition, clerkship directors customarily teach, supervise, advise and advocate for students, and anticipate and field problems. They may participate in educational research and in psychiatry clubs and may implement educational programs for faculty and residents on teaching and evaluation.

The director's job is made immeasurably more pleasant and productive

Table 13–1. Duties of the clerkship director

1. Establish and convey standards for student participation in patient care at clinical training sites.
2. Determine (with departmental and school input) and implement the didactic curriculum.
3. Organize schedules and assignments.
4. Monitor and respond to the effectiveness of clinical sites, faculty, and the clerkship as a whole in achieving its goals.
5. Serve as a liaison with clinical training sites, the department and chair, the Office of Medical Education (OME), other departments' clerkship directors, and medical school education and evaluation committees.
6. Recruit faculty to teach.
7. Obtain and convey feedback to students and teachers.
8. Set standards and evaluation procedures for student performance.
9. Summarize and transmit grades and evaluations to the dean's office.

by a supportive, accessible chair or vice-chair for education. It is crucial that the chair believes that student teaching is a vital departmental mission, allocates the resources and time necessary—approximately 25% FTE for the clerkship director (Fincher 1996, p. 2)—and encourages and rewards excellent teaching. An education budget should cover direct student costs (e.g., printed and audiovisual materials, books, computer programs, National Board of Medical Examiners [NBME] subject exams, standardized patients), faculty needs (faculty development and the director's professional development), and administrative support costs (e.g., computers and software, funding for a psychiatry club, awards) (Fincher 1996, pp. 88–91). During regular meetings of the director and the chair, the broad goals of the clerkship, the teaching program, and outcome measures should be discussed. They should also inform each other of educational issues in the medical school that may affect the clerkship and may occasionally require the chair's intervention.

Another indispensable requisite for the clerkship is a competent, organized, pleasant full-time administrative assistant, whose responsibilities are listed in Table 13–2.

A clerkship committee that sets goals, policies, and standards; informs and advises; monitors performance; and shares responsibility for decisions can keep faculty involved in the medical student program and keep the director from becoming isolated. In programs with associate directors, communication regarding philosophy and expectations must be particularly clear, and the director must delegate some responsibility and authority. Relationships with the school's other clerkship directors foster exchanges of

Table 13–2. Duties of the administrative assistant (clerkship coordinator)

1. Schedules classes, reserves classrooms, and obtains audiovisual and other equipment.
2. Makes clinical assignments.
3. Prepares written materials.
4. Distributes keys and meal tickets, fields questions, relays messages, and handles emergencies.
5. Proctors and grades exams.
6. Keeps track of evaluations and maintains student records and databases for research and evaluation.
7. Communicates with the dean's office, the OME, and other clerkship administrators.
8. Provides a sympathetic ear to students and information to the director.

information, coordination of the curriculum, and moral support. Offices of medical education (OMEs) may provide technical assistance (e.g., automated examination grading and statistical analyses), advice, and resources for educational innovation (e.g., computer-assisted learning, objective structured clinical exams) and research.

Also of interest is the director's role on student evaluation committees, where two problems may occur. The first is the blurring of the psychiatrist's roles as educator and clinician, as in "please explain this student's problem." Although the director may need to educate committee members on aspects of psychopathology that may affect a student's performance, from learning disabilities to suicide potential, the educator and clinician roles must be separated. Second, some faculty still hold the idea that psychiatry has little content and therefore is less deserving of time, is less rigorous, and certainly cannot be failed. Tactful but firm explanations may help to alter these attitudes.

Goals of the Clerkship

Psychiatric clerkship directors share broad agreement on the goals of clerkships (Brodkey et al. 1997). Given both the high prevalence and deficiencies in recognizing and treating psychiatric disorders in primary care populations, the most important purpose is to impart basic skills and knowledge to future generalist physicians, most of whom will have minimal further training in psychiatry. This encompasses the ability to (1) conduct, record, and present an initial psychiatric interview, (2) use the history and mental status examination to identify psychopathology, and (3) know the differential diagnosis, evaluation, and management of the most common and emergent psychiatric disorders. Moreover, attitudes and skills vital to practitioners of any specialty are reinforced in psychiatry. These include interviewing proficiently; developing attitudes of professionalism, caring, empathy, tolerance, and comfort with a wide variety of patients; communicating effectively, working in teams, and making a referral; knowing one's own limitations and biases; understanding the psychosocial aspects of illness, including the process of psychological adaptation; and utilizing holistic models of causation, discouraging the mind-brain split, and tolerating ambiguity. Finally, the clerkship should teach about psychiatry as a specialty, including the spectrum of psychiatric practice, the mental health system, and various treatment modalities. Clerkship goals and objectives are discussed in detail elsewhere (Brodkey et al. 1997).

Other goals include decreasing prejudice against the field and its patients, emphasizing both the validity of diagnosis and the efficacy of treatments, preparing students for the psychiatry portion of the United States Medical Licensing Examination (USMLE) Step 2, and assisting in the recruitment of students interested in psychiatry. A long-term study at one school showed that better USMLE scores were correlated with a longer clerkship and more interactive teaching (Schottstaedt et al. 1991). The clerkship is probably the most important medical school influence on recruitment, and higher rates are associated with excellent educational programs in departments that give priority and resources to teaching (Sierles and Taylor 1995).

Evaluation of the Clerkship

Evaluation of how well the clerkship meets its goals is essential. Students' perceptions can be solicited informally during the clerkship, individually and in groups. The director should maintain frequent contact and sincerely encourage feedback. Medical students are often unwilling to rock the boat with criticisms unless they perceive they will be taken seriously and there will be no retribution. An open door policy for both faculty and students is essential to staying on top of immediate problems. In addition, the coordinator is well positioned to hear and convey timely information.

Logs

Student logs of required learning objectives (Hudziak et al. 1995) or clinical experiences (Links et al. 1988; Weissberg 1996) can provide feedback about the extent to which the clerkship's objectives are met. Students may be given a log at the beginning of the clerkship and asked to indicate if and when the objective or experience is attained.

Student Evaluations

Formal evaluation is obtained at the end of the clerkship. The dean's office usually uses a standardized form, which is often computerized. These evaluations have the advantages of greater honesty (due to their preservation of students' anonymity) and comparability with other clerkships.

A supplementary departmental evaluation can be designed to answer questions not asked on the dean's form; these may be available much sooner. The director should ensure that all students complete these forms by collecting them at the final examination or by withholding grades until they are received. Assurance of protection from retaliation, by ensuring anonymity and by returning the results to faculty only after grades are given, is essential. All aspects of the clerkship, including overall experience, clinical experiences (including night call), courses, lecturers, attendings, residents, texts and other learning resources, and examinations should be rated on an ordinal scale with ample room for narrative comments. Other facets of the clerkship, such as students' opinions about its success in preparing them for future practice, clarity of objectives, inclusion of the student on the team, and how often the student was observed interviewing, can be incorporated. These ratings, which have demonstrated validity (Fincher 1996, p. 45), can be summarized periodically for review by the chair and the clerkship committee. The department can use these ratings as part of the periodic performance review with faculty and residents. Finally, ratings of the clerkship and of individual faculty can be used as documentation for promotion decisions.

Direct Observation

Another valuable evaluation component is the director's observation of clinical and classroom teaching. Because it is so time-consuming, this effort may be restricted to new faculty or faculty whom there is reason to believe are having difficulty in their teaching role. Feedback should emphasize positive aspects of performance as well as areas for improvement and should focus on specific, modifiable behaviors (Table 13–3). It must be emphasized that effective teaching is a skill to be mastered, not a judgment of character. The director may also coteach with faculty or invite them to observe his or her teaching. It is important to meet with all teaching faculty on an as-needed basis to review student ratings and teaching objectives and solicit feedback.

Examination Performance

Data about the clerkship is also obtained through assessment of student performance on departmental examinations and USMLE Step 2 scores "Evaluation of Students" (Templeton). By specifying the educational objectives of the clerkship and ensuring that these objectives are taught and tested on departmental examinations, the director can to some extent esti-

Table 13–3. Principles of giving and receiving feedback

1. Feedback is constructive, specific, and descriptive, never humiliating.
2. It concerns observable and changeable behavior.
3. Positive feedback is given before suggestions for change.
4. Feedback is given in a timely fashion.
5. Subjective data is labeled as such.
6. The recipient of the feedback listens carefully and then evaluates its quality and helpfulness.

mate the achievement of the goals of the clerkship. Since broad areas of learning (e.g., assessment of psychopathology, interviewing skills, and knowledge base) are acquired separately (Goldney and McFarlane 1986), it is important to assess them independently. Utilizing USMLE scores to measure the effectiveness of the clerkship is less straightforward; scores are determined by multiple variables, including characteristics of the student body, clerkship length, and discrepancies between what is taught in a clerkship and what is tested. For a given department, strong upward or downward trends in scores over several years is noteworthy. To control for characteristics of the student body, scores on the psychiatry section may be compared with those achieved in other specialties.

Orientation to the Clerkship: Structuring Students' Expectations and Responsibilities

Conveying Guidelines

Clear communication of expectations and responsibilities to students, residents, and faculty is essential to reduce anxiety, achieve the goals of the clerkship, and avoid the problems that result from failure to meet unclear standards. Written guidelines should be distributed to and verbally reviewed with incoming students at their orientation session. Typically, third-year students will not remember much of what they hear about the details of the organization of the clerkship; hence, the need for written guidelines. Explicit instructions regarding clinical responsibilities, including number of assigned patients, hours of attendance, directions for chart documentation, night call schedules and duties, rounds participation, responsibilities in the assessment of new patients (including the physical examination), what to do in case of absence, and any dress codes should be covered.

A schedule of classes and conferences is distributed and reviewed, along with guidelines on what to do about conflicts between clinical duties and class attendance. Expectations for written assignments, such as patient assessments and logs, should be distributed along with guidelines and examples. Goals and objectives of the clerkship, textbooks and other learning resources, and evaluation standards and procedures are discussed. Examinations and evaluations are potent motivators of students, most of whom believe their residency matches depend on their clerkship grades. The grading system must be described explicitly, orally and in writing, and standards must remain the same throughout each academic year.

Students must be told what to expect of faculty, residents, and staff. Guidelines for supervision and teaching, feedback, and general participation by clerks should be reviewed, with directions to report deviations to the director. For example, if clerks are assigned two new inpatients per week, they should report if they are overloaded, inadequately supervised, or given too few patients. Orientation is an opportune time to review the importance and principles of giving and receiving feedback (Table 13–3) and to encourage students to solicit it.

Student Concerns

Students beginning the clerkship are often anxious about certain issues; preclerkship anxiety is associated with negative attitudes and is best addressed explicitly at this initial meeting. The director may begin by eliciting students' ideas of how psychiatric patients may resemble or differ from other types of patients. Concerns about patient assaultiveness should be addressed by a discussion of the assessment and management of agitated patients, followed up during the first week by a presentation on psychiatric emergencies. Misperceptions may include that psychiatric patients are more chronically ill or less treatable than other patients, that psychiatrists use only one type of treatment for all problems (e.g., psychotherapy or medication), or that psychiatrists (and, therefore, medical students on rotation in psychiatry) should maintain a blank facade when dealing with patients. Beginning students may need the director to raise these myths. It is useful to (1) review some of the real differences they can expect with some patients, such as increased difficulty in communicating, greater likelihood of unconventional behavior, the stigma and denial associated with psychiatric illness, the involuntary status of some of the patients, and the greater reliance on the history and mental status exam to make a diagnosis, and (2) to remind students of the importance of observing and understanding their own reactions to patients.

It is helpful to tell students that they may have distressing emotional responses to some patients that they should discuss with a faculty supervisor or colleague. It is also prudent to discuss maintaining professional boundaries with patients; students should be specifically instructed that they may not date or befriend patients during or after the clerkship. Orientation also provides an opportunity to discuss the high prevalence of psychiatric disorders seen in all specialties.

During this first meeting the director must convey openness, warmth, respect, a sincere desire for communication, and excitement about this mutual endeavor. Because some students believe that the psychiatry clerkship is a "vacation," expectations that they will be involved in patient care, meet high standards in their learning, and develop important professional skills and attitudes should be apparent.

Nuts and Bolts Items

Nuts and bolts items like phones and beepers, storage of personal items, office space, transportation, parking, keys, meal tickets, and student memberships to the American Psychiatric Association can be addressed by the coordinator. There must be a system of prompt communication between the clerks and the administrator to handle cancellations and rescheduling of classes and other "crises" that inevitably occur. An old-fashioned posting board, pagers, or electronic mail may be used.

The Clerkship Curriculum

A major responsibility of the director, establishing and implementing the curriculum, is complex and sometimes intimidating. Although lack of time and resources may forestall a department-wide, comprehensive review and revision of its current educational program and outcomes, the director must proceed based on the clerkship's overall goals and specific learning objectives and the resources available to achieve them. This planning is crucial, both for the achievement and measurement of desired outcomes, and for the education and cooperation of the teaching faculty, who may otherwise view student teaching as watered-down residency training.

Model Clerkship Objectives

Formulating goals and objectives has been made considerably easier by the introduction of model clerkship objectives by the Association of Directors of Medical Student Education in Psychiatry (ADMSEP) (Brodkey et al. 1997) (Appendix 13–A). These were explicitly based on an assessment of what generalists need to know and do to adequately diagnose and treat or refer the psychiatric problems they are likely to encounter. The objectives address behaviorally defined knowledge, skills, and attitudes to facilitate selection of learning experiences and evaluation of student competencies and of the clerkship (Tyler 1949). They include "enabling" and "terminal" objectives; the former term describes skills such as patient interviewing or relating to a treatment team that are necessary to achieve the desired terminal outcomes of effective diagnosis and treatment. The ADMSEP objectives could be a starting point for a department to define its curriculum in light of its priorities and resources. Not all the objectives can be mastered during the clerkship; some can be taught in preclinical courses and other clerkships. What is crucial is engaging key faculty in curriculum development to generate a sense of ownership and enthusiasm (Brodkey et al. 1997). A thorough departmental review of the teaching program should occur every 4 or 5 years, and it helps to involve trainees in the process.

Implementation

Establishing goals and objectives is but the first step in producing a "curriculum," which is Latin for "path." Fundamental to curriculum development is implementation, guiding the student down the path. Equating curriculum with formal classroom teaching splits what students learn in class from what they do clinically. Although some prior knowledge is essential, clinical learning requires discovery and reflection that cannot be captured didactically. It involves exercising judgment in unique and uncertain situations (Schon 1987). Integrating idealized and compartmentalized objectives with rich and complicated experiences with patients and coworkers focuses educators on the learning process.

In some settings, education is moving toward specifying minimal competency standards based on "critical incidents" that are essential to the clinician's development at each level of training. Weissberg (1996) developed 11 psychiatric "screens"—questions to facilitate the diagnosis of common problems like depression, substance abuse, and violence—that can be assigned to students. These are in the appendix to the ADMSEP objectives. Since there is a limit to how well clinical experience can be controlled, standardized patient formats and structured case-based seminars (Ende et al. 1986) can fill in the gaps. The didactic program should be evaluated for its success in addressing the immediate clinical skills and problems faced by students in the context of the clerkship objectives.

The Hidden Curriculum

Sometimes overlooked is the "hidden curriculum," an important aspect of student socialization related to the culture of medicine (e.g., attitudes toward patients, organizing work, obtaining good grades, political opinions, dealing with hierarchy, managing affective responses). If directors are aware of such ideas, it may be possible to address them explicitly. For instance, they can discuss hostility toward substance abusers or the inadequacy of certain unassigned textbooks.

Certain curricular topics deserve special mention. Surveys of primary care practitioners indicate that they feel underprepared in such areas as substance abuse, suicide risk, sexual history-taking, child abuse, depression, health behavior change, somatization and chronic pain, interviewing, psychopharmacology, doctor-patient relationship skills, compliance, community resources, and counseling and referral techniques (Callen 1980; Holmes et al. 1990). Although not all of these topics may be addressed in a psychiatry clerkship, particularly on an inpatient service, some offer opportunities for collaborative interdisciplinary teaching "Educational Collaboration with other Specialties" (Weissberg et al).

It is important to balance education (scientific enquiry, critical thought, understanding, values) and training (mastery of specific, practical knowledge and skills through mnemonics, algorithms, competency-building exercises). Though the latter have a time-honored place in the clerkship, there is a danger of reducing the complexity and richness of psychiatry to a simple cognizance of diagnostic criteria. The idea that this constitutes knowledge of psychiatry may be comforting, but ultimately detracts from the intellectual and emotional challenge of understanding and integrating specific biological and psychosocial aspects of illness and treatment, which is uniquely attractive to many students (Kaltreider et al. 1994).

Didactic Components of the Clerkship

Broad areas of learning, such as identification of psychopathology, mastery of interpersonal skills, acquisition of knowledge, and attainment of professional attitudes are acquired independent of each other and should be taught using the most appropriate methods (Goldney and McFarlane 1986).

It helps to map the clerkship objectives onto available teaching opportunities, including clinical experiences. Didactic formats include lectures, journal clubs, interactive group discussions based on case material (live, role-played, videotaped, written, or standardized patient), computer-assisted instruction, and self-study such as reading, viewing videotapes, case assessments, and writing papers. Covering important topics with a variety of teaching formats is an adaptation to different learning styles and developmental levels of students. The best repetitions are between classroom teaching and clinical care. Excellent guides for lecture and small-group teaching exist (Whitman 1982a, 1982b).

Lectures and Case Discussions

Eighty-six percent of psychiatry clerkships offer lecture series; over 70% include psychopharmacology, history and mental status, major psychiatric disorders including substance abuse, and suicide, while a smaller number cover emergency, child and adolescent and geriatric psychiatry, sleep disorders, and sexuality (Abrams et al. 1987). Clerkship lectures should differ from those typically given in second-year psychopathology courses in placing greater emphasis on practical aspects of differential diagnosis, assessment, and management. Although much may be learned from reading, well-designed lectures put information into a coherent, developmentally appropriate framework.

The major problem with lectures is audience passivity, which discourages the deep learning necessary to successful understanding, critical thinking, and clinical reasoning (Newble and Entwistle 1986). Most lecturers tire quickly of giving the same speech every 6 or 8 weeks, although some are adept at keeping students interested. Serious consideration should be given to alternative formats. For example, students can be assigned written case vignettes or videotapes designed to elicit learning of specific objectives along with readings prior to a class using a problem-solving format (Barrows and Tamblyn 1980; Ende et al. 1986; Wilkerson and Feletti 1989). This format stimulates curiosity and resourcefulness, forces students to integrate facts, and increases their feelings of competence. One study shows that this strategy, although it requires advanced preparation, results in greater learning of targeted material and better standardized test scores (Ende et al. 1986). Faculty may also use a Socratic teaching style, in which the teacher's questions elicit students' answers.

Psychiatric Interviewing

Many clerkships offer a course that covers psychiatric interviewing, clinical reasoning, and diagnosis; this recognizes that clerks are learning the basics and are often at a loss to explain, let alone imitate, their supervisor's ability to elicit information efficiently, make diagnoses, and formulate treatment plans. Student acquisition of these skills can be accelerated if it is explicitly addressed, demonstrated (by having experts "think aloud"), and practiced (Nurcombe and Fitzhenry-Coor 1987). In such a course, either students (preferably) or faculty or residents (less often) may interview patients.

The need for improving physician interview skills is well documented, and several studies indicate that the performance of medical students may deteriorate from the first year to the fourth (Craig 1992). A number of formats for teaching this subject, including lecture/discussion, live demonstrations, practice interviews, direct feedback, and programmed demonstration videotapes (Enelow et al. 1970), can improve students' skills and are described in the literature (Carroll and Monroe 1980). Basic principles and functions of interviewing and the mental status examination should be covered at the beginning of the clerkship, followed by opportunities for clerks to observe and perform interviews. Students and faculty can utilize one of the many available checklists to specify the skills to be learned, practiced, and evaluated (Appendix 13–B). Review and critique of videotaped student interviews is particularly effective. Alternatively, a student can interview a live or simulated patient, followed by a group critique of the interview, the interviewer's reactions to the experience, and a discussion of the patient's diagnosis and treatment. This provides an opportunity to review and practice giving and receiving feedback collegially (Table 13–3).

In addition, the teacher should also use these sessions to identify and discuss attitudes and reactions to patients, help students identify psychopathology, demonstrate clinical reasoning, or discuss other relevant topics (e.g., ethics, psychiatry and medicine, health care financing). Videotapes or role plays can also be used to teach students how to handle emotionally charged or otherwise difficult interviews that may be troublesome for physicians. All students *must* be directly observed and given immediate feedback (Carroll and Monroe 1980). Though time-consuming, teaching this course involves the director with students and permits evaluation of the achievement of many clerkship objectives.

Other Formats

Computer-assisted instruction (CAI) affords the advantages of independent scheduling and interactive formats. Aside from software produced for their own use by several schools, CAI is still rare in psychiatry. However, widespread availability of the necessary technology predicts development of interactive programs to teach diagnosis, clinical management, and even interviewing skills.

Other assignments include written patient assessments with case formulations, case conference presentations, and papers on topics of special interest to the student. Clerks should be taught how to conduct a literature search and can be assigned to do one. Such assignments can be done after hours or during unplanned slack time. Ideally, early in the clerkship every student should be assessed for and encouraged to pursue personal goals. Written assignments must be perceived by students to be useful to their development as clinicians, not as busy work.

Logistical details of the didactic curriculum, such as reserving rooms and learning to run equipment, should be attended to carefully. Scheduling of classes is often difficult due to the different routines of various services and to transportation difficulties. Some programs, especially those with widely dispersed sites, give all classes during the first several days, rather than throughout the clerkship. This requires intensive faculty time and cooperation and must be a "good show" lest it bore students not yet involved with patients. Classes should not be scheduled during times when large numbers of patients are seen. Since some attending physicians will be inconvenienced by whatever schedule is chosen, they should be consulted in creating it.

Clinical Components of the Clerkship

A consensus exists regarding the characteristics of clinical experiences most valued by students. These include exposure to patients with more acute and clear psychopathology, observing improvement in patients, having well-defined roles, and experiencing considerable patient responsibility along with enthusiastic, accessible supervision (Sierles and Taylor 1995). For students who eventually selected psychiatry as their specialty, one study showed that the two most appealing clerkship features cited were the intellectual challenge of understanding patients and positive experiences talking to them (Weissman and Bashook 1986). Other factors include good residents who enjoy their work, a variety of clinical experiences, positive relationships with supervisors and fellow students, and a busy workday.

Clinical Teaching

Students should be oriented on their first day at their clinical placements about site-specific expectations for performance, including daily work schedules, unit conferences, teaching by residents, and exact duties. Junior clerks simultaneously crave and fear patient care responsibility; too little or too much direction will frustrate them. Some newer or more anxious students may do better "shadowing" a resident or attending awhile before seeing patients independently, whereas others thrive on more responsibility. Faculty and resident preceptors must identify and respond to these differences.

Both students and residents learn diagnosis and therapeutics in part by observing experienced clinicians think out loud. More details about patient-centered teaching are presented elsewhere (Weinholtz et al. 1992).

Because a student's performance during rounds or on examinations may bear little relation to his or her skills in obtaining a history, assessing psychopathology, or having professional behaviors, clinical teaching and evaluation require direct observation and feedback. As well, observing supervisors model interactions with patients is immensely helpful. Guidelines should be established for these activities, specifying, for example, the number of observed interviews and amount of individual supervision expected.

Residents as Teachers

Students receive considerable instruction from residents; because of their closeness in age and professional development, they are often more comfortable with them than with attendings. Residents are role models in their attitudes toward patients, staff, and clinical work and must be reminded of the importance of their interactions with students. Minimally, each group should be oriented to the clerkship schedule, the clinical expectations and didactic objectives, and to their roles in educating students. The director should attend residents' meetings periodically to review the role and performance of the residents in the medical student education program. Like faculty, residents vary in skill and inclination for teaching. They are often anxious about their knowledge and skills, their effectiveness as teachers, and their obligations toward students. They may be unsure how the students' role differs from theirs and may feel competitive with them. These issues are best addressed openly, empathetically, and practically. The value of teaching, both in learning to explain clearly and in stimulating further learning, should be presented to them. A useful exercise is to ask residents to recall attributes of effective and ineffective teachers they have experienced in the past. It should be stressed that students care much more about the enthusiasm with which they are taught and being a valued part of the team than they do about their resident knowing everything. Indeed, part of teaching is demonstrating how to handle ambiguous situations despite not knowing. Students' needs for clear explanations of clinical decisions, organized supervision, and an active role in patient care should be reviewed. The director, as well as the students' primary supervisors, should be available to residents with questions or problems about teaching students.

Only 13% of psychiatric residents receive formal training in teaching (Painter et al. 1987). Teaching workshops improve skills but need to be reinforced regularly (Edwards et al. 1988; Katzelnick et al. 1991). Another option is the introduction of didactic sessions in instructional methods and teaching supervision into the residency curriculum. Like faculty, residents should have their teaching evaluations reviewed periodically with the clerkship director or residency training director.

Identifying residents who are particularly good teachers is very helpful. Such residents can be assigned more students or particular students (e.g., those interested in psychiatry) while more advanced residents may assume such responsibilities as giving lectures, supervising students in enrichment experiences, remediating students with specific deficits, or helping new residents learn to teach. These residents should be recognized with teaching awards. At the other end of the spectrum are residents who neglect or abuse students or patients. Such reports by students should be investigated, and, when warranted, the clerkship director or residency director should counsel the involved resident. Cases of ethical violations should be presented to the residency director. Examples of abuses include asking a student for personal services (e.g., "pick up my dry cleaning") or for a date and making insulting comments about patient gender or ethnic group.

Clerkship Sites

Clerkship sites may include child, adolescent, geriatric, and adult inpatient units; consultation-liaison, emergency, and substance abuse services; outpatient clinics; and community mental health centers. Ideally, settings are chosen based on clerkship objectives, but external constraints are often limiting. The literature is mixed as to which rotations are preferable. There is some suggestion that consultation-liaison and outpatient sites are rated better than inpatient units, perhaps because the patients are higher functioning or students perceive greater relevance of these experiences to their future practices. However, we maintain that good results are based more on enthusiastic teaching and close attention to students' needs for supervised responsibility than on the place where it occurs. Until recently, inpatient units had the advantages of providing continuity of patient care, exposure to patients with marked psychopathology who clinically improve during their hospital stay, working with a multidisciplinary team, observation of the details of clinical decision making, and direct patient responsibility under close supervision. However, as lengths of stay decrease and third-party payers demand more care by attendings, and as medical education increasingly focuses on training future generalists, inpatient services will be less attractive as sole training sites. Ambulatory sites have the advantage of more patients with a wider variety of common clinical problems, but educators need to find ways to integrate students into these settings and ensure that effective education takes place. Clinics in which new patients are assessed, and specialty (e.g., mood disorder) clinics in which patients are already diagnosed, lend themselves well to student participation.

Therefore, if possible, several services should be involved in training each student. Assigning students to services in sequential short blocks (e.g., 2 or 3 weeks) deprives them and their supervisors of the continuity and familiarity necessary for real investment on either side. Thus, it is preferable to utilize several services concurrently, exposing students to a variety of patients and settings while affording the chance to settle in. For instance, students could be assigned primarily to an inpatient unit, do night or occasional daytime call on an emergency service, and spend several afternoons each week in outpatient settings. Continuity of care and supervision can be maximized in a "principal care" or "firm" model in which the physicians care for their patients in all settings (Greenfield 1995; Sierles et al. 1996). If possible, students should have experiences evaluating patients in consultation and child and adolescent settings and observing ECT. When multiple primary services are available, students should be given their preference through a fair system like a lottery.

Occasionally it becomes apparent, usually through student complaints, that a clerkship rotation is unsatisfactory. Most often this is due to inadequate supervision, unclear student roles, or abuse of students for their value in delivering service over their need for education. In such cases, the director must promptly and energetically advocate for the students.

Multisite Clerkships

In many medical schools, increased enrollments, decreased funding and faculty time for teaching, and a shift to ambulatory environments have required adding clerkship sites. All training sites must provide adequate teaching and supervision, learning resources, experiences that meet the clerkship's goals and objectives, and sufficient numbers and types of patients. Office and conference space, transportation, housing, and security are also factors. The director must evaluate, monitor, and coordinate diverse sites to secure comparability of experience and outcome. Factors critical to the success of geographically dispersed clerkships include frequent communication between the clerkship director and on-site coordinators, a core clerkship curriculum operationalized for each site, commitment from on-site staff and administration, faculty development and support, and continuous systematic program evaluation (Fincher 1996, pp. 95–113). The site coordinator and director should develop a teaching plan that specifies how and when objectives will be learned. Students must have clear roles and direct patient responsibilities; they must be integral members of the team.

The Didactic Curriculum in Multisite Clerkships

Another challenge is delivery of the didactic curriculum. Centrally located classes avoid duplication of effort but rely on proximity and transportation unless condensed into an initial or terminal period or given once per week. Structured case-based formats are suitable for small-group learning in diverse sites. Another possibility is videoteleconferencing of lectures and case presentations; however, this requires expensive equipment and faculty participation at all sites. Independent study modules using print, video, or CAI are also exportable. Computer-based technologies, such as electronic mail, information databases and the Internet, and case simulations, lend themselves to the communication and educational needs of students at geographically dispersed sites but are currently rarely used.

Site Evaluation

Student-compiled logs of clinical encounters can monitor achievement of certain clerkship objectives, such as experience with adequate numbers and types of patients or performance of critical procedures, and can thus help to evaluate comparability of clerkship sites. Problems associated with their use include ambiguity of requested information and purpose (some departments obtain them perfunctorily to please the dean's office), inadequate instruction, and student fatigue, leading to underreporting; in addition, converting voluminous amounts of handwritten information into usable data is time-consuming. Devices like handheld Personal Data Assistants permit easy entry of patient data, which can then be transferred to a centralized computer (Fincher 1996, p. 110). Other methods of evaluation include verbal and written student feedback, student performance on examinations, and visits by the director.

Prior to the clerkship, students should receive a description of each site. They may need reassurance that core experiences and outcomes are comparable in terms of test scores and grades.

Special Problems

Students on the psychiatry clerkship may be anxious for reasons apart from feeling that they know nothing and are being judged constantly. They are exposed, perhaps for the first time, to extreme emotions posed as unendurable or insoluble (e.g., suicidal thoughts), unpredictable behavior (e.g., assaultiveness), and intimate details of patients' lives. These may touch on difficult aspects of their own lives. At the least, students may have very little idea of how to respond. It is not unusual for their reactions to include exhaustion, depression, anxiety, sleeplessness, and overeating. Forewarning, support, supervision, and attention to students' perceptions, as well as adequate preparation in preclinical courses, will suffice for most.

Troubled and Troublesome Students

The literature suggests that students who may be particularly vulnerable during the clerkship include those with a family history of psychiatric disorder, those who have suffered abuse, and those whose own psychopathology resembles that of their patients. On the other hand, having an ill family member or having previously successfully managed personal problems may enhance empathy and motivation. Troubled students often make themselves known through repeated lateness or absence, failure to complete work, unusually intense affective responses, extreme overidentification with or rejection of patients, or inappropriate interactions with staff and supervisors. In such instances, the director should investigate promptly and take steps, which may include a conversation, a psychiatric referral, or notification of the student affairs dean.

In addition to troubled students, there are troublesome ones. Some come to the clerkship with skeptical or negative attitudes toward psychiatry; these are best handled by increasing their understanding and mastery of the field and by presenting them with good role models. Misunderstandings should be corrected, but it is best not to argue with or criticize them. Students who are disruptive or personally abusive must have limits reinforced and should be counseled and redirected toward their clerkship assignments. They are often well known to the dean's office and to evaluations committees, and their behaviors should be reported to the dean's office. Students whose interpersonal abilities are extremely poor despite adequate examination performance present a particular dilemma. Approaches to this problem may include repetition of all or part of the clerkship, remediation of specific skills, passing the issue on to the dean's office, or psychiatric evaluation if indicated. Finally, some students will ask to have their grade raised; they should be told to write a detailed memo stating their reasons, and this memo should be reviewed by the student's supervisors. Students should not be permitted to approach their former supervisors to discuss grades.

Recruitment of Students into Psychiatry

Psychiatry's "recruitment crisis" may place directors in positions of ethical compromise when there is a conflict between acting as the students' educator and adviser and acting as a recruiter. This tension may be felt when the director feels the urge to give a better grade to a student who has expressed interest in the field, or makes curriculum decisions on the basis of student popularity. Like the boundary between educator and therapist, that between educator and recruiter must be firmly maintained. And although the director will inevitably like some students better than others, open favoritism will impair his or her credibility.

Future Challenges

The future of psychiatric education is inextricably tied to the future of psychiatry and medicine as determined by social, economic, political, and scientific forces. Three changes are particularly pertinent and are already having an impact. First, moving students to ambulatory (including primary care) clerkship sites will presumably better prepare them for roles as generalists. However, ambulatory education poses a number of as yet unresolved problems (Irby 1995). These include identifying sites, defining appropriate, active student roles, providing sufficient numbers of patients, affording continuity of care, ensuring adequate supervision and patient acceptance, developing appropriate instructional methods, supporting faculty development, and obtaining funding for this labor-intensive, expensive type of training.

It is likely that medical student education will focus increasingly on interdisciplinary functioning in integrated settings. This development could illustrate to students the importance of psychiatry in medicine and enlighten faculty from other disciplines.

Second, managed care and its attendant financial stresses on academic departments has jeopardized funding and protected time for medical education. Indeed, a recent survey of the perceptions of psychiatric educators found that managed care had negatively impacted every feature of the teaching program examined, with marked effects on teacher recruitment, quality of directors' lives, and students' clerkship experiences (Brodkey et al. 1998). Students could well become the last priority of departments struggling to survive. New funding sources for medical education must be developed if old ones (e.g., Medicare) cannot be retained.

Third, the future of the clerkship may become tied to technological developments in medical education. Computerized simulations using interactive software have been shown to be effective instructional tools and may, with the availability of CD-ROM imaging, be particularly suitable for teaching interpersonal processes. CAI allows students discretion as to the time, place, and pace of instruction; this can help ensure comparable learning at diverse sites. "Adaptive testing," in which a computer determines the level of performance of a student at the beginning of the clerkship and prescribes an appropriate study program, may occur in the future (Piemme 1988). Videoconferencing, computerized records, enhanced communication, availability of curricula on the Internet, and ready access to information databases and decision supports at the point of patient care will have a profound impact.

Conclusion

Like all roles, that of clerkship director encompasses difficulties and delights. However skilled directors are at middle management, they inevitably come up short in serving all constituencies (the chair, the faculty, residents, students, the medical school). Changes in health care financing have resulted in the need to make do with increasingly inadequate time and support for teaching at the very time when profound changes in clinical education are occurring. In addition, in some institutions, extensive, skillful teaching (especially without publication) may fail to enhance prospects for promotion.

The good news is that most clerkship directors view their role as fulfilling and many want to direct the clerkship for the rest of their careers (Sierles and Magrane 1996). The educational importance of the clerkship is unquestionable. The pitfalls of the position are compensated by the satisfactions of teaching and nurturing the next generation of physicians, the challenge of continued self-education and maintaining a comprehensive perspective, and the gratification of working with colleagues.

References

Abrams HL, Dralle PW, Wallick MM: Psychiatry clerkships at U.S. medical schools. J Med Educ 62:55–57, 1987

Barrows HS, Tamblyn RM: Problem-Based Learning: An Approach to Medical Education. New York, Springer, 1980

Brodkey AC, Van Zant K, Sierles FS: Educational objectives for the junior psychiatry clerkship: development and rationale. Academic Psychiatry 21(4):179–185, 1997

Brodkey AC, Weiner CL, Sierles FS: unpublished data, 1998

Callen KE: Psychiatric education of nonpsychiatrists: is it relevant to medical practice? Psychosomatics 21(1):43–54, 1980

Carroll JG, Monroe J: Teaching clinical interviewing in the health professions: a review of empirical research. Evaluation and the Health Professions 3(1):21–45, 1980

Craig JL: Retention of interviewing skills learned by first-year medical students: a longitudinal study. Med Educ 26:276–281, 1992

Edwards JC, Kissling GE, Brannan JR, et al: Study of teaching residents how to teach. J Med Educ 63:603–610, 1988

Ende J, Pozen JT, Levinsky NG: Enhancing learning during a clinical clerkship: the value of a structured curriculum. J Gen Intern Med 1:232–237, 1986

Enelow AJ, Adler LM, Wexler M: Programmed instruction in interviewing: an experiment in medical education. JAMA 212(11):1843–1846, 1970

Fincher RME (ed): Handbook for Clerkship Directors. Washington, DC, AAMC, 1996

Goldney RD, McFarlane AC: Assessment in undergraduate psychiatric education. Med Educ 20:117–122, 1986

Greenfield D: Organizing psychiatric training around "firm models." Newsletter of the American Association of Directors of Psychiatric Research Training Fall, 1995

Holmes GR, Muster JS, Wright HH, et al: How recent medical school graduates evaluate the clinical relevancy of their behavioral science curriculum. Academic Psychiatry 14(1):17–20, 1990

Hudziak JJ, Waterman GS, Coletti G: UVM procedure book for the psychiatry clerkship, from the Association of Directors of Medical Student Education in Psychiatry Study Guide, 1995

Irby DM: Teaching and learning in ambulatory care settings: a thematic review of the literature. Acad Med 70(10):898–931, 1995

Kaltreider NB, Lu FG, Thompson TL: Student education and recruitment into psychiatry: a synergistic proposal. Academic Psychiatry 18(3):154–161, 1994

Katzelnick DJ, Gonzales JJ, Conley MC, et al: Teaching psychiatric residents to teach. Academic Psychiatry 15(3):153–159, 1991

Links PS, Foley F, Feltham R: The educational value of student encounter logs in a psychiatry clerkship. Med Teach 10(1):33–40, 1988

Newble DI, Entwistle NJ: Learning styles and approaches: implications for medical education. Med Educ 20:162–175, 1986

Nurcombe B, Fitzhenry-Coor I: Diagnostic reasoning and treatment planning: I. Diagnosis. Aust N Z J Psychiatry 21:477–483, 1987

Painter AF, Rodenhauser PR, Rudisill JR: Psychiatric residents as teachers: a national survey. Journal of Psychiatric Education 11:21–26, 1987

Piemme TE: Computer-assisted learning and evaluation in medicine. JAMA 260(3):367–372, 1988

Schon DA: Educating the Reflective Practitioner. San Francisco, CA, Jossey-Bass, 1987

Schottstaedt MF, O'Boyle M, Gardner R, et al: Long-term evaluation of a psychiatry clerkship. Academic Psychiatry 15(3):137–145, 1991

Sierles FS, Magrane D: Psychiatry clerkship directors: who they are, what they do, and what they think. Psychiatr Q 67:153–162, 1996

Sierles FS, Taylor MA: Medical student career choice of psychiatry: the U.S. decline and what to do about it. Am J Psychiatry 152:1416–1426, 1995

Sierles FS, Fichtner CG, Garfield DAS, et al: The "firm model" of patient care and postgraduate and undergraduate training in psychiatry at a Veterans Affairs Medical Center, in Proceedings of the 48th Institute of Psychiatric Services of the American Psychiatric Association, APA Institute on Psychiatric Services, Washington, DC, 1996, p 166

Tyler R: Basic Principles of Curriculum and Instruction. Chicago, IL, University of Chicago Press, 1949

Weinholtz D, Edward JC, Mumford LM: Teaching During Rounds, A Handbook for

Attending Physicians and Residents. Baltimore, MD, The Johns Hopkins University Press, 1992

Weissberg M: Less is more: the case for "basic" psychiatry and the Colorado medical student log. Psychiatr Q 67(2):139–151, 1996

Weissman SH, Bashook PG: A view of the prospective child psychiatrist. Am J Psychiatry 143:722–727, 1986

Whitman NA: There Is No Gene for Good Teaching: A Handbook on Lecturing for Medical Teachers. Salt Lake City, UT, The University of Utah School of Medicine, 1982a

Whitman NA: A Handbook for Group Discussion Leaders: Alternatives to Lecturing Medical Students to Death. Salt Lake City, UT, The University of Utah School of Medicine, 1982b

Wilkerson L, Feletti G: Problem-based learning: one approach to increasing student participation, in The Department Chairperson's Role in Enhancing College Teaching. New Directions for Teaching and Learning, No 37. Edited by Lucas A. San Francisco, CA, Jossey-Bass, 1989

Objectives for the
Junior Psychiatry Clerkship

**Members of the Association of Directors of Medical Student
Education in Psychiatry's Clerkship Objectives Committee:**
Amy C. Brodkey, M.D., Chairperson
Irwin Hassenfeld, M.D., Myrl R. S. Manley, M.D.,
Deborah C. Roth, D.O., Kristin Van Zant, M.D.,
Michael Weissberg, M.D., Frederick S. Sierles, M.D. ex officio

I. PSYCHIATRIC HISTORY, PHYSICAL, AND THE MENTAL STATUS EXAMINATION

Overall Goal

By the end of the clerkship, the student will demonstrate the ability to obtain a complete psychiatric history, recognize relevant physical findings, and perform a complete mental status examination.

Specific Objectives

The student will be able to

1. elicit and clearly record a complete psychiatric history including the identifying data, chief complaint, history of the present illness, past psychiatric history, medications (psychiatric and nonpsychiatric), general medical history, review of systems, substance abuse history, family history, and personal and social history;
2. recognize the importance of, and be able to obtain and evaluate, historical data from multiple sources (family members, community mental health resources, old records, etc.);
3. discuss the effect of developmental issues on the assessment of patients;
4. elicit, describe, and precisely record the components of the mental status examination including: general appearance and behavior, motor activity, speech, affect, mood, thought processes, thought content, perception, sensorium and cognition (e.g., state of consciousness, orientation, registration, recent and remote memory, calculations, capacity to read and write, abstraction), judgment, and insight;
5. use appropriate terms associated with the mental status examination;

6. for each category of the mental status exam, list common abnormalities and their common causes;
7. make a clear and concise case presentation;
8. assess and record mental status changes, and alter hypotheses and management in response to these changes;
9. recognize physical signs and symptoms that accompany classic psychiatric disorders (e.g., tachycardia and hyperventilation in panic disorder);
10. appreciate the implications of the high rates of general medical illness in psychiatric patients, and state reasons why it is important to diagnose and treat these illnesses;
11. assess for the presence of general medical illness in psychiatric patients, and determine the extent to which a general medical illness contributes to a patient's psychiatric problem; and
12. recognize and identify the effects of psychotropic medication in the physical examination.

II. DIAGNOSIS, CLASSIFICATION, AND TREATMENT PLANNING

Overall Goal

By the end of the clerkship, the student will be able to identify psychopathology, formulate accurate differential and working diagnoses, and develop appropriate assessment and treatment plans for psychiatric patients.

Specific Objectives

Using his or her knowledge of psychopathology, diagnostic criteria, and epidemiology, the student will

1. discuss the advantages and limitations of using a diagnostic system like the DSM-IV;
2. use the DSM-IV in identifying specific signs and symptoms that comprise a syndrome or disorder;
3. use the five axes of the DSM-IV in evaluating patients;
4. state the typical signs and symptoms of the common psychiatric disorders, such as major depression, anxiety disorders, bipolar disorder, dementia, delirium, schizophrenia, personality disorders, and substance use disorders;
5. formulate a differential diagnosis for major presenting problems;
6. formulate a plan for evaluation;
7. assess changes in clinical status, and alter hypotheses and management in response to changes;
8. develop an individualized treatment plan for each patient; and
9. discuss the prevalence and barriers to recognition of psychiatric illnesses in general medical settings, including variations in presentation.

III. INTERVIEWING SKILLS

Overall Goal

By the end of the clerkship, the student will conduct an interview in a manner that facilitates information-gathering and formation of a therapeutic alliance.

Specific Objectives

The student will

1. explain the value of skillful interviewing for patient and doctor satisfaction and for obtaining optimal clinical outcomes;
2. demonstrate respect, empathy, responsiveness, and concern regardless of the patient's problems or personal characteristics;
3. identify his or her emotional responses to patients;
4. identify strengths and weaknesses in his or her interviewing skills;
5. discuss the preceding perceptions (objectives 3 and 4) with a colleague or supervisor to improve interviewing skill;
6. identify verbal and nonverbal expressions of affect in a patient's responses and apply this information in assessing and treating the patient;
7. state and use basic strategies for interviewing disorganized, cognitively impaired, hostile/resistant, mistrustful, circumstantial/hyperverbal, unspontaneous/hypoverbal, and potentially assaultive patients;
8. demonstrate the following interviewing skills: appropriate initiation of the interview; establishing rapport; the appropriate use of open-ended and closed questions; techniques for asking "difficult" questions; the appropriate use of facilitation, empathy, clarification, confrontation, reassurance, silence, summary statements; soliciting and acknowledging expression of the patient's ideas, concerns, questions, and feelings about the illness and its treatment; communicating information to patients in a clear fashion; appropriate closure of the interview;
9. state and avoid the following common mistakes in interviewing technique: interrupting the patient unnecessarily; asking long, complex questions; using jargon; asking questions in a manner suggesting the desired answer; asking questions in an interrogatory manner; ignoring patient verbal or nonverbal cues; making sudden inappropriate changes in topic; indicating patronizing or judgmental attitudes by verbal or nonverbal cues (e.g., calling an adult patient by his or her first name, questioning in an oversimplified manner, etc.); incomplete questioning about important topics; and
10. demonstrate sensitivity to student–patient similarities and differences in gender, ethnic background, sexual orientation, socioeconomic status, education, political views, and personality traits.

IV. DIAGNOSTIC TESTING

Overall Goal

By the end of the clerkship, the student will use laboratory testing, imaging tests, psychological tests, and consultation to assist in the diagnosis of persons with neuropsychiatric symptoms.

Specific Objectives

The student will

1. state the indications for, and limitations of, the tests that are used to evaluate the neurophysiologic functioning of persons with neuropsychiatric symptoms (e.g., TFT, EEG, RPR, DST, toxicologies, HIV testing);
2. discuss the use of, and indications for, neuroimaging in psychiatry;
3. summarize the similarities and differences between neuropsychological and other psychological testing, and state indications for each;
4. list the psychiatric medications that require blood level monitoring, and discuss the indications for blood level monitoring for these medications; and
5. state the EEG correlates of neuropsychiatric disorders.

V. PSYCHIATRIC EMERGENCIES

Overall Goal

By the end of the clerkship, the student will assess and begin emergency management and referral of a person with neuropsychiatric symptoms.

Specific Objectives

The student will

1. identify the clinical and demographic factors associated with a statistically increased risk of suicide in general and clinical populations;
2. develop a differential diagnosis, conduct a clinical assessment, and recommend management for a patient exhibiting suicidal thoughts or behavior;
3. recognize the clinical findings that might suggest a general medical cause for neuropsychiatric symptoms such as hallucinations, delusions, confusion, altered consciousness, and violent behavior;
4. discuss the clinical features, differential diagnosis, and evaluation of delirium, including emergent conditions;
5. recognize the typical signs and symptoms of common psychopharmacologic emergencies (e.g., lithium toxicity, neuroleptic malignant syndrome, anticholinergic delirium, MAOI-related hypertensive crisis), and discuss treatment strategies;
6. recognize signs and symptoms of potential assaultiveness;
7. develop a differential diagnosis, conduct a clinical assessment, and state

the principles of management of a person with potential or active violent behavior;

8. discuss classes, indications, and associated risks of medications used for management of acutely psychotic, agitated, and combative patients;

9. discuss the nonpharmacologic components of management of acute psychosis, agitation, and combativeness;

10. identify the indications, precautions, and proper use of restraints;

11. state the prevalence, morbidity, mortality, and risk factors associated with adult domestic violence in clinical and nonclinical populations;

12. discuss the physician's role in screening, diagnosing, managing, documenting, reporting, and referring victims of child abuse, adult domestic violence, and elder abuse;

13. list the psychiatric problems that are frequently seen in battered women and child abuse victims;

14. outline the emergency management of a rape victim;

15. discuss the indications for psychiatric hospitalization, including the presenting problem and its acuity, risk of danger to patient or others, community resources, and family support;

16. identify the problems associated with the use of the terms "medical clearance" and "psychiatric clearance";

17. discuss the clinical and administrative aspects of the transfer of a patient to another facility; and

18. summarize the process of admission to a psychiatric hospital; specifically
    a. the implications of voluntary versus involuntary commitment status;
    b. the principles of civil commitment; and
    c. the process of obtaining a voluntary or involuntary commitment, and the role of the physician in obtaining it.

VI. DELIRIUM, DEMENTIA, AND AMNESTIC AND OTHER COGNITIVE DISORDERS

Overall Goal

By the end of the clerkship, the student will recognize the psychiatric manifestations of brain disease of known etiology or pathophysiology and will state the evaluation and initial management of these neuropsychiatric disorders.

Specific Objectives

The student will

1. recognize the cognitive, psychological, and behavioral manifestations of brain disease of known etiology, anatomy, or pathophysiology;

2. compare, contrast, and give examples of the following: delirium, dementia (including treatable dementia), dementia syndrome of depression (pseudodementia), cortical dementia, and subcortical dementia;

3. discuss the clinical features, differential diagnosis and evaluation of delirium, including emergent conditions;
4. state the prevalence of delirium in hospitalized elderly patients;
5. discuss the behavioral and pharmacologic treatments of delirious patients;
6. discuss the epidemiology, differential diagnosis, clinical features, and course of Alzheimer's disease, vascular dementia, substance-induced persisting dementia, Parkinson's disease, and HIV encephalopathy;
7. list the treatable causes of dementia and summarize their clinical manifestations;
8. summarize the medical evaluation and clinical management of a patient with dementia;
9. discuss the diagnosis, differential diagnosis, and treatment of amnestic disorder due to general medical conditions (e.g., head trauma) and substance-induced conditions (e.g., Korsakoff's syndrome due to thiamine deficiency);
10. employ a cognitive screening evaluation to assess and follow patients with cognitive impairment, and state the limitations of these instruments;
11. state the neuropsychiatric manifestations of HIV-related illnesses; and
12. state the neuropsychiatric manifestations of seizure disorders, strokes, and head injuries.

VII. SUBSTANCE-RELATED DISORDERS

Overall Goal

By the end of the clerkship, the student will identify, clinically evaluate, and treat the neuropsychiatric consequences of substance abuse and dependence.

Specific Objectives

The student will

1. obtain a thorough history of a patient's substance use through empathic, nonjudgmental, and systematic interviewing;
2. list and compare the characteristic clinical features (including denial) of substance abuse and dependence;
3. discuss the epidemiology (including the effects of gender), clinical features, patterns of usage, course of illness, and treatment of substance use disorders (including anabolic steroids);
4. identify typical presentations of substance abuse in general medical practice;
5. list the psychiatric disorders that share significant comorbidity with substance-related disorders, and discuss some criteria for determining whether the comorbid disorder should be treated independently;
6. discuss the role of the family, support groups, and rehabilitation programs in the recovry of patients with substance use disorders;
7. list the questions that comprise the CAGE questionnaire and discuss its use as a screening instrument;

8. discuss the genetic, neurobiological, and psychosocial explanations of the etiology of alcoholism;
9. list the psychiatric and psychosocial complications of alcoholism;
10. know the clinical features of intoxication with, and withdrawal from cocaine, amphetamines, hallucinogens, cannabis, phencyclidine, barbiturates, opiates, caffeine, nicotine, benzodiazepines, and alcohol;
11. state the treatments of intoxication and withdrawal induced by the substances listed above;
12. list patient characteristics associated with benzodiazepine abuse;
13. state guidelines for prescribing benzodiazepines; and
14. discuss the difficulties experienced by health care personnel in providing empathic, nonjudgmental care to substance abusers.

VIII. SCHIZOPHRENIA AND OTHER PSYCHOTIC DISORDERS

Overall Goal

By the end of the clerkship, the student will demonstrate proficiency in the recognition, evaluation, and management of persons with psychosis associated with schizophrenic, affective, general medical, and other psychotic disorders.

Specific Objectives

The student will

1. define the term psychosis;
2. develop a differential diagnosis for a person presenting with psychosis, including identifying historical and clinical features which assist in the differentiation of general medical, substance-induced, affective, schizophrenic and other causes;
3. state the neurobiologic, genetic, and environmental theories of etiology and pathophysiology of schizophrenia;
4. summarize the epidemiology, clinical features, course, and complications of schizophrenia;
5. name the clinical features of schizophrenia that are associated with good and poor outcome, and explain the significance of negative symptoms;
6. summarize the treatment of schizophrenia, including both pharmacologic and psychosocial interventions; and
7. list the features that differentiate delusional disorder, schizophreniform disorder, schizoaffective disorder, and brief psychotic disorder from each other and from schizophrenia.

IX. MOOD DISORDERS

Overall Goal

By the end of the clerkship, the student will recognize, evaluate, and state the treatments for patients with mood disorders.

Specific Objectives
The student will

1. discuss evidence for neurobiological, genetic, psychological, and environmental etiologies of mood disorders;
2. state the epidemiologic features, prevalence rates, and lifetime risks of mood disorders in clinical and nonclinical populations;
3. compare and contrast the epidemiologic and clinical features of unipolar depression and bipolar disorders;
4. state the common signs and symptoms, differential diagnosis (including general medical and substance-induced disorders), course of illness, comorbidity, prognosis, and complications of mood disorders;
5. contrast normal mood variations, states of demoralization, and bereavement with the pathological mood changes that constitute depressive illness;
6. identify the difference in the presentation, treatment, and prognosis of major depression with and without melancholic features, psychotic features, atypical features, catatonic features, seasonal pattern and postpartum onset;
7. compare and contrast the clinical presentations of mood disorders in children, adults and the elderly;
8. describe some common presentations of depressive disorders in nonpsychiatric settings, define the term "masked depression," and develop an approach to evaluating and treating mood disorders in a general medical practice;
9. discuss the increased prevalence of major depression in patients with general medical/surgical illness (e.g., myocardial infarction, diabetes, CVAs, hip fractures) and the impact of depression on morbidity and mortality from their illnesses;
10. discuss the identification and management of suicide risk in general medical settings;
11. outline the recommended acute and maintenance treatments for dysthymia, major depression, and bipolar disorders (manic and depressive phases); and
12. state the characteristics and techniques of the nonpharmacological treatments for depression, including psychotherapy, cognitive therapy, couple's therapy and phototherapy.

X. ANXIETY DISORDERS

Overall Goal

By the end of the clerkship, the student will recognize, evaluate, and state the treatments for patients with anxiety disorders.

Specific Objectives
The student will

1. summarize neurobiological, psychological, environmental, and genetic etiologic hypotheses for the anxiety disorders;
2. discuss the epidemiology, clinical features, course, and psychiatric comorbidity of panic disorder, agoraphobia, social phobia, specific phobias, generalized anxiety disorder, posttraumatic stress disorder, acute stress disorder, and obsessive compulsive disorder;
3. distinguish panic attack from panic disorder;
4. list the common general medical and substance-induced causes of anxiety, and assess for these causes in evaluating a person with an anxiety disorder;
5. outline psychotherapeutic and pharmacologic treatments for each of the anxiety disorders;
6. compare and contrast clinical presentations of anxiety disorders in children and adults; and
7. discuss the role of anxiety and anxiety disorders in the presentation of general medical symptoms, the decision to visit a physician, and health care expenditures.

XI. SOMATOFORM AND FACTITIOUS DISORDERS

Overall Goal
By the end of the clerkship, the student will diagnose and discuss the principles of management of patients with somatoform disorders.

Specific Objectives
The student will

1. state the clinical characteristics of somatization disorder, conversion disorder, pain disorder, body dysmorphic disorder, and hypochondriasis;
2. list the psychiatric disorders that have high comorbidity with somatoform disorders;
3. discuss the implications of the high rate of underlying general medical/ neurologic illness in patients diagnosed with pain disorder and conversion disorder;
4. list the characteristic features of factitious disorder and malingering, and compare these with the somatoform disorders;
5. discuss the frequency and importance of physical symptoms as manifestations of psychological distress;
6. summarize the principles of management of patients with somatoform disorders; and
7. discuss difficulties physicians may have with patients with these diagnoses.

XII. DISSOCIATIVE AND AMNESTIC DISORDERS

Overall Goal

By the end of the clerkship, the student will define dissociation, state its psychological defensive role, and discuss the clinical syndromes with which it is associated.

Specific Objectives

The student will

1. list a differential diagnosis of psychiatric, substance-induced and general medical conditions that may present with amnesia, and discuss the evaluation and treatment of persons with amnesia;
2. state the clinical features of dissociative amnesia, dissociative fugue, depersonalization disorder, and dissociative identity disorder;
3. discuss the hypothesized role of psychological trauma, including sexual, physical and emotional abuse, in the development of dissociative disorders (and posttraumatic stress disorders);
4. discuss the etiologic hypotheses, epidemiology, clinical features, course, and treatment of dissociative identity disorder; and
5. state the indications for an amobarbital interview and for hypnosis.

XIII. EATING DISORDERS

Overall Goal

By the end of the clerkship, the student will summarize the distinguishing clinical features, evaluation, and treatment of patients with eating disorders.

Specific Objectives

The student will

1. summarize the etiologic hypotheses, clinical features, epidemiology, course, comorbid disorders, complications, and treatment for anorexia nervosa;
2. summarize the etiologic hypotheses, clinical features, epidemiology, course, comorbid disorders, complications, and treatment for bulimia;
3. discuss the role of the primary care physician in the prevention and early identification of eating disorders; and
4. list the medical complications and indications for hospitalization in patients with eating disorders.

XIV. SEXUAL DYSFUNCTIONS AND PARAPHILIAS

Overall Goal

By the end of the clerkship, the student will summarize the process of evaluation and treatment of persons with sexual dysfunctions or paraphilias.

Specific Objectives
The student will

1. discuss the anatomy and physiology of the male and female sexual response cycles;
2. obtain a patient's sexual history, including an assessment of risk for sexually transmitted diseases, especially HIV;
3. state the implications of the high prevalence of sexual dysfunctions in the general population, and particularly in the medically ill;
4. list the common causes of sexual dysfunctions, including general medical and substance-related etiologies;
5. summarize the manifestations, differential diagnosis, and treatment of hypoactive sexual desire disorder and sexual aversion disorder; male erectile disorder and female sexual arousal disorder; female and male orgasmic disorders and premature ejaculation; and dyspareunia and vaginismus;
6. define the term paraphilia;
7. list and define each of the common paraphilias;
8. review the management of the paraphilias; and
9. discuss the prevalence, manifestations, diagnosis, and treatment of gender identity disorder.

XV. SLEEP DISORDERS

Overall Goal
By the end of the clerkship, the student will evaluate, and refer or treat, persons with sleep problems.

Specific Objectives
The student will

1. describe normal sleep physiology, including sleep architecture, throughout the life cycle;
2. obtain a complete sleep history;
3. discuss the manifestations, differential diagnosis, evaluation, and treatment of primary sleep disorders, including dyssomnias and parasomnias;
4. describe typical sleep disturbances that accompany psychiatric and substance use disorders;
5. summarize the effect(s) of psychotropic medications on sleep; and
6. describe sleep hygiene treatment.

XVI. PERSONALITY DISORDERS

Overall Goal
By the end of the clerkship, the student will recognize maladaptive traits and interpersonal patterns that typify personality disorders, and discuss strategies

for caring for patients with personality disorders.

Specific Objectives
The student will

1. explain how the DSM IV defines personality traits and disorders, and identify features common to all personality disorders;
2. list the three descriptive groupings (clusters) of personality disorders in the DSM IV, and describe the typical traits of each personality disorder;
3. summarize the neurobiological, genetic, developmental, behavioral, and sociological theories of the etiology of personality disorders, including the association of childhood abuse and trauma;
4. discuss the biogenetic relationships that exist between certain Axis I and Axis II disorders (e.g., schizotypal personality disorder and schizophrenia);
5. discuss the epidemiology, differential diagnosis, course of illness, prognosis, and comorbid psychiatric disorders in patients with personality disorders;
6. list the general medical and Axis I psychiatric disorders that may present with personality changes;
7. identify difficulties in diagnosing personality disorders in the presence of stress, substance abuse, and other Axis I disorders;
8. discuss the concepts of hierarchical levels of defense and regression under stress, and list typical defense mechanisms used in various personality disorders;
9. list the psychotherapeutic and pharmacologic treatment strategies for patients with personality disorders;
10. discuss the management of patients with personality disorders in the general medical setting; and
11. summarize principles of management of patients with personality disorders, including being aware of one's own response to the patient, soliciting consultations from colleagues when indicated, and using both support and nonpunitive limit setting.

XVII. CHILD AND ADOLESCENT PSYCHIATRY

Overall Goal
By the end of the clerkship, the student will summarize the unique factors essential to the evaluation of children and adolescents and will diagnose the common child psychiatric disorders.

Specific Objectives
The student will

1. compare and contrast the process of psychiatric evaluation of children and adolescents at different developmental stages with that of adults;

2. state the value of obtaining data from families, teachers, and other non-physicians in the evaluation and treatment of children and adolescents;
3. state the indications for psychological assessment in children and list some of the common tests in a psychometric evaluation;
4. list a differential diagnosis and outline the evaluation of academic performance and behavioral problems in children;
5. summarize the etiologic hypotheses, clinical features, epidemiology, pathophysiology, course, comorbid disorders, complications, and treatment for attention deficit hyperactivity disorder and conduct disorder;
6. discuss the etiologies, epidemiology, clinical features, and psychiatric comorbidity of mental retardation;
7. name the major clinical features of autism;
8. differentiate developmentally based anxiety (e.g., stranger, separation anxiety) from pathological anxiety disorders in childhood;
9. describe typical clinical features of anxiety disorders at different developmental stages;
10. compare and contrast the clinical features of mood disorders in children with those of adults;
11. discuss the epidemiology and clinical features of suicide risk in adolescents;
12. state when and how a physician must protect the safety of a child who may be the victim of physical or sexual abuse or neglect; and
13. identify signs and symptoms of child sexual and physical abuse, and discuss its short and long-term psychiatric sequelae.

XVIII. GERIATRIC PSYCHIATRY

Overall Goal

By the end of the clerkship, the student will evaluate and begin neuropsychiatric management of elderly patients

Specific Objectives

The student will

1. employ a cognitive screening evaluation to assess and follow patients with cognitive impairment, and state the limitations of these instruments;
2. compare and contrast the clinical presentation of depression in elderly patients with that of younger adults;
3. summarize the special considerations in prescribing psychotropic medications in the elderly;
4. appreciate that multiple medications can cause cognitive, behavioral, and affective problems in the elderly;
5. compare, contrast, and give examples of the following: delirium, dementia

(including treatable dementia), dementia syndrome of depression (pseudo-dementia), subcortical and cortical dementia;

6. state the prevalence of delirium in hospitalized elderly patients;
7. discuss the differential diagnosis, etiological hypotheses, epidemiology, clinical features, and course of Alzheimer's disease, vascular dementia, and Parkinson's disease;
8. summarize the assessment and treatment of a patient with dementia;
9. discuss the physician's role in diagnosing, managing, and reporting elderly victims of physical or sexual abuse; and
10. discuss the role of losses in the etiology of psychiatric disorders in the elderly.

XIX. COMMUNITY AND FORENSIC PSYCHIATRY

Overall Goal

By the end of the clerkship the student will discuss the structure of the mental health system, as well as legal issues important in the care of psychiatric patients.

Specific Objectives

The student will

1. define the term catchment area;
2. list the psychiatric services each community mental health center must provide;
3. define deinstitutionalization, and discuss its effects on patients and on the community;
4. discuss the process of admission to a psychiatric hospital; specifically
    a. the implications of voluntary versus involuntary commitment status;
    b. the principles of civil commitment; and
    c. the process for obtaining a voluntary or involuntary commitment, and the physician's role in obtaining it;
5. summarize the elements of informed consent, determination of capacities (e.g., to consent to treatment, to manage funds), and the role of judicial or administrative orders for treatment;
6. discuss the duty to warn;
7. define the right to treatment and right to refuse treatment;
8. discuss when and how a physician must protect the safety of a child or an elderly person who may be the victim of physical or sexual abuse or neglect;
9. discuss the economic impact of chronic mental illness on patients and their families, including the effect of discriminatory insurance coverage; and
10. discuss the financial and psychosocial burden of chronic mental illness to family members.

XX. PSYCHOPHARMACOLOGY

Overall Goal

By the end of the clerkship, the student will summarize the indications, basic mechanisms of action, common side effects and drug interactions of each class of psychotropic medications, and demonstrate the ability to select and use these agents to treat mental disorders.

Specific Objectives

Anxiolytics—The student will discuss

1. the indications, mechanism of action, pharmacokinetics, common side effects, signs of toxicity, and drug interactions of the different benzodiazepines and sedative-hypnotics;
2. the consequences of abrupt discontinuation;
3. patient characteristics associated with benzodiazepine abuse;
4. guidelines for prescribing benzodiazepines; and
5. the differences (mechanism of action, onset of effect, and indications) between buspirone and benzodiazepines.

Antidepressants—The student will summarize

1. the indications, mechanisms of action, pharmacokinetics, common or serious side effects (including overdose potential), signs of toxicity, and drug interactions of tricyclics, second generation (atypical) antidepressants, monoamine oxidase inhibitors, and serotonin reuptake inhibitors;
2. the pretreatment assessment and strategies of antidepressant use, including ensuring adequacy of trial and blood level monitoring;
3. the effect of antidepressants on the cardiac conduction system and EKG;
4. dietary and pharmacologic restrictions in prescribing an MAOI; and
5. advantages of serotonin reuptake inhibitors.

Antipsychotics (neuroleptics)—The student will discuss

1. the indications, mechanisms of action, pharmacokinetics, common or serious side effects, signs of toxicity, and drug interactions of antipsychotics;
2. differences between high-potency and low-potency antipsychotics, including the side effects common to each group;
3. diagnosis and management of extrapyramidal side effects including acute dystonia, parkinsonism, akathisia, tardive dyskinesia, and neuroleptic malignant syndrome; and
4. the indications and special considerations in using clozapine and resperidone.

Mood Stabilizers—The student will discuss

1. the indications, mechanism of action, pharmacokinetics, side effects, signs of toxicity (neurological, gastrointestinal, renal, endocrine, cardiac), and drug interactions of lithium;

2. the pretreatment assessment and strategies of use of lithium, including blood level monitoring; and
3. the indications, mechanisms of action, pharmacokinetics, common and serious side effects, toxicity, drug interactions, and plasma level monitoring for carbamazepine, valproic acid, and calcium channel blockers.

Anticholinergics—The student will discuss
1. the indications, mechanisms of action, pharmacokinetics, common and serious side effects, signs of toxicity, and drug interactions of antiparkinsonian agents;
2. which antidepressants and antipsychotics have a higher incidence of anticholinergic side effects;
3. special considerations in prescribing these medications in the elderly; and
4. the high prevalence of anticholinergics in over-the-counter medications.

Electroconvulsive therapy (ECT)—The student will summarize
1. indications, physiologic effects, and side effects of ECT;
2. clinical situations in which ECT may be the treatment of choice;
3. pretreatment assessment, including conditions requiring special precautions; and
4. the medical care of the patient before, during, and after ECT treatment.

Other topics—The student will discuss
1. the use of beta blockers in psychiatry; and
2. the indications for and side effects of stimulants.

XXI. PSYCHOTHERAPIES

Overall Goal
By the end of the clerkship, the student will understand the principles and techniques of the psychosocial therapies sufficient to explain to a patient and make a referral when indicated.

Specific Objectives
The student will

1. state the characteristics and techniques of, and common indications and contraindictions for psychodynamic psychotherapy, psychoanalysis, supportive psychotherapy, cognitive and behavioral therapies, group therapies, couples and family therapy, and psychoeducational interventions;
2. describe behavioral medicine interventions (e.g., relaxation training, assertiveness training, contingency management, stimulus control, relapse prevention, biofeedback), and know for which medical problems they are effective (e.g., smoking cessation) and ineffective;

3. define and begin to recognize transference, countertransference, and commonly used defense mechanisms; discuss the concepts of hierarchical levels of defense and regression under stress; and list some typical defense mechanisms used in various personality disorders;
4. state the major findings of studies of the efficacy of psychosocial interventions in the treatment of psychiatric and general medical disorders and in reducing health care costs; and
5. discuss techniques for increasing the likelihood of successful referral for psychotherapy.

XXII. COLLABORATION

Overall Goal

By the end of the clerkship, the student will work effectively with other health professionals.

Specific Objectives
The student will

1. participate as a member of a multidisciplinary patient care team;
2. summarize the special skills of a psychiatric nurse, psychologist, psychiatric social worker, and physician assistant;
3. demonstrate respect for, and appreciation of, the contributions of others participating in patient care;
4. participate in a family meeting with other members of the treatment team;
5. participate in discharge planning and referral of a patient to an ambulatory setting or to another inpatient facility;
6. request a consultation, in writing or by phone, from a practitioner of another specialty; and
7. work collaboratively in the care of a patient with nonpsychiatric physicians and health care teams from other specialties.

XXIII. ATTITUDES, PERSPECTIVES, AND PERSONAL DEVELOPMENT

Overall Goal

By the end of the clerkship, the student will demonstrate maturation in clinical and personal development.

Specific Objectives
The student will

1. summarize his or her strengths and weaknesses in interviewing skills, assessment, and management of persons with psychiatric disorders;
2. solicit, utilize, and provide constructive criticism;
3. demonstrate respect and empathy for patients, colleagues, and supervisors;

4. request consultation and supervision when knowledge, attitudes, or skills are insufficient for a given patient's care;
5. accept that some patients and colleagues are not cooperative and likable, and that some patients and colleagues will not like the student;
6. perform clinical tasks (including soliciting assistance) under the pressure of difficult situations;
7. demonstrate comfort, concern, and responsibility in the care of psychiatrically ill persons;
8. obtain information from the psychiatric and general medical literature;
9. refute myths about psychiatric illness, psychiatric patients, psychiatric treatments, and mental health practitioners;
10. comment on the value of prompt and enthusiastic response to requests for consultation; and
11. discuss a patient incorporating multiple perspectives (i.e., biological, psychological, developmental, and social).

Appendix: Sample psychiatric screens

Introduction

Attitudes toward psychiatry and psychiatric patients are often enhanced when students develop competence in interviewing patients about sensitive issues. The following psychiatric "screens" are useful in general medical practice. The psychiatry clerkship would be an appropriate time for students to learn these (or other) sets of questions. Some screens may be more appropriate in different clinical sites such as psychiatric emergency departments, consultation services or outpatient departments. However, the sites where they are practiced are less important than the fact that students achieve familiarity and comfort with using them.

THE PSYCHIATRIC WORKUP

Seven questions should be asked about any psychiatric patient:

1. Why is the patient here *now*?
2. What does the patient want/expect?
3. Is a general medical illness contributing to the patient's difficulties?
4. How lethal is the situation?
5. In what ways are the patient's relationships helping or exacerbating the problem?
6. What are the patient's cultural expectations/explanations/treatments for their illness?
7. What is the psychiatric diagnosis?

Sample Psychiatric Screens

1. *Mini-Mental State Examination:* **Note—This is a test of cognitive functioning, *not* a complete Mental Status Examination.**

Folstein MF, Folstein SE & McHugh PR: Mini-mental state: A practical method for grading the cognitive state of patients for the clinician, *J Psychiatr Res* 12: 189–198, 1975.

2. *Alcohol and Drug Abuse Screen*

Have you ever had a drinking or drug problem? (Yes: 70% of alcoholics, 1% of nonalcoholics; JAMA 259:51, 1988.)

Has anyone else ever worried that you had a drinking or drug problem?

Did you ever use sleeping pills, weight loss medications, or painkillers?

CAGE questions (JAMA 252:1905, 1984).

(A positive answer on two or more will identify the majority of people with alcohol abuse or dependence)

When is the last time you used any tobacco?

How much are you using now (were you using then)?

Have you used any other forms of tobacco (chew, cigarettes, cigars, pipes)?

3. *Sexual Screen*

A. General Screen

Are you sexually active at the present time?
If NO, have you ever been?

Are (were) your partners men, women, or both?
If BOTH, which do you prefer?

What means of birth control do you (have you) use(d)?
Ask both males and females

Do you have any concerns or problems with your sexual life?

Have there been any changes in your sexual activity?
Changes in level and frequency of interest?
Changes in type of interest?
Do you or have you ever engaged in anal intercourse?

Are there any ways in which you would like your sexual life to be different?

Have any bad or frightening things ever happened to you sexually? For example: rape, sexual abuse, or molestation? (See Abuse Screen)

Have you had any sexually transmitted diseases such as herpes, chlamydia, gonorrhea, syphilis, or AIDS? (See HIV Screen)

Have you ever been treated for a sexually transmitted disease?

B. HIV Risk Factors

Do you worry about getting AIDS? Why? or Why not?

Do you practice safe sex? (Explain)

Have you ever injected (or shot up) drugs into your veins?

(If male) Have you ever had sexual contact with another man or with someone who used IV drugs?

(If female) Have you ever had sexual contact with someone who was bisexual or someone who used IV drugs?

How many sexual partners have you had in the last 10 years?

Have you ever needed a blood transfusion? What year?
(1979–1985 is risk period)

4. *Suicide and Violence Screen*

Have you ever had thoughts that life is not worth living?

Have you ever had thoughts of killing yourself? (Now?)

How would you do it?

Have you taken steps to carry out your plan? (collected weapons, pills, etc.)

Patients who are suicidal may also be homicidal and vice versa, so ask:

Have you ever had thoughts of hurting anyone else? (Now?)

Have you ever hurt anyone else?

What plans do you now have to hurt anyone?

5. *Screens for Family Violence*

   A. **Child Abuse** (Modify for male perpetrators)

      How did you feel during your pregnancy?

      Has your child lived up to your expectations?

      At what age do you think children know right from wrong?
      (Abusers often have unrealistically high expectations of children)

      How do you feel when your child behaves badly? What do you do?

      Is there anyone you can turn to for help?

      Have you ever been concerned that anyone would hurt your child?

      Have you been frightened with thoughts of hurting your child?

      Have you or anyone else hurt your child?

   B. **Sexual Abuse Victims**

      Are there things going on in your home that you are uncomfortable with or ashamed to talk about?

      Has there been any sexual contact between family members in your home besides your parents?

      Have you been involved sexually with any adult, including either of your parents?

   C. **Partner/Elder Abuse Victims**

      I know that you may be ashamed of what happened (or might have happened), but could it be that this injury did not happen by accident?

Is your family under a lot of stress?

What happens when you and your partner argue?

Do either of you have trouble with your temper?

Have you ever fought physically with your partner? How badly have you been hurt?

Is there a weapon in the house?

Are you afraid to go home?

D. Abuse History

Did you ever witness any violence in your home when you were growing up?

How were you disciplined as a child?

Were you ever physically hurt by a family member?

During your childhood or adolescence:

Did a relative, family friend or stranger ever touch your body, or have you touch them, in a sexual way?

Did anyone attempt or succeed in having sexual intercourse with you?

Did you ever have an unwanted sexual experience of any kind?

6. *Trauma Screen*

Have you ever had anything happen to you where you thought you would be seriously injured or might die?

Have you ever been in a life-threatening accident? Fire? Disaster?

Have you ever been attacked or raped?

Have you ever seen these things happen to someone else?

7. *Screen for Sleep Disorders*

Are you content with your sleep pattern?

Are you excessively tired during the day?

Does your bed partner complain about your sleep pattern?

8. *Screen for Depression/Hypomania*

How would you describe your mood?

A. In the past month, have you felt down, depressed, or hopeless most of the day nearly every day?

If yes: Describe what that is like for you.

Do you feel that way now?

How long have you felt depressed?

If no: When did you last feel down, depressed, or hopeless?

How long did you feel depressed?

B. Have you lost interest or pleasure in doing things you used to enjoy?

If yes: What do you usually enjoy doing?

When was the last time you did one or more of those things? Was it enjoyable?

How long have you had difficulty getting interested in or enjoying activities?

If no: What do you enjoy doing?

When was the last time you did one or more of those things?

If A or B is positive:

Sleep, increase or decrease

Interest (previously determined)

Guilt, hopelessness, helplessness

Energy, decreased

Concentration, decreased

Appetite, increased or decreased

Psychomotor, retardation or agitation

Suicidality, active vs. passive

C. **Hypomania Screen**

Have you had periods of needing very little sleep and not feeling tired?

Has anyone ever worried that you were excessively happy or so energetic that you were not your normal self?

Have your thoughts ever raced and you could not control them?

Have you ever had periods of greatly increased energy when you felt you could accomplish almost anything?

Have you had periods of thrill seeking when you took physical risks, such as speeding or doing other dangerous things?

9. *Screen for Anxiety Disorders*

Do you feel nervous or tense?

Have you ever felt extremely frightened, physically uncomfortable, or worried that something terrible was going to happen?

If yes: Tell me about that.

Did you expect to feel that way?

Are there situations or activities that cause you a lot of anxiety or that you are more afraid of than most people would be?

If yes: What happens when you _____?

Do you avoid that/those situations/activities?

Do you worry a lot or have trouble getting things off your mind?

If yes: What do you worry about?

What do you have trouble getting off your mind?

Is there anything you have to do over and over again and cannot stop
yourself from doing?

If yes: Tell me about that.

10. *Screen for Eating Disorders*

Have you lost or gained weight in the last year? How much?

How many times have you started a diet in the last year?

Have you ever felt that your eating was out of control? Have you gone on
eating binges?

Have you ever vomited or spit out food after eating to get rid of it?

Have you ever used diuretics or laxatives? How often?

Have people ever given you a hard time about being too thin?

11. *Screen for Psychosis*

Have you ever had trouble with your thinking?

Has your thinking ever been so confused that you lost track of your ideas?

Have any of your thoughts seemed frightening or disturbing to you?

Have you ever felt like people were watching or following you, or that they
wanted to hurt you?

Have your eyes or ears ever played tricks on you?

Have you ever had the experience of hearing a voice when nobody else
was around, or of seeing things that weren't there?

*From Brodkey AC, Van Zant K, Sierles FS: Educational objectives for the junior psychi-
atry clerkship: development and rationale.* Academic Psychiatry *21(4), 1997.*
Used with permission of American Psychiatric Press Inc. and the authors.

Medical Student Interview Evaluation Form

STUDENT _____ DATE _____

	YES	NO
In beginning the interview did the student		
1. Introduce him/herself appropriately?	_____	_____
2. Explain why he/she was here?	_____	_____
3. Elicit patient concerns regarding the purpose of the interview, privacy and physical comfort?	_____	_____
4. Establish rapport by asking the patient about him/herself?	_____	_____
In the initial phase of the interview did the student		
1. Allow patient to tell his/her own story of present illness?	_____	_____
2. Use open-ended questions?	_____	_____
3. Use the patient's statements to guide flow of interview?	_____	_____
During the interview did the student appropriately utilize		
1. Nonverbal communications?	_____	_____
2. Facilitating, supportive, and empathic comments?	_____	_____
3. Interviewer silence?	_____	_____
4. Acknowledge and allow expression of patient's feelings?	_____	_____
5. Appropriate reassurance?	_____	_____
6. Summary statements?	_____	_____
7. Open and close-ended questions?	_____	_____
8. Confrontation and clarification?	_____	_____
9. Patient's own words (and clarify their meaning)?	_____	_____
10. Techniques to structure hyperverbal patients?	_____	_____
11. Techniques for asking difficult/embarrassing questions?	_____	_____
During the interview did the student avoid		
1. Interrupting the patient inappropriately?	_____	_____

2. Asking long, complex questions? _____ _____
3. Asking questions suggesting answer he/she wanted? _____ _____
4. Asking directive or yes/no questions too early or too often (interrogative-like manner)? _____ _____
5. Sudden, inappropriate changes of topic? _____ _____
6. Asking the patient for information he/she had already mentioned? _____ _____
7. Using jargon? _____ _____
8. Judgmental, patronizing, overly familiar or disdainful, or otherwise unprofessional attitudes? _____ _____

In ending the interview did the student
1. Indicate a few minutes ahead that the interview was going to end? _____ _____
2. Provide feedback and summation and inform the patient about what's next? _____ _____
3. Ask whether the patient had anything further to mention? _____ _____
4. Ask whether the patient had questions he/she wanted to ask? _____ _____
5. Thank the patient? _____ _____

In general, did the student
1. Follow up verbal and nonverbal leads offered by the patient? _____ _____
2. Handle emotionally laden material well? _____ _____
3. Communicate ideas clearly? _____ _____
4. Explore the patient's ideas of why he/she got ill? _____ _____
5. Elicit the patient's feelings about being ill and in the hospital? _____ _____
6. Explore effects of the illness on patient's work, home life, leisure activities? _____ _____
7. Delineate psychosocial setting associated with onset or exacerbation of symptoms? _____ _____
8. Demonstrate respect, concern, empathy, sensitivity, responsiveness? _____ _____
9. Identify and analyze strengths and weaknesses in his/her own interviewing skills? _____ _____

History, Mental Status Exam, and Diagnosis

Did the student demonstrate
1. An adequate knowledge base of psychiatric symptoms and diagnosis? _____ _____

2. The ability to elicit necessary and relevant
   historical data, including the chief complaint,
   history of present illness, past personal and
   psychiatric histories, medical history, and family
   history?   _____ _____
3. An understanding of the key features of the
   mental status exam, including the cognitive
   exam?   _____ _____
4. The ability to reason clinically from the data to a
   differential diagnosis, workup, and treatment
   plan?   _____ _____

How difficult was the patient to interview?

Very Easy   Easy   Moderately Hard   Hard   Very Hard

Additional Comments:

Overall rating of Interview:

Honors   **High Pass**   **Pass**   **Borderline Pass**   **Fail**

SIGNATURE _____ **DATE:** _____

14

Undergraduate Electives and Special Activities

Theodore B. Feldmann, M.D.

This chapter focuses on the importance of psychiatric electives and other educational programs in medical student education. These activities complement the required core curriculum and help to stimulate student interest in psychiatry. The development and implementation of these programs is discussed, and guidelines for their creation are presented.

Before proceeding, however, it is useful to ask: Why is this area important? The answer to that question lies in an examination of the characteristics of successful medical student programs in psychiatry. These programs all share certain characteristics (Feldmann 1994). Obviously, *curriculum strength* is essential. The quality and variety of teaching programs enables students to gain a *positive view of psychiatry* as a medical specialty and career choice. All courses must have a strong clinical emphasis. By *stressing what we do* with patients, students get a realistic view of psychiatry, which helps to overcome the stigma of mental illness and the students' discomfort with emotional and behavioral problems. The "hands-on" experience that students receive increases their awareness of the effectiveness of psychiatric therapies. The importance of seeing psychiatrists every day cannot be underestimated in shaping student attitudes about psychiatry as a viable medical specialty. Thus, maintaining a *high visibility* within the medical school is also important. This, in turn, creates an atmosphere in which students feel they have *access to the department*. The result is that *personalized contacts and mentoring* of students are established. When students are identified as having an interest in psychiatry, an *aggressive outreach* to them helps to solidify their commitment. The *tracking of interested students* may make a difference in their career choices. Although these areas overlap to a great degree, the common thread is that students gain an in-depth exposure to us not just as teachers but as people who are interested in their well-being and professional future (Table 14–1).

The development of high-quality electives and special programs allows psychiatry departments to address many of the areas just listed. One of psychiatry's greatest strengths is its *diversity.* Unfortunately, it is often difficult to present this to students within the constraints of preclinical core courses and clerkships with limited time. The development of electives and other special programs helps students to gain a better appreciation of our field. This, in turn, heightens their educational experience and improves the perception of psychiatry. Thus, the goals of both education and recruitment are fostered (Weissman 1993).

Support for psychiatric education must literally come from the top! It is essential, therefore, that the *department chair* establish an environment conducive to and supportive of psychiatric education. This encompasses much more than simply encouraging faculty and residents to teach students. The chair must also be willing to actively participate in student teaching and other special activities (Pardes 1989). An example is Chairman's Rounds, a regularly scheduled activity during the clerkship in which the chair meets with students for a case conference and discussion. The chair should also be available to talk with students interested in psychiatry. Tak-

Table 14–1. Characteristics of successful medical student programs

1. A strong core curriculum
2. Commitment to education
3. Diversity of educational experiences
4. High visibility within the medical school
5. Aggressive outreach to students
6. Projection of a positive view of psychiatry
7. An emphasis on what we do
8. Personalized contacts and mentoring
9. Tracking of interested students
10. Special activities for students

ing the time to meet with students makes a powerful impression and often makes a critical difference in recruitment.

The key figure in the development of a quality program is the *director of medical student education*. This is the person who sets the overall tone for the psychiatric medical student curriculum. He or she is also the person having the most consistent contact with medical students. This person must be dynamic, outgoing, and able to foster an atmosphere in which students feel comfortable coming forward with their educational and career concerns. It is also imperative that this person possess the organizational skills required to develop and implement a high-quality curriculum (Table 14–2).

Another important person in the medical student curriculum is the *residency training director*. As stressed earlier, as more senior faculty are involved in teaching, students come to see us as mentors and role models. This enhances the perception of psychiatry as a vibrant and expanding specialty and also projects the image of psychiatrists as concerned about medical education. Involvement of the residency training director in teaching activities serves two additional functions. Students interested in psychiatry will naturally have many questions about residency programs. The training director is in the best position to provide information useful to students. At the same time, direct contact with students allows the residency director to get to know those students who wish to pursue psychiatric training. It also gives the training director an opportunity to identify and track students who display an aptitude for psychiatry. It is essential that the residency training director and the director of medical student education work together closely. These two positions share much in common, but the people who hold these positions often work in isolation due to time constraints, pressure for clinical service, or "turf issues." When this occurs, the department chair should intervene to maximize communication and cooperation between the two offices.

Table 14–2. Roles of the director of medical student education

1. Determines the educational philosophy of the medical student curriculum
2. Organization and coordination of the curriculum
3. Balances student needs versus educational needs (i.e., makes sure the curriculum is both student-friendly and academically sound)
4. Works with residency training director on recruitment issues
5. Liaison between students and the department

Finally, the importance of resident involvement in student teaching cannot be underestimated. Residents often get to know medical students before faculty. The common bond between residents and students of being "in training" often allows students to feel more comfortable approaching residents about academic or career issues. There is also less "formality" between residents and students, leading to more of a peer relationship. Thus, residents are a tremendous asset in the recruitment of medical students into psychiatry. As such, departments should actively encourage resident teaching and provide the training and resources (e.g., the American Psychiatric Association [APA] pamphlet "The Resident as Teacher") necessary for resident involvement.

The Development of Electives in Psychiatry

It was stressed earlier that diversity of educational experiences is an important component in the overall quality of a psychiatric curriculum. Although the preclinical core courses and the junior clerkship form the foundation of a department's educational programs, electives also play an important role. The basic functions of electives in psychiatry are to (1) increase student awareness of the diverse nature of our specialty, (2) expose students to specialized areas of psychiatry not necessarily covered in core courses, (3) allow students to pursue study in their own areas of special interest, and (4) foster creativity in education through nontraditional methods of education. Electives also allow for an interface between psychiatry and primary care fields; examples include behavioral medicine electives taught jointly by psychiatrists and family physicians, and consultation-liaison rotations.

Although there is much variability in curriculum structure from one medical school to another, most U.S. schools offer elective time at both the preclinical and clinical levels. A variety of strong courses aimed at students through all 4 years of medical school increases the overall quality of the curriculum. The goal, once again, is to give students the broadest possible exposure to psychiatric issues and practice. This, in turn, may lead to increased recruitment into psychiatry (Weintraub et al. 1996).

Preclinical Electives

The target audience for preclinical electives consists of first- and second-year medical students. To develop electives for this group, it is necessary to understand the unique needs of preclinical students. One of the most important concerns for students at this level is mastery of the extensive basic science material presented in the core curriculum. Another involves adjusting to life in medical school and the pressures that go along with medical education. Beginning students also struggle with the identity issues in becoming a physician. Finally, students begin their medical education with unique individual and interpersonal issues. These personal variables must be acknowledged and addressed for students to maximize the educational experience (Table 14–3).

With these needs and concerns in mind, it is possible to identify three broad categories of psychiatric electives: (1) those that integrate psychiatry into the basic sciences; (2) courses presenting an introduction to clinical psychiatry; and (3) examinations of lifestyle issues that affect health and illness. Electives can easily be developed to address each of these areas (Table 14–4).

Two areas of psychiatry lend themselves particularly well to the interface of psychiatry and basic science: neuroscience and behavioral medicine. Electives in neuroscience allow students to integrate such basic science courses as anatomy, biochemistry, and pharmacology into a clinical framework. Given the tremendous advances in our knowledge of the brain and behavior, neuroscience courses provide an exciting and stimulating environment in which students can apply their basic science knowledge to clinical situations. Behavioral medicine electives facilitate a better understanding of the interaction of anatomy, physiology, and pathology in disease pro-

Table 14–3. Concerns of preclinical students

1. Passing required courses
2. "Surviving" medical school
3. Developing a professional identity
4. Forming and maintaining relationships

Table 14–4. Categories of preclinical electives

1. Basic science correlation
2. Clinical and professional issues
3. Interpersonal issues in health

cesses. Health and wellness issues are also stressed through behavioral medicine (Table 14–5).

Electives focusing on an introduction to clinical psychiatry serve a variety of functions. They help students to view psychiatrists as physician mentors and role models, clinicians, and medical specialists. In addition, they contribute to the development of students' professional identities as physicians. Not only do these courses provide introductory clinical material, they also give students a better understanding of what psychiatrists do. Examples include physician-patient relationship electives, courses focusing on clinical issues (e.g., depression), and subspecialty areas such as child development and behavioral science and the law (Table 14–6).

Perhaps the most diverse and creative group of electives relate to lifestyle issues. These are more likely to address the personal concerns or interests of students. Included in this group are stress management courses, electives dealing with HIV and AIDS, social and cultural issues in medical practice, and the psychology of women and men. Student should also be encouraged to pursue their own creative interests during medical school. At the University of Louisville, for example, an elective called "Physicians and the Arts" allows students to develop special projects based on their own personal interests (Table 14–7).

Special Considerations in Electives

A number of elements must be considered in the development of preclinical electives. These include course structure, evaluation, faculty recruitment, and resident involvement.

Table 14–5. Sample electives to integrate basic science

1. The Brain and Behavior: Clinical Neuroscience
2. Research Advances in Psychiatry
3. Behavioral Medicine: The Mind–Body Connection

Table 14–6. Electives introducing clinical issues

1. The Doctor–Patient Relationship
2. Advanced Interviewing Skills
3. AIDS and the Health Care Provider
4. Behavioral Science and the Law

Table 14–7. Electives dealing with lifestyle issues

1. Physicians and the Arts
2. Health Awareness Workshop
3. The Psychology of Women and Men

The traditional lecture or seminar format can be applied to any pre-clinical elective. You must remember, however, that this is how most basic science courses are taught. Students often look for something different in their electives. An innovative approach, then, may make your elective more attractive. Small-group discussions of preassigned readings, problem-based learning exercises, preceptorships in clinical settings, independent study, research, or computer-based learning are some of the alternative instructional methods that can be utilized.

The *evaluation* of student performance in preclinical electives is often problematic. The most important initial consideration is to remember that these are electives, and, therefore, they will be viewed quite differently by students than the core courses. Course requirements and evaluation procedures must be set up with more flexibility that the core courses. Faculty must also be aware of the pressure and time constraints of the core curriculum. The bottom line is this: students will *not* sign up for electives that are perceived as too intense or time-consuming when compared with the core courses. Although we all like to think that our courses are the most important, that is an extremely unrealistic view. It also demonstrates a lack of empathy with the students' experience.

With those considerations in mind, the instructor must find inventive methods of evaluation. Those that involve the active participation of the student are preferable. Thus, final examinations are to be discouraged. Completion of a special project, independent study program, brief research paper, learning objective checklist, or experiential report are some of the evaluation instruments that can be utilized (Kay 1981). Self-evaluation by students is another useful method. Again, the more creative the evaluation methodology is, the greater the overall educational experience. Whatever method is chosen, however, don't forget that your elective will have a relatively low priority for students compared with anatomy, physiology, and other major courses.

Faculty recruitment for electives usually occurs in one of two ways.

First, faculty may submit elective proposals based on their particular academic interests. As an alternative, an educational need may be identified by the director of medical student education, or the department's education committee. Faculty are then identified to develop the course. Regardless of the method, however, the essential requirements are that the instructor be *enthusiastic* and *committed* to developing a top-flight course. A dynamic and charismatic teacher can often make the difference between an elective's success or failure. Clearly, someone who simply lectures and does not attempt to actively engage students will not attract a great deal of interest. Students expect to have fun in electives in addition to acquiring a body of knowledge or skills. With that in mind, it is important to remember one of the cardinal rules of good teaching: *Whatever you do, don't be boring!*

Clinical Electives

At most medical schools, students take clinical electives during the fourth year. These students have very different concerns than their preclinical colleagues. Most senior students select electives to broaden their clinical knowledge base in a specific area. Others look for rotations that will help them to clarify their career choice. Finally, there are many students who want to pursue areas of special interest, regardless of residency plans. Clinical electives should be developed with sufficient diversity to meet the needs of all three groups (Table 14–8).

Most clinical electives will be comprised of intensive clinical experiences, such as adult inpatient, outpatient, consultation-liaison, or emergency psychiatry. Specialized rotations may also be developed, such as rotations in child, adolescent, or forensic psychiatry (Table 14–9). Each of these areas gives students an in-depth look at psychiatry, helps to clarify career goals, and acquaints students with what a psychiatry residency is really like.

In addition to clinical electives in traditional academic settings, a wide range of alternative practice environments should be included. Medicine is increasingly moving away from the traditional hospital-based practice. To-

Table 14–8. Key elements of clinical electives

1. Diversity of clinical settings
2. Subspecialty exposure
3. "Acting-intern" level of responsibility
4. Intensive supervision

Table 14–9. Examples of clinical electives

---

1. Advanced Inpatient Rotations
2. Child Psychiatry
3. Ambulatory Care Electives
4. Community Mental Heatlh Centers
5. Forensic Psychiatry
6. Rural/Underserved Rotations
7. Combined Clinical Rotations

---

day's students will find themselves working more in ambulatory care settings, rural and underserved areas, community psychiatry, and managed care (Gabbard 1992). Thus, electives with private psychiatrists or in rural mental health clinics, for example, are useful in broadening the training experiences of the students. Finally, electives combining two or more clinical activities, such as emergency psychiatry and consultation-liaison, are effective in maximizing the student's educational experience.

Successful clinical electives incorporate a high degree of clinical responsibility coupled with intensive supervision. Senior students should be expected to perform at an *acting-intern level.* They should also participate in seminars and case conferences along with first-year residents. This added level of responsibility not only challenges students to acquire advanced clinical skills but also helps students entering psychiatric residencies to get a head start on the PG-I year. *Supervision* must be available on two levels: daily clinical supervision and regular process supervision. The latter form, ideally occurring twice a week throughout the rotation, allows for more in-depth examination of psychodynamic issues and also provides an opportunity for students to reflect on their experience with patients.

Evaluation of student performance will generally be done according to a standardized instrument used by the medical school. Additional feedback from supervisors about strengths and weaknesses is invaluable for senior students. The fourth year of medical school is really a transitional period bridging the gap between required medical school courses and residency. An open and candid relationship with supervisors is important in maximizing the educational benefit of the elective. An alternative and useful evaluation tool involves having the student keep a *daily log* of patient encounters, psychodynamic impressions, and general observations. The contents of the log will often serve as a useful discussion point for process-oriented supervision. If the elective involves research work, a brief summary paper also provides an effective evaluation method.

A final type of clinical elective is the *senior honors program in psychiatry*. This format has been used by other specialties, particularly surgery, to provide in-depth clinical experience for senior students. These programs are generally longer (e.g., 8 to 12 weeks) and more intensive than other clinical electives, and they are designed primarily for students interested in pursuing academic careers. A variety of formats can be utilized in developing honors programs. One method involves designating two tracks for the rotation: clinical and research. The student then chooses one track in consultation with the faculty adviser or program director. The clinical track involves more extensive responsibility and supervision than other electives, and the research track allows the student to work on established research with a faculty member or develop research activities suited to the student's particular interest. The honors program ideally is a *selective,* rather than elective course, with the director of medical student education interviewing students to determine their suitability for the rotation. Honors programs are exciting ways for students interested in psychiatry to prepare for residency training.

Special Activities for Medical Students

Although the academic curriculum constitutes the most important facet of the medical student program in psychiatry, a number of other activities can be developed to give our specialty greater exposure. There are two major objectives of these special activities. The first is to provide students with a better understanding of what psychiatry is, free of the constraints of traditional academic courses. A second, and related, outcome is to increase recruitment. Although a tension always exists between education and recruitment, and many psychiatric educators feel that recruitment is unrelated to education, it is nevertheless naive to think that these areas are mutually exclusive. The survival of psychiatry depends not only on educating physicians but also on recruiting the best medical students into our ranks.

Psychiatry Clubs

The Psychiatry Club is an organization for all medical students who have an interest in psychiatry, psychology, mental health issues, and/or human behavior (Kay 1984). The clubs generally have monthly meetings during which presentations or panel discussions on important issues in psychiatry are held. Meetings should be informal and open to any students wishing to attend; students should be told that interest in a psychiatric career is not a prerequisite to participation. Pizza, or other food, and soft drinks are usually served at each meeting.

The club serves as a course of information for students interested in psychiatry as a career, or for students who simply have an interest in the study of human behavior. It also functions to assist students in learning more about psychiatry and provides an opportunity to become acquainted with faculty and residents. The emphasis of the club is collegial with frequent social events designed to acquaint students with the department. New friendships and lasting professional relationships will be one result of this endeavor. A newsletter can also be published every month, or whenever there is important news or information about the club or the department.

Initially the club should be organized by a faculty member willing to be responsible for all of the club's activities. Active participation by residents should also be encouraged. Eventually, however, students must be encouraged to take ownership of the group, including the election of student officers or the creation of a steering committee to oversee activities. It must be remembered that a successful psychiatry club requires a great deal of nurturing by the department. The demands on medical students for time is very great; the faculty adviser, therefore, must be willing to make a commitment to keep the club going, even if student interest is slow to develop.

Health Awareness Week:
The University of Louisville Program

A unique student activity, the Health Awareness Week, has been developed by Leah Dickstein, M.D., at the University of Louisville (Dickstein and Elkes 1987). It consists of a weeklong series of programs given to incoming freshman students immediately before the official start of classes. The primary objective of the Health Awareness Week is to assist students in making the transition to medical school. Programs are aimed at maintaining a healthy lifestyle while dealing with the rigors of medical school, managing stress effectively, developing effective study habits, and initiating the development of a professional identity. Many social activities are also planned for students and their spouses or partners. These facilitate the acquisition of a strong social support system. Community outings are held to familiarize students with the city. Included are trips to the zoo, picnics, a riverboat cruise, and exposure to the area's cultural and recreational activities. The final day of Health Awareness Week includes the formal medical school orientation. Thus, first-year students receive exposure to the Department of Psychiatry before any other.

A great many faculty and residents are involved in this activity. One of the unique aspects of the program, however, is that sophomores actually coordinate and organize most of the events. They thus serve as mentors who share their own experiences and insights into medical school. Each freshman unit lab, of approximately 16 students, is assigned two second-year advisers along with two faculty advisers. Regular contact is maintained throughout the academic year by monthly lunches with each unit lab. This ongoing contact helps to ensure that freshmen feel supported and serves to diminish feelings of isolation.

Literature and Film Seminars

Another interesting and useful activity is literature or film seminars focus-ing on medically related themes (Fritz and Poe 1979; Schneider 1977; Sond-heimer 1994). These sessions may utilize a variety of sources, including films, novels, short stories, or plays, to illustrate behavioral, affective, or cognitive aspects of human behavior. For example, the film *The Doctor* is a useful vehicle for exploring reactions to illness as well as issues of em-pathy and physician sensitivity. The story focuses on a physician, played by William Hurt, who develops throat cancer. As a result of his own ex-periences, the doctor learns much about illness and what it is like to be a patient. There are countless literary and cinematic works that lend them-selves to this type of seminar. It can be offered as either an elective for academic credit, or as a department-wide activity. Faculty facilitators may be chosen to lead the group discussion, or outside speakers from drama departments or local theater companies may be invited to participate. Ses-sions may be held on campus or at faculty homes. The overall goal is to stimulate thought and discussion about human behavior in a nontraditional format while also fostering a sense of camaraderie and collegiality between students and the department.

Student Participation in Departmental Functions

A relatively easy, yet important, component of a psychiatric curriculum for medical students involves inviting them to special departmental activities. These include parties, picnics, grand rounds, journal clubs, and special seminars or conferences (Yager et al. 1991). For the latter two activities, students should be offered a reduced registration fee, or, ideally, the fee should be waived completely. Doing this allows students with an interest in psychiatry to maintain contact with the department. This type of outreach is very important, but it is one that psychiatrists have been slow to adopt. Other specialties, such as surgery, have been much more aggressive in identifying potential residents early in medical school and then linking them up with faulty in an ongoing way throughout medical school. Announcements of special activities can be made in the psychiatry club newsletter, by the director of medical student education, or from the chairman's office.

Utilizing the APA

Finally, resources from the APA should be utilized and made available to medical students. The benefits of student membership in the APA should be explained at Psychiatry Club meetings, behavioral science courses, and at the beginning of each clerkship. Membership forms can easily be distributed to all interested students. The APA Office of Education is also an important resource for educational materials or information about careers in psychiatry. Coordination of special seminars or activities with the APA district branch is another useful activity. Mentoring programs, for example, connect interested students with psychiatrists in the community and give students a different perspective about psychiatric practice outside an academic environment.

Summary

A comprehensive program of medical student electives in psychiatry, coupled with special activities such as a psychiatry club, greatly increases the strength of a department's curriculum. Students come to see psychiatry as a diverse and vibrant specialty and gain a greater appreciation of the psychiatrist's role as a physician. Students entering psychiatric residencies also have a greater knowledge base as a result of elective experiences. Finally, diverse exposure to our field stimulates student interest in psychiatry, ultimately fostering our recruitment efforts.

References

Dickstein L, Elkes J: Extraordinary program prepares students for stresses of medical school. Psychiatric Times 4(6):9–10, 1987

Feldmann TB: The generalist initiatives: a challenge for psychiatric educators. Medical Student Education in Psychiatry Newsletter 6(1):3–4, 1994

Fritz GK, Poe RO: The role of a cinema seminar in psychiatric education. Am J Psychiatry 136(2):207–210, 1979

Gabbard GO: The big chill: the transition from residency to managed care nightmare. Academic Psychiatry 16(3):119–126, 1992

Kay J: The independent psychiatry project: a model exercise in student learning. J Med Educ 56(4):347–351, 1981

Kay J: The psychiatry club: enhancing career choice of psychiatry. J Med Educ 59(1):62–63, 1984

Pardes H: Educating psychiatrists for the 1990's. Academic Psychiatry 13(1):3–12, 1989

Schneider I: Images of the mind: psychiatry in the commercial film. Am J Psychiatry 134(6):613–620, 1977

Sondheimer A: The literature and medicine seminar for medical students: a potential recruitment tool. Academic Psychiatry 18(1):38–44, 1994

Weintraub W, Plaut SM, Weintraub E: Medical school electives and recruitment into psychiatry: a 20-year experience. Academic Psychiatry 20(4):220–225, 1996

Weissman SH: Recommendations from the May 1992 conference to enhance recruitment of U.S. medical graduates into psychiatry. Academic Psychiatry 17(4):180–185, 1993

Yager J, Linn LS, Winstead DK, et al: characteristics of journal clubs in psychiatric training. Academic Psychiatry 15(1):18–32, 1991

15

Evaluation of Students

Bryce Templeton, M.D., M.Ed.

Linking Evaluation to Objectives

After determining programmatic objectives and designing a curriculum, the instructor's next task is to develop an evaluation program. The goals of the evaluation program involve assessing student progress and determining the effectiveness of the training program. This chapter outlines recommendations regarding evaluating student progress.

Concepts and Terminology

In discussing evaluation procedures, there are a number of useful terms (Thorndike 1971). For example, *formative evaluation* refers to ongoing assessments that are typically used to help guide the trainee and/or the course director as seen in the use of quizzes and midclerkship reviews of a student's progress. In contrast, *summative evaluation* is designed to make major decisions about a student, for example, the determination of readiness for progression from one year to the next or for receiving a license to practice.

Another set of terms concerns reliability and validity. *Reliability* is essentially the reproducibility of a measurement and is usually specified as a correlation coefficient ranging from 1.0 (perfect correlation) to 0.0 (random correlation) to -1.0 (extreme negative correlation). Thus, if a written exam were to have a reliability of 1.00, giving the same exam to a student 2 or 3 weeks later would result in an identical score. Interrater reliability is used in discussing observers' judgments about performance such as interviewing skills or responses in an oral exam.

319

Validity concerns the degree to which an assessment procedure measures what it is intended to measure. Important forms of validity include the following: (1) *face validity,* that is, how valid the evaluation appears to be in the eyes of a faculty member or student (testing experts and the courts give it little credence because it is unsystematic and too subjective; however, the lack of face validity of an examination in the eyes of students can have a demoralizing impact on the latter); (2) *content validity,* for example, how well the assessment systematically samples from a well-designed content outline or from a listing of important skills; (3) *criterion validity* or predictive validity, for example, how well the assessment of clinical skills during an examination setting will predict performance with patients in other settings in the weeks or months to come; and (4) *construct validity,* a more complex concept that, in medical training, is usually measured by demonstrating a growth in scores during the course of training (e.g., a gradual gain in in-training examination scores during residency training).

Evaluation procedures must be reliable and valid to have credibility with students, colleagues, and, if necessary, the courts (Helms and Helms 1991). The latter takes on great importance when a student fails a course or clerkship, and especially if the resulting course or clerkship failure results in dismissal from medical school for poor academic performance.

With a growing cutback of funds to support medical education, the need to operate evaluation programs in a more cost-effective manner will be increasingly important. Methods of reducing costs include the sharing of evaluation materials among academic centers and being sure to delegate evaluation responsibilities to the least costly staff member who can carry out the task effectively.

Evaluation must be employed within a setting of *due process,* which requires that a school describe in writing, what is required of a student, how a student is to be evaluated, and, if a student fails to meet performance standards, how and to whom the student may appeal (Irby et al. 1981). Generally, due process procedures are determined by the dean's office in collaboration with attorneys and are described in the school's student handbook. Keep a copy of the current student handbook close to your desk and be familiar with your school's due process guidelines.

Useful Resources

In developing an evaluation program for medical students, there may be several useful resources within an institution: (1) an office of medical education (OME); (2) the clerkship directors in the other major disciplines; and (3) the residency training directors. If your school is fortunate enough to have an OME, find out who has the best expertise in various aspects of evaluation, such as multiple-choice testing, assessing interviewing skills, and assessing day-to-day performance. Other useful resources include many good monographs (Muslin et al. 1974; Neufeld and Norman 1985; Templeton 1980) and articles in various educational journals including *Academic Medicine, Academic Psychiatry, Medical Education* (a British journal), *Medical Teacher, Teaching and Learning in Medicine,* and so on (Templeton and Selarnick 1994).

A great deal of useful information can be obtained by attending the annual meetings of the Association of Directors of Medical Student Education in Psychiatry (ADMSEP), the Association of Academic Psychiatry (AAP), and the American Association of Directors of Psychiatric Residency Training (AADPRT), and the regional and national meetings of the Association of American Medical Colleges' (AAMC) Group on Medical Education.

Written Examinations

Written exams are very helpful in tracking a student's acquisition of essential knowledge and, despite various critics, will continue to prove useful to both instructors and trainees (Hubbard et al. 1978; Weaver et al. 1979). For most medical schools, a class size of more than 50 students will require the instructor to make use of multiple-choice examinations. Essay questions or other non-multiple-choice formats are simply too time consuming to grade for such large classes. The use of frequent quizzes during preclinical courses and, if logistically feasible, during the clerkship, can help to keep students up-to-date on their reading and help students become better prepared for intramural finals as well as the United States Medical Licensing Examinations (USMLE).

An important question for each department concerns the decision about developing its own examinations versus using the *subject examinations* provided by the National Board of Medical Examiners (NBME). Use of NBME subject exams (often called "shelf exams") provides a reliable assessment of student knowledge of the field and data, which helps instructors compare their own students with those from other medical schools. In addition, shelf exams help maintain credibility of the course among other departments and may help students feel better prepared for Step 1 and/or Step 2 of the USMLE. The major disadvantages of NBME exams concern their cost, which might run $3,000 to $5,000 per year. Advantages of administering your own intramural examinations include ensuring a close link between your teaching objectives and the assessment and the relative ease of reexamining the student who fails the first test.

Writing Multiple-Choice Test Items

The best way to become a proficient preparer of multiple-choice examinations is to get some training. Several types of training are available. The first is to become a member of a test committee for one of the major testing groups: the NBME, the Educational Commission for Foreign Medical Graduates (ECFMG), Psychiatric Residency In-Training Examination (PRITE), or the American Board of Psychiatry and Neurology (ABPN). Another form of training is to attend workshops on exam preparation such as those held at national education meetings (e.g., at ADMSEP, AAMC, or the AAP meeting). Occasionally medical schools will sponsor such item-writing workshops. Finally, the use of written manuals can be extremely helpful. Examples include the booklet of sample questions or CD-ROM provided by the NBME.

Linking Objectives and Exams

To establish a link between the course objectives and the content of the examination, the instructor must prepare a content outline. Various approaches are used. Probably the simplest approach involves taking the units of instruction (e.g., the assigned chapters and/or the scheduled lectures) and preparing a given number of test items per unit of instruction to achieve an examination of sufficient length (e.g., 120 test items divided by 16 chapters = 7–8 items/chapter. If the instructor had sufficient time, it might be advisable to review the content of an examination from the perspective of a series of dimensions, each of which contains mutually exclusive components (Muslin et al. 1974). For example, for a second-year or end-of-clerkship examination in clinical psychiatry, it would be useful to assess the student's knowledge of various physician tasks (e.g., use of the patient's history, results of the physical examination, mental status, and ancillary studies; differential diagnosis; and various forms of therapy). In addition, it would be useful to review the examination content from the perspective of various diagnoses to be certain that the examination samples from a wide variety of important clinical disorders. Other important content dimensions include the age of the patient, etiologic factors, and so on.

Format of Test Items

The three formats used most widely today include the one-best answer; the a/b/both/neither; and the full matching set. Although the one-best-answer format is very useful, in the hands of inexperienced writers, it is associated with the largest number of inadvertent clues to the correct answer. The most common errors that help give away the correct answer include the following:

1. Making many of the correct answers the longest of the options.
   (a) XXXXXX XX XXXXXX XXX XXXX   ← Correct answer
        XXXX X XXXXXX XXXXXXX XXXX
   (b) XXXXX XXXXX XXXXXX   ← Length of all other options
2. Making the correct answer different in some manner, such as the only option containing an eponym, the only option containing both a generic and a brand name, etc.
   (a) XXXXXXXX (XXXXX XXXXX)   ← Correct option
   (b) XXXXXXX XXXXXXXXXXX XXX   ← Incorrect
   (c) XXXXXXXXXXX XXXXXXXXXXX   ← options

    A useful design of multiple-choice exams questions has included questions with *stems* stating "Characteristics of [disorder XYZ] include..." and "Complications of [drug XYZ] include . . ." These questions worked well with the so-called K-type item (a multiple, true-false format), which the NBME no longer uses. One alternative to the K-type approach is to write an *EXCEPT stem* such as "Each of the following is a DSM-IV characteristic of [disorder XYZ] EXCEPT . . .". As a second alternative, the author has devised a *chart-option* format, which is illustrated as follows:

DSM-IV criteria for schizophrenia include

	A	B	C	D	E
avolition	X		X		
delusions	X	X	X	X	X
disorganized speech	X	X	X		
hallucinations	X	X	X	X	X
indifference to praise				X	X
odd beliefs	X	X		X	X

ANSWER = C; DSM-IV-QR, p. 147. The chart-option technique is a one-best answer format and lends itself well to making multiple equivalent forms, so-called "item modeling."

Most medical schools have an optical-scan scoring machine that provides a method of efficiently scoring multiple-choice examinations. Find out who runs the system, and learn how to make the best use of the system. These machines will provide instructors with valuable information about the overall test and will generate *item statistics* that give crucial information about the effectiveness of individual questions. When these data come from an end-of-clerkship examination involving only 15 to 25 students, their utility will be very limited. But if these data come from a full class of 100 to 250 students, the resulting information will be quite valuable. For example, the mean percentage correct for the overall examination tells you the number of test items typically answered correctly by the average student. These data can be evaluated as follows:

Mean percentage correct:
85–100%   Too easy; it will be hard to get reliable scores.
70–85   Just about right; students will feel they are being tested on things they need to know.
<70   Students will feel the exam is too difficult, has too much minutia, and so on.

Many school op-scan scoring systems will also give an estimate of the overall reliability of an exam. The reliability of a written exam used for pass-fail purposes should probably be above .80. If your final examination has a lower reliability, at its next administration, you should increase its length.

Other important data concerning individual test items include the *P value,* that is, the percentage of students who answered the item correctly:

95–100%   Probably too easy for the level of student being tested
70–95   Satisfactory
50–70   A bit difficult, but don't throw them out
<50   Probably too difficult; save for a higher level trainee or discard

For each test item, you will also receive an *r value,* which essentially is a correlation coefficient that tells you how well the item differentiates between the top group of examinees (e.g., top 25%) in comparison to the bottom group (e.g., bottom 25%). The math is more complicated. Interpret these data as follows:

>.15	A good item; the higher the r value, the better; will rarely go above .30 to .40.
.05–.15	The item is not helping you very much in getting reliable scores; you probably should modify or discard it from the pool.
<.00	Any item with a negative r value should probably be discarded before final scoring.

The reliability of an examination is highly correlated with its length—the longer the examination, the more reliable the score. To have a reliable assessment of your students, you should probably base a grade on at least 120 test questions. This can be achieved in two ways: by having one or more short quizzes and a longer final exam and adding up the scores for each student for the entire course: Quiz # 1—20 items; Quiz # 2—18 items; Final Exam—100 items; TOTAL = 138 items. Alternatively you can have a single final examination of more than 120 questions.

If you want to keep the examination *secure* so that you can use it again, you need to label each exam book with a student's name taken from a class roster and then pass out exam papers by name to the appropriate student. Then you must be certain that you get an examination booklet from each student before each student leaves the exam room. In spite of doing this, using the same examination repeatedly will eventually cause you major problems when a group of students complain to the dean that some students had prior access to major portions of the exam and others did not.

During the exam, you should give students guidelines about how you wish to receive comments or concerns about specific test items. If you let students keep the exam, posting one copy and requesting that all comments be placed on the posted copy within 48 hours will provide you with the easiest method of reviewing student concerns. If you collect the exams, ask students to write comments on the exam with a note about each page of concern on page 1.

Following completion of the examination, send the answer sheets for preliminary scoring. While it is being scored review the students' written complaints, and make a tentative decisions about whether or not to keep the item based on a review of the assigned text or by consulting with other faculty. Then review the item statistics, paying special attention to items where the P value is less than 30%; and those items with negative r values. Be sure that the latter are correctly keyed. Based on a synthesis of the preceding, decide which items should be deleted from final scoring. As part of your request for final scoring, be sure to ask for a histogram showing the distribution of raw scores.

Testing experts have had a long-standing debate about the utility of *norm-referenced* testing, in which you look at the bell curve and fail a percentage of the lowest scorers; and *criterion-referenced* testing, in which you set a pass-fail standard in advance of the exam. Although I am very sympathetic with the arguments in favor of criterion-referenced testing, I do not think it is practical. I tend to de-emphasize the word *failure* and simply notify students that those students getting below a certain score must be reexamined. In my view, passing 100% of students is unwise. I find that a pass rate of 92% to 96% keeps the course credible in the eyes of the students; with this failure rate, the students conclude that they must study the material to satisfy the department requirements. In addition, this type of standard setting approach also helps keep students, as a group, from performing poorly on the USMLE Step 1 and Step 2 examinations.

Credibility of a written examination in the eyes of students can be enhanced by the following: letting students know about the nature of the assessment (format and content) at the very beginning of the course or rotation; ensuring broad sampling among the information presented; ensuring that difficulty level is appropriate (see preceding comments about the "mean percentage correct"); and avoiding a we-never-fail-anyone philosophy. A sloppy approach to testing can have a major adverse effect of a class's view of the course and the department. Anecdotal reports suggest that frequent (possibly weekly) quizzes combined with an NBME shelf examination works very well.

Medical student directors would benefit greatly from a test item banking system. The system would require the deposit of new test items on a periodic basis and would permit the instructors to use the resulting pool of materials. At the time of this writing, ADMSEP has helped to sponsor such a bank. Test item banks require periodic deposits of new items, must be administered by sound accounting principles, and cannot allow more assets to be withdrawn than are deposited. Users of the bank must be prepared to submit new, thoughtfully written questions, and to pay reasonable fees to the sponsoring institution for costs associated with maintenance and the provision of the service.

The USMLE Step 1 and Step 2 examinations can have an important impact on your instructional program and on your job. If the mean scores on the Step 1 behavioral science component or the Step 2 psychiatry component fall much below the mean scores for the other discipline scores for your students (e.g., the mean scores for biochemistry or internal medicine), your chair will receive a note from the dean's office and you, in turn, will be called in by your chair. You can plead for more curriculum time, but this approach often falls on deaf ears. If your mean scores are low and you want to retain your job, you better change something: Get some new lecturers; set up more quizzes; make the pass-fail level somewhat higher; try to instill more enthusiasm into both classroom teachers and the students; and so on.

The *Hawthorne effect* is a concept drawn from industrial psychology that was derived from a study in which both increases *and* decreases in industrial lighting produced more worker productivity as long as the changes appeared to be designed to help the workers. Figure out some way to make sure that whatever instructional changes you employ are carried out with enough enthusiasm to help ensure that the Hawthorne effect will work in your favor and help bring those Step 1 and 2 scores back up to a level that will be deemed acceptable in the eyes of the chair and the dean.

Evaluating Interview Skills

Interviewing skills represent one aspect of assessing noncognitive attributes. Departments vary greatly in the extent to which they participate in interviewing instruction (Lipkin et al. 1995). The range of approaches varies from schools in which the department's role may be directed primarily, during third year, to the mental status exam and related aspects of a psychiatric assessment to other schools in which the department may take a major role in the school's overall medical interviewing instruction.

In any case, evaluating interviewing skills is difficult (Kalet et al. 1992). Getting a sufficient number of faculty to observe just one interview for each medical student is often hard to accomplish. Some instructors resist the use of any structured evaluation forms and prefer to simply watch an interview and provide a trainee with verbal feedback in an unsystematic manner. Many programs rely on the use of global ratings scales by a single instructor who observes a single student with a patient; these forms include such questions as "followed leads appropriately" and "used language that was appropriate to the patient's level of education." Both the unstructured approach and the use of global rating forms by an instructor are associated with very poor reliability (Templeton and Allen 1990).

Checklists appear to provide more reliable data. Checklists usually focus primarily on the data requested and/or collected by students. But some checklists also try to focus on certain process measures: for example, the student introduced himself or herself in an acceptable manner. Figure 15–1 illustrates a generic checklist that can be used in assessing a medical student's initial interview with a psychiatric inpatient or outpatient. If the checklist data are to be used for formal evaluation, the faculty would need to determine how many items would reflect meeting minimal standards.

Standardized patients (SPs), once call *simulated patients,* are individuals who are hired to portray a patient and the patient's medical or psychiatric problems at a specific point in the patient's life. Some are trained just for history-taking skills, whereas others help train both history and physical examination skills. A growing number of schools are developing SP programs for teaching and evaluating medical interviewing and physical examination skills. These programs are usually administered by an OME or the dean's office, have their own budget, and have personnel with considerable sophistication in training SPs in devising methods of evaluating student performance in a reliable and valid manner.

Observed structured clinical examination (OSCE) is an evaluation procedure involving a series of 6 to 18 *stations,* each of which requires the student to demonstrate some form of clinical performance. At each OSCE station, a student is usually required to perform some aspect of the medical history, the physical examination, or patient education. Usually each station includes an SP. OSCEs provide another mechanism of assessing some noncognitive attributes under fairly standardized conditions.

If your school has such an SP and/or OSCE program, your efforts at instruction in and evaluation of interviewing skills might be spent more efficiently by collaborating with the SP program. Your goals then should be to ensure that the bank of cases employed in that program include an appropriate number of well-designed psychiatric cases (e.g., the assessment of patients with alcoholism, anxiety, bereavement, somatoform disorders, etc.), that the evaluative instruments include attention to important aspects of psychiatry as it applies to medical student instruction, and that you and your colleagues are able to get feedback about how the students handle those aspects of interviewing skills that are of special importance to the department.

Tape #_____   Date of Taping _____ 19_____

Date of Coding: _____ 19_____   Reviewer's Initials _____

Patient age: _____   Patient sex: M   F

Interview length: _____ minutes.

[Instructions: check each item reflecting an inquiry by the physician trainee and/or giving of information by the patient.]

PRESENT ILLNESS

_____ Onset, time of
_____ Symptoms (Ss)
_____ Course of Ss (e.g., sudden onset, intermittent, steadily worse, etc.)
_____ Did some event precipitate hospitalization/ambulatory visit

PAST MEDICAL HISTORY

_____ Allergies
_____ Drug reactions
_____ Medications, recent/current
_____ Past illnesses (nonsurg)
_____ Past operations
_____ Other hospitalizations
_____ Alcohol use/abuse
_____ Substance use/abuse, other

FAMILY MEDICAL HISTORY

_____ Mother (Living vs Dead; L/D)
_____ Mother, state of health
_____ Nature of relationship or feelings about
_____ Father (L/D)
_____ Father, state of health
_____ Nature of relationship or feelings about
_____ Siblings (L/D)
_____ Siblings, state of health
_____ Nature of relationship or feelings about (mention of one or more)
_____ Marital status
_____ Nature of relationship or feelings about spouse (if married)
_____ Children, state of health
_____ Nature of relationship or feelings about (mention of one or more)
_____ Family members do/don't have same problem as patient's admission
_____ Diabetes in other family members
_____ Hypertension in other family members

_____ Heart disease, other type, in other family members
_____ Kidney problems in other family members
_____ Liver problems in other family members
_____ Psychiatric problems in other family members
_____ Seizures/epilepsy in other family members

REVIEW OF SYSTEMS

_____ GEN   Fever
_____ GEN   Weight change
_____ SKIN   Bruising
_____ HEAD   Headaches
_____ HEAD   Passing out
_____ EYES   Double vision
_____ EYES   Other impairment
_____ EARS   Pain
_____ NOSE   Nosebleeds
_____ NOSE   Sinus problems
_____ MOUTH   Any problems
_____ NECK   Thyroid/node enlargement
_____ CV   Chest pain
_____ CV   Palpitations
_____ CV   Edema (ankles, hands, etc)
_____ CV   Murmurs
_____ CV   Shortness of breath
_____ RESPT   Asthma/wheezing
_____ RESPT   Cough
_____ RESPT   Coughing up blood
_____ RESPT   Sputum
_____ GI   Swallowing difficulty
_____ GI   Nausea/vomiting
_____ GI   Abdominal pain
_____ GI   Food intolerance
_____ GI   Gall bladder attacks
_____ GI   Diarrhea/constipation
_____ GI   Blood in bowel movements
_____ GI   Black bowel movements

(*continued*)

Figure 15–1. Initial interview evaluation—generic checklist

REVIEW OF SYSTEMS (continued)

_____ GU   Increased frequency
_____ GU   Urinating at night
_____ GU   Blood in urine
_____ GU-Male   Pain
_____ GU-Male   Discharge (VD)
_____ GU-Male   Prostate problems
_____ GU-Male   Urinary stream
_____ GU-FEMALE   Pain
_____ GU-FEMALE   Discharge
_____ GU-FEMALE   Menstrual pattern
_____ GU-FEMALE   Venereal Disease
_____ GU-FEMALE   Contraception use
_____ GU-FEMALE   Obstetrical hx
_____ GU-FEMALE   Recent breast exam
_____ MUSC   Joint pain
_____ NMUSC   Joint swelling
_____ NMUSC   Weakness of
                   extremities
_____ UMUSC   Circulation problems

MENTAL STATUS

_____ Assaultive feelings
_____ Date of month (orientation)
_____ Day of week (orientation)
_____ Delusions
_____ Depressed mood
_____ Highs (euphoria, racing thoughts, etc.)
_____ Nervousness
_____ Hallucinations
_____ Suicidal thoughts

PSYCHOSOCIAL

_____ Recent life crisis
_____ Closest person, opposite sex, relationship
       to
_____ Other people (e.g., friends, pastor, rabbi,
       etc. providing support)
_____ Employment
_____ Education, extent of
_____ Housing, current satisfaction with
_____ Financial status
_____ Major surgery, reaction to
_____ Major illnesses, reaction to
_____ Sleep patterns
_____ Sexual life/problems
_____ Hobbies; other pleasurable activities.

CLOSURE OF INTERVIEW

_____ Warned patient >1 min before ending
       interview
_____ Notified patient of ending
_____ Provided some note of encouragement
       (e.g., "I hope things go well with. . . .")
_____ Thanked patient

Figure 15–1. Continued

Video Examinations

A few instructors become enamored with video examinations in which a patient is portrayed for 1 to 8 minutes and then students are asked to answer written questions, usually multiple-choice questions, about the patient portrayed in the video. From my experience of reviewing a number of these video examinations, usually only 5% of questions require a video signal. Another 10% to 35% of questions could be answered with a written text of the interview. Typically 65% to 90% of video-based questions do not require a video or text presentation. In addition, problems in case-to-case variability make sampling and therefore content validity a major problem; space limitations of this chapter, however, preclude detailed explanation. In my view, an instructor is best advised not to employ video examinations.

Evaluating Students During Small-Group Instruction

Many departments include small-group instruction as part of their course in behavioral science or introductory psychiatry during the first two years of medical school. These groups are usually designed to include discussion about topics related to lectures and/or readings. Instructors who serve as group leaders are often able to provide meaningful evaluations of certain noncognitive attributes for those students at the extremes of performance: (1) those students who are especially good participants, who take leadership roles in the group, who appear very knowledgeable, and who are thorough and timely in assignments; and (2) those few students who stand out because they are excessively shy and/or inhibited, come late or miss sessions, don't relate to or get along well with peers, and so on. However, instructors often feel at a loss in grading the remaining students even if the group has met weekly for 4 to 9 months. To obtain the valuable data about the 4two outlier groups, I encourage faculty to simply record, for the remaining students, "performed acceptably within the group" without much additional detail in order to obtain useful data about the high and low performers.

Including senior residents as coleaders is an effective method of providing residents with some hands-on instruction in teaching and evaluating students.

Oral Examinations

Studies of question-and-answer oral examinations generally show the following deficiencies: most of the questions require primarily recall of information and not "problem solving" as many examiners contend; sampling of content varies widely among examiners unless the exam is highly structured; oral examiners have difficulty achieving good interrater reliability; and the hidden cost per student examined is very high. Based on available research, the popularity of this technique among some instructors seems unfounded.

Performance Assessment of Noncognitive Traits

Assessing student's day-to-day performance provides an important approach in evaluating many noncognitive characteristics and is an important aspect of student evaluation especially during the clinical assignments of the third and fourth year. Here again, problems of poor interrater reliability are rampant. For example, McLeod (1986) has shown the wide variation in faculty judgments regarding medical student case write-ups. Most medical schools have adopted clinical skills rating forms that each department is required to use. Recommendations as to how these forms can be employed in the most reliable, valid, and cost-effective manner are outlined in Table 15–1.

Effective evaluation of day-to-day performance is positively correlated with the following: synthesizing information for a given student from a number of instructors and ancillary personnel; conducting an end-of-clerkship group meeting of instructors to discuss the proposed evaluations; having photographs of students available when the preceding ratings are being completed; and managing the system to ensure the collection of evaluations within 10 days of the end of each clerkship. Some faculty members are substantially tougher or easier graders than their colleagues, which causes morale problems among students; providing faculty members, every year or so, with a summary of their distribution of grades and the distribution of the grades for the department may help to bring outliers closer to the mean.

Some schools encourage departments to avoid inflating grades by strictly limiting the number of students getting honor grades. Although there are good reasons to comply with the dean's office request, if a department's distribution of grades falls too far to the left of other clinical departments, students may become unduly critical of the department for adhering too strictly to schoolwide policies.

Training Faculty and Residents to Give Feedback to Students

The effectiveness of the faculty and residents in evaluating students can probably be enhanced through both formal and informal mechanisms. In an informal approach, maintaining contact with the faculty and residents

Table 15–1. Methods of ensuring effective assessment of day-to-day performance

Synthesize information for each student from several sources: instructors, residents, and ancillary personnel.
Conduct end-of-clerkship group meeting of instructors and ancillary personnel.
Have photographs available at the above sessions.
Collect the evaluation forms within 10 days of the end of the clerkship.

in order to be aware of their concerns about all aspects of the teaching program will help to maintain their interest in providing thoughtful and valid feedback about student performance. More formal approaches include meeting with faculty or residents periodically. Alternative approaches include devoting a regular faculty meeting to review these concerns or periodically to attend divisional meetings (e.g., divisional meetings of the inpatient service or the consultation service). Consider distributing copies of the APA's most recent addition of the brochure, *The Resident as a Teacher.*

Promotions Committee Participation

Serving on a basic science or clinical science promotions committee is an important faculty responsibility and provides an opportunity to get to know other faculty and to learn how other departments handle their teaching and evaluation responsibilities. In my experience, it is surprising that these committees often find themselves struggling with difficult summative decisions about individual students about whom relatively little is known other than the fact that they are in academic difficulty. Although the committee may request psychiatric evaluation for selected students, there may be value in attempting to obtain a relatively standard database on all students having academic difficulty, including the presence of medical problems, family crises, evidence of alcohol or substance abuse, apparent motivation for continuing medical studies, evidence of a learning disability and so on.

If a formal psychiatric consultation is requested, questions that should be posed by the committee to the consultant should include the following: Are there any reasons why the student should be discouraged from continuing medical school on a temporary or long-term basis? Does the consultant recommend some form of ongoing treatment? Are there any other suggestions for the committee that might help the student succeed? Students may feel a greater degree of comfort with issues of confidentiality if the assessment is carried out by a part-time faculty member, and if they are aware of the specific questions that the consultant has been asked to answer.

Conclusion

Evaluation plays an important role in medical education. If performed in a reliable manner with valid techniques, we have the capability of determining the readiness of students to progress in training, and to determine the overall effectiveness of our educational efforts. For evaluation to work successfully, we must apply the same degree of care exercised in diagnosing and treating patients to the selection and application of evaluative procedures in our work with students.

References

Helms LB, Helms CM: Forty years of litigation involving medical students and their education: I. General educational issues. Acad Med 66:1–7, 1991

Hubbard JP, Andrew BJ, Chase RA, et al: Measuring Medical Education: The Tests and the Experience of the National Board of Medical Examiners, 2nd Edition. Philadelphia, PA, Lea & Febiger, 1978, pp 1–17

Irby DM, Fantel JI, Milam SD, et al: Legal guidelines for evaluating and dismissing medical students. N Engl J Med 304:180–184, 1981

Kalet A, Earp JA, Kowlowitz V: How well the faculty evaluate the interviewing skills of medical students. J Gen Intern Med 7:499–505, 1992

Lipkin M Jr, Putnam SM, Lazare A (eds): The Medical Interview; Clinical Care, Education, and Research. New York, New York, Springer-Verlag, 1995

McLeod PJ: Faculty assessments of case reports of medical students. J Med Educ 62:673–677, 1987

Muslin HL, Thurnblad RJ, Templeton B, et al: Evaluation Methods in Psychiatry. Washington, DC, American Psychiatric Association, 1974

Neufeld VR, Norman GR: Assessing Clinical Competence. New York, Springer, 1985

Templeton B. Evaluation in the continuum of psychiatric education, in Comprehensive Textbook of Psychiatry, 3rd Edition. Edited by Kaplan HI, Freedman AM, Sadock BJ. Baltimore, MD, Williams & Wilkins, 1980, pp 2181–2189

Templeton B, Allen MM: Interrater reliability in evaluating trainee interviewing skills. Academic Psychiatry 14:188–196, 1990

Templeton B, Selarnick HS: Evaluating consultation psychiatry residents. Gen Hosp Psychiatry 16:326–334, 1994

Thorndike RL: Educational Measurement, 2nd Edition. Washington, DC, American Council on Education, 1971

Weaver FJ, Ramirez AG, Dorfman SB, et al: Trainees' retention of cardiopulmonary resuscitation; how quickly they forget. JAMA 241:901–903, 1979

16

Educational Collaboration With Other Specialties

**Michael Weissberg, M.D., Steven Kick, M.D.,
Emily Borus McCort, M.D., and Gwyn Barley, Ph.D.**

Collaborating with other medical school educational programs allows the influence of psychiatry to spread beyond the boundaries of the discipline. Clearly, collaboration flies in the face of guild and turf issues and for such collaboration to be fully successful psychiatry must have a place—however small—"under the educational tent." Such inclusion is not always the case in some schools. It has been our experience that "frontline teachers" more easily see the benefits of collaboration; it is the remote administrators who worry about adverse "political," and not educational, consequences.

However, persistent and collegial attempts at engaging other "guilds" in mutual educational activities often help undo psychiatry's isolation in those medical school settings that are less than hospitable. Hopefully, collaboration can be "official," aboveboard and obvious and, therefore, successful from the outset. In other settings, collaboration must be bootlegged and minimal. For example, such bootlegged collaboration may start small by frontline educators sharing evaluation methodologies, outside speakers, or participating in combined case-conferences. Sometimes, frontline teachers from different departments will work together on research projects of mutual interest and generate chapters, books, or articles. In all cases, collaboration depends on the maintenance of mutually respectful personal relationships with educators in other specialties.

Collaboration is not a synonym for capitulation nor a euphemism for relegating the responsibility for psychiatric education to others in other disciplines. In fact, it takes even more effort to collaborate effectively, not less. In all cases, psychiatric educators must *enthusiastically* insinuate themselves into the various educational structures and venues of their schools. No medical school committee should be left unexplored, especially if that committee has anything to do with the school's curriculum, the development of new courses, or the use of standardized patients and cases designed for problem-based learning (PBL).

Clearly, it will be impossible to fruitfully work with all people in all departments at all times. The best strategy is to find the most welcoming colleagues, proceed to identify areas of mutual interest and benefit, and then begin. So, if psychiatric educators are initially rebuffed by one discipline or department, they should move on to another. We have found, for instance, surgery to be open to collaboration while other departments may be more wary. If collaboration proves to be successful, then the more reticent may eventually come along.

Therefore, how and where to attempt collaboration depends on the idiosyncrasies of each educational site, on the strengths of the department, and, certainly, on the interests and duties of the medical student director/ educator. Collaboration takes time, commitment, and enthusiasm; different departments approach student affairs with differing levels of effort. However, medical student directorships should be considered full-time academic positions; anything less makes the possibilities of collaboration much more challenging.

Collaboration can be successfully accomplished at any one of three junctures of medical training: in the preclinical years, during the clinical clerkships, or during postgraduate training. In addition, collaboration may involve any one of the three separable elements of educational programs: There may be collaboration at *sites of practice,* when *a mixture of disciplines or specialties* teach, or when *curricular goals are shared* with those of other disciplines.

In most cases, psychiatric education will be enhanced when psychiatric educators look for ways to collaborate with other specialties. Collaboration at its best exposes students to psychiatry while they are in courses or on clinical rotations not typically labeled as "psychiatry." For example, there can be collaboration in traditional medical school courses, for example, in medical interviewing, often the responsibility of psychiatry but which utilizes both psychiatric and nonpsychiatric faculty. Collaboration can occur in clinical sites, for example, pain clinics. Specialties currently collaborate on the graduate level in the relatively uncommon multiple-boarded programs such as Psychiatry-CAP-Pediatrics, Psychiatry-Family Practice, Psychiatry-Internal Medicine, and Psychiatry-Neurology.

We suggest, therefore, that, when done well, interspecialty collaboration is desirable in medical schools and residencies, in different clinical venues and utilizing a variety of curricular formats. Psychiatry as a specialty will benefit by seeking ways of working with other specialties in the clinical setting either during the undergraduate or graduate years. (Patients will also benefit when care is better integrated). Although undergraduate education will be the primary focus of this chapter, we will, however, briefly discuss postgraduate education as well.

The Advantages of Collaboration

Psychiatry accrues at least two clear educational advantages by seeking ways to collaborate with other specialties. In addition, a third reason for collaboration—especially with primary care specialties—is that the types of problems—and patients—seen in primary care practices are so typically "psychosocial" and "psychiatric."

1. The first benefit is educational. Students (and physicians) often have difficulty applying what they *know* about psychiatry to their patients in the clinical setting. The relationship between cognitive mastery and clinical behavior is the core conundrum of medical education.

   Students, for example, have difficulty "generalizing" their knowledge and applying what they learned on their psychiatry rotation while they are on another medical or surgical service. In other words, in some students knowledge and clinical competence is "state" specific, not a trait, and is defined by the service that they are on.

   Students "forget" to ask their patients about depression or suicide, for instance, while on surgery. Information learned in one state is best recalled in that state. If medical students learn psychiatry in psychiatric settings but practice later in different settings, then recall of clinical psychiatry will be hindered (McKegney and Weiner 1976). *Therefore, breaking down the educational walls between departments will encourage students to think holistically and not by categories, for example, surgically on surgery and psychiatrically on psychiatry.*

2. A second benefit of collaboration is that it *functionally increases psychiatric preclinical and clinical curriculum time.* In addition to fostering more realistic clinical attitudes in students taught in more naturalistic settings, collaboration allows psychiatric departments to expand the field on which their curriculum is played out. Traditionally, departments have focused their educational efforts on their average of approximately 100 hours of preclinical teaching time and their 4- to 6-week clerkships. But collaboration can provide other venues—and therefore additional hours—for psychiatric education.

    Therefore, psychiatric education need not be limited by the amount of curriculum time labeled "psychiatry." With a clearly articulated curriculum (see the following) as the cornerstone of collaboration, psychiatric education need not be limited by the number of hours or weeks in the classroom or spent on specific sites of practice.

    For example, students can appropriately be taught about the mental status examination, the evaluation of drug or alcohol abuse, depression, anxiety and suicide while they are on a primary care service such as internal medicine or family practice. The same educational goals can be met in medical emergency departments, as well.

3. A third strong argument in favor of collaboration is that it *benefits similar clinical populations in psychiatry and primary care.* It is well accepted that 30% to 70% of patients seen in general medical practice suffer from a psychiatric diagnosis or are in some form of psychosocial difficulty. Conversely, many psychiatric patients suffer from concurrent medical conditions. In addition, a variety of medical problems may present with psychiatric symptoms. Therefore, physicians in nonpsychiatric practice need psychiatric training and psychiatrists must have a solid medical background to practice psychiatry effectively. Interspecialty collaboration makes sense because the clinical population seen by, for example, primary care specialists and psychiatrists are often so similar.

Where Should the Educational Focus Lie?

Major collaborative efforts should be focused in the undergraduate years. It is notoriously difficult to train physicians to recognize psychiatric problems in their patients, for example, depression, once they have left medical school.

In addition, many residencies only give lip service to even the most rudimentary psychiatric training such as the identification and emergent treatment of patients who are suicidal or involved in some form of child or spouse abuse. This lack of training persists despite the fact that such problems are likely to be seen in most medical practices (Weissberg 1990).

Therefore, medical school is the first and likely the last place where the groundwork for effective psychiatric care will be laid. Medical school has been called the last occasion of formal training in psychiatry (Voineskos et al. 1981); it is here that we should begin to concentrate our educational energies. We will focus on sites and programs where medicine and psychiatry can interact for the benefit of both.

The Development of Collaborative Efforts

Undergraduate medical education is usually structured along one of two models: programmatic (which cuts across departments), and the more traditional departmental organization. Interdepartmental, programmatic efforts (besides medical interviewing) are found mainly in schools that utilize problem-based learning methodologies. But most undergraduate medical education continues to be organized along more traditional, departmental, not programmatic, lines.

No matter the organization, however, in order to take full advantage of the benefits of collaboration (less state-dependent learning, expanded venues and time in which to teach psychiatry), medical schools will be well served if each department develops core curricula that can then inform their educational efforts. At its most functional, such a curriculum should be *vertically integrated so that the preclinical years are tied to the clinical activities in sequence and content.* This curriculum will then guide students no matter the clinical site. *The need for a clearly articulated curriculum cannot be overemphasized.*

When core curricula are clearly articulated, students can take coresponsibility for its mastery no matter the clinical training site. For example, the identification and emergent evaluation of the suicidal patient may best be accomplished in any one of a number of clinical settings. But, for this to happen, each department, in this case psychiatry, *must clearly state the learning objectives and what the student is to master.*

Developing core curricula, however, can be difficult given the relentless expansion of psychiatric knowledge. DSM-IV (American Psychiatric Association 1994) is 300 pages longer than the DSM-III-R (American Psychiatric Association 1987); a new synopsis of psychiatry is more than 1,200 pages; the last edition was 800 pages—and had larger print (Weissberg 1996). Despite the difficulties, as educators, we should be expected to parse out the *minimum* learning objectives we wish our students to learn from all that we teach.

It is counterproductive to develop "pie in the sky curricula" in which students are expected to cover "everything" but master little. Such exhaustive laundry lists reassure teachers but do not represent realistic or effective education. As educators we have not yet honestly identified what we, in John Romano's words, consider "basic and fundamental" psychiatric knowledge necessary for the practice of medicine. Since we have not done that, we list nearly everything (Weissberg 1996).

These core curricula can follow the students through their preclinical and clinical experiences and not just be confined to their psychiatric rotations. In this way, psychiatry can be inserted into a number of educational venues.

At Colorado, we developed the menu and method of *The Colorado Medical Student Log* to articulate the minimal educational goals for our students: 10 core clinical experiences and 10 core psychiatric screens (see Appendix 16–A). The log also provides a simple method by which we can be satisfied that some of our minimal educational goals are being met. Students are now given the log during their preclinical years during Primary Care I, another example of the benefits of collaboration since students, while in primary care practices, will also begin their march through their psychiatric curriculum.

Examples of Collaboration

Preclinical Years

Medical interviewing is an excellent place for collaboration, especially when psychiatrists, as is often the case, direct or codirect medical interviewing or are involved with small-group teaching. The use of standardized patients in medical interviewing presents ample opportunities to encourage students to conceptualize patients utilizing the biopsychosocial approach, which is a true collaborative model. It is always easy, for instance, to insert the issues of depression, grief, anxiety, sleep disorders, somatoform disorders, nonadherence, chemical dependency, abuse, or suicide into scripts describing patients who suffer from the panoply of chronic medical or surgical illness.

Longitudinal, primary care sequences provide another ideal opportunity for collaboration with medicine, family medicine, and pediatrics by inserting psychiatry into nonpsychiatric curricula. At the University of Colorado, our clinical sequence, The Primary Care Curriculum, meets one afternoon each week beginning the first year of medical school. Students spend 3 out of 4 afternoons in a primary care practitioner's office. These practitioners are part of our volunteer faculty. The didactic curriculum has become primarily problem based and takes place on the fourth afternoon throughout the 3 years.

In such settings, there are ample opportunities to design PBL cases, small-group exercises and standardized patient scripts with psychosocial problems in mind. These cases, exercises, and standardized patients may form part of a course's curriculum or be part of an evaluation strategy such as an Objective Standardized Clinical Examination (OSCE). An example of a useful small-group exercise is to ask each student to relate where their grandparents are from and then to describe a home remedy. This exercise demonstrates that what looks like a monoethnic group is really culturally diverse and also begins to sensitize students to differing cultural explanations, expectations, and treatments for illness (see Seven Diagnostic Questions in Appendix 16–A).

The design of such cases and exercises depends on the educational structure of each course or sequence. Hopefully, a psychiatrist is already part of the curriculum team; if not, the psychiatric educator can submit a case or script to the powers that be. Therefore, when not officially asked, psychiatrists must volunteer to actively participate in the design of these cases and exercises. We have not found it difficult to be certain that the issues of depression, grief, anxiety, sleep disorders, somatoform disorders, nonadherence, chemical dependency, abuse, or suicide are present in the scripts or case reports of patients who suffer from the panoply of chronic medical or surgical illness. For instance, our primary care sequence uses a standardized patient script, which has within it issues of grief, depression, dementia, and drug dependence, as part of a patient's evaluation.

Collaboration can occur between nonpsychiatric and psychiatry preclinical courses. At Colorado, medical students in Human Behavior (MSII) are asked to write up two patients from their Primary Care sequence. This *Psychiatry in Primary Care Psychiatric Case Report* stimulates students to think "psychiatrically" in medical settings. Furthermore, students are encouraged to bring their patients to their small groups. In addition to allowing students to further improve their interviewing, diagnostic, and formulation skills, this exercise also exposes students to a collaborative—psychiatric and primary care—approach to their patient. It is important to contact the primary care preceptors so that they can understand the nature of this exercise. For this, we write a yearly letter to all preceptors and ask them to contact us if they have questions; many of them do.

Collaboration occurs in PBL. Problem-based learning provides an excellent vehicle for interspecialty collaboration. If cases are developed realistically, psychiatric issues will be represented by necessity (see earlier comments).

Clinical Collaboration

Educational collaboration can occur on consultation services and other clinical sites. Consultation-liaison services provide a time-honored site for interspecialty collaboration and are, along with psychiatric emergency services, one of the oldest sites for teaching psychiatry in nonpsychiatric settings to medical students and residents. *Specialty services* such as hospice, cancer units, pain clinics, detoxification units, burn units, transplant services, and HIV clinics also are places for interspecialty collaboration and, therefore, education. How psychiatric input is paid for on such services can be problematic, and salary support often has to be cobbled together from clinical earnings, grants, and contracts. Use the services where psychiatric faculty already have research or clinical interests for the education of students.

Collaboration can occur in emergency psychiatry and walk-in clinics. Emergency psychiatric dervices that are *based in general hospital emergency* rooms offer the opportunity to work with nonpsychiatric trainees, medical students, and residents. Such services lose their educational utility if they are isolated from other medical services. When psychiatric emergency services are part of a general hospital emergency department, however, students and residents will have many opportunities to see the relationship of medical and psychiatric illness and to observe, it is hoped, useful collaboration between specialties.

Collaboration in establishing minimal clinical curricular goals can be achieved on a variety of rotations via "patient sharing." Where departmental lines are tightly demarcated and the clinical training is guild driven and not programmatic, the possibility still exists to identify overall clinical curricular goals for medical students. Thus, while students rotate through individual specialties, they may master an overarching goal even when that goal is not particularly associated with the rotation they are on currently. For example, students are likely to encounter more examples of grieving patients on pediatrics or medicine than on psychiatry. Conversely, students will be faced with many primary care medical issues when dealing with the chronically mentally ill while they rotate on psychiatry.

Where there is agreement between directors of the cognate departments, such "patient sharing" can become a fruitful educational resource. Such planning also forces medical schools to articulate a core, overarching clinical curriculum with clearly stated, achievable goals.

Collaboration in Educational Research and Faculty Development

Interdepartmental research is an ideal vehicle to generate educational collaboration. Departments can also collaborate in faculty development. For instance, education experts can be brought in by groups of faculty to help them develop their teaching techniques, curriculum, or evaluation strategies. The development of *joint faculty appointments* is another, more administrative way to acknowledge and, therefore, promote, interdepartmental collaboration.

Collaboration in Postgraduate Training

Medicine/Neurology Training for Psychiatrists

Despite the fact that psychiatrists are trained as physicians, several reviews of practice demographics and attitudes among psychiatrists have suggested that medical training may often be inadequate. Physical illness among psychiatric patients ranges as high as 4 in 10 among inpatients and outpatients. In a substantial proportion of these patients, the medical illnesses either caused or exacerbated the psychiatric disorders and were considered important in the psychiatric differential.

Several settings are available for providing the necessary training for psychiatry residents in medicine. Although interns often rotate on inpatient medical services, the following settings might be more useful:

1. Continuity outpatient medicine clinics
2. Consultation-liaison services
3. Subspecialty medicine clinics
4. Inpatient combined medical/psychiatry services
5. Combined medical psychiatric emergency department observation units

Broadening the clinical settings for psychiatry residents would augment their medical training in a way most useful to them in later practice. The majority of medical problems seen among psychiatric patients are similar to those medical problems seen in medical outpatients, such as diabetes, hypertension, and heart disease. The diagnosis, management, and psychiatric complications of these illnesses would be better taught in outpatient settings where psychiatric residents could follow patients longitudinally and collaboratively with their medical colleagues. Some psychiatric training programs are planning to train their psychiatric residents to treat the "top 10" medical problems in psychiatric patients typically seen in public settings (personal communication).

Psychiatry Training in Nonpsychiatric Training Programs

Training in psychiatry for nonpsychiatrists, particularly primary care specialists, is essential for obvious reasons. Cross-sectional studies have indicated that the prevalence of psychiatric disorders in primary care settings ranges from 30% to 50%. Most of these patients suffer from depressive, anxiety, or substance use disorders.

Failure to diagnose psychiatric problems in medical patients is typically blamed on doctors' personality deficiencies such as decreased altruism, inadequate compassion, or a deep-seated need to deny psychological problems. But there is little evidence that physicians really learn "to do" basic psychiatry in medical school or beyond. For example, physicians reported that their medical training had not done well in preparing them to assist heavy drinkers to modify their behavior or to identify depression in their patients (Cantor et al. 1993). Another study found that during their residencies few physicians are taught anything about the identification and acute treatment of patients who are "suicidal, homicidal, child- or spouse abusing, or violent" (Weissberg 1990).

Therefore, more attention must be paid to training nonpsychiatrists in psychiatry. As with psychiatry residents, a move from more inpatient-based training to more outpatient-based training is more likely to yield better results. One particular way to meet this need is to have psychiatry attendings available in primary care outpatient clinics for teaching collaborative evaluations. This model provides the primary care resident with immediate help in learning about psychiatry in a medical setting and is likely to be more useful than separate psychiatry rotations. Teaching sessions facilitated by these psychiatry attendings can also be used to cover important topics in psychiatry amenable to didactic sessions. For residents interested in more complex patients, a rotation on a consultation-liaison service could provide more intensive experiences in psychiatry.

Dual-Boarded Programs

For residents interested in both psychiatry and another specialty, a number of residencies offer programs leading to board eligibility in both areas of study. These programs typically integrate psychiatry and a primary care specialty (internal medicine, family practice, pediatrics), or neurology. Dual-boarded programs must meet the requirements for both specialties. In the case of internal medicine and psychiatry, there are approximately 20 residency programs offering dual programs (Accreditation Council on Graduate Medical Education 1996).

Although these programs do provide the additional training experience, it is not clear that residents completing one of these programs actually end up practicing both specialties. Although the conventional wisdom is that graduates of such programs ultimately will choose to practice one or the other, many graduates appear to choose academic careers (personal communication). Whether the additional board-certification enhances a practitioner's skills is unknown.

The main drawback of these programs is the additional time spent in training. However, for those persons entering academic fields, and for those small number of persons who intend to have an integrated practice, dual residencies may make sense. As of now, we are not aware of any data on this question.

A Tool for Enhanced Collaboration: A Basic Psychiatric Curriculum

A Psychiatric Core Curriculum

A clearly articulated core curriculum enhances and expands the possibilities of collaboration. Such a curriculum also allows for a *vertically as well as a horizontally* integrated curriculum. Therefore, the curriculum can be inserted repetitively in more than 1 year of medical school in a variety of venues, not just in psychiatry courses or psychiatry rotations. An example of such a minimal, basic curriculum is summarized in *The Colorado Medical Student Log* (Weissberg 1996). In outline, it consists of the following 10 core experiences and screens and seven diagnostic questions.

I. Ten Core Clinical Experiences

Students interview appropriate patients with faculty or residents and fulfill specific cognitive goals concerning:

1. Cognitive Disorders
2. Psychosis
3. Depression/Grief
4. Anxiety Disorders including PTSD
5. Substance Abuse
6. Sleep Disorders
7. Sexual Dysfunctions
8. Psychiatric Aspects of Medical Patients (at least five patients)
9. Child Psychiatry (at least two children)
10. Emergency Psychiatry

II. Ten Core Psychiatric Screens

Students are observed doing each screen at least twice:

1. The Mini-Mental State Examination
2. Substance Abuse (CAGE)
3. Sexual History for Dysfunction and High-Risk Behaviors
4. Suicide, Homicide
5. Family Violence: Child Abuse/Incest/Spouse Abuse
6. Trauma: Rape, Accidents, Disasters
7. Sleep Disorders
8. Depression/Hypomania
9. Anxiety
10. Eating Disorders

III. Seven Diagnostic Questions
Seven diagnostic questions must be asked about all patients. The medical and lethality questions must be asked right away; the others can wait:

1. Why is the patient here now?
2. What does the patient want/expect?
3. Is a general medical illness contributing to the patient's difficulties?
4. How lethal (suicide, violence, etc.) is the situation?
5. Are family/friends part of the problem or the solution?
6. What are the patients cultural expectations/explanations/treatment for their illness?
7. What is the psychiatric diagnosis?

Medicine for Psychiatric Residents
A medical curriculum for psychiatry residents should not only include knowledge objectives but also attitudinal and skill objectives. The following is a summary list of these objectives.

Attitudinal
1. Understand the importance of medical evaluations of psychiatric patients.
2. Learn the importance of psychiatrist-nonpsychiatrist alliances in the primary care setting.
3. Learn to deal with the stigma of being a psychiatrist in a primary care setting.

Knowledge Objectives
1. Recognition and maintenance treatment of common and uncomplicated medical conditions, for example, hypertension.
2. Guidelines for prevention and health maintenance of psychiatric patients.
3. Components of the history, examination, and laboratory tests that help differentiate general medical from psychiatric disease.
4. Psychiatric manifestations of patients with medical illness or symptoms.
5. Medical manifestations in patients with psychiatric illness, for example, hepatic encephalopathy, amenorrhea secondary to anorexia nervosa, and so on.
6. Psychiatric complications due to nonpsychiatric medications.
7. Medical complications of psychiatric medications.
8. The use of psychiatric medications in altered physiological conditions.
9. Competence assessments in medical patients.

Skill Objectives
1. The physical examination.
2. The use of laboratory and X ray in psychiatry.
3. Medical evaluation prior to psychiatric procedures, for example, ECT.
4. When to ask for a consultation and when to refer.

References

Accreditation Council on Graduate Medical Education: The 1996–97 Directory of Graduate Medical Education Programs. Chicago, IL, American Medical Association, 1996

American Psychiatric Association: Diagnostic and Statistical Manual of Mental Disorders, 3rd Edition, Revised. Washington, DC, American Psychiatric Association, 1987

American Psychiatric Association: Diagnostic and Statistical Manual of Mental Disorders, 4th Edition. Washington, DC, American Psychiatric Association, 1994

Cantor JC, Baker MA, Hughes RG: Preparedness for practice; young physicians' views of their profession. JAMA 270:1035–1040, 1993

McKegney FP, Weiner S: A consultation-liaison psychiatry clinical clerkship. Psychosom Med 38(1):45–54, 1976

Voineskos G, Greben SE, Lowy FH, et al: The psychiatric training of medical students. Can J Psychiatry 26:301–308, 1981

Weissberg MP: The meagerness of physicians' training in emergency psychiatric intervention. Acad Med 65:747–750, 1990

Weissberg MP: Less is more: the case for "basic" psychiatry and the Colorado Medical Student Log. Psychiatr Q 67(2):139–150, 1996

17

Administration of Residency Programs

David Bienenfeld, M.D.

The biopsychosocial model of human behavior, with which all psychiatrists are familiar, is a special application of *general systems theory*. General systems theory provides a framework for the derivation of administrative systems and the understanding of administrative dynamics (Figure 17–1). In this model, all systems are (1) *sets of interrelated objects* in (2) *an environment*. (3) *Inputs* from the environment enter the system and are utilized in (4) *processes* that perform the work of the system, yielding (5) *output*. The effect of that output on the environment provides (6) *feedback*. Viewing the residency training program as such a system allows for a coherent picture of its administration (Mann 1975).

The structure and function of the system are most productively determined by looking first at its output. The output of a residency program is well-trained and well-educated psychiatrists. With that goal in mind, the training director can analyze, design, implement, and assess the training process; the structure necessary to implement that process; the resources and ingredients on which the process operates; the environment that must be accommodated; and the feedback mechanisms of quality control.

The Process

The education of residents is a venture that demands flexibility, responsivity, and collaboration. Since there are numerous participants and stakehold-

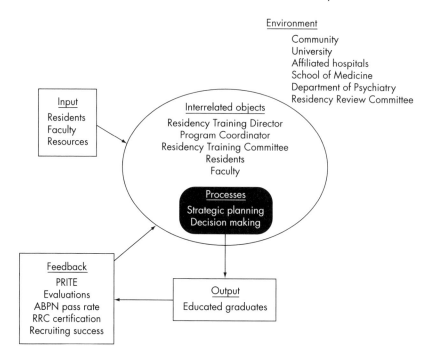

Figure 17–1. General systems outline of residency training.

ers in the educational process, and since the pressures and demands on the system are in constant flux, change and adaptability are essential characteristics of the successful program. Training directors, however, must be wary of losing sight of the program's broader purposes in the face of acute pressures. They must discriminate between the processes of *planning* and *governance,* between goal setting and problem solving.

Strategic planning is the process of setting long-range goals for the organization. The training program that has a clear and constant sense of mission will be best suited to accommodating short-term issues. Arriving at long-term goals requires consensus among the major participants: residents, faculty, and administrators. Typically, the derivation of a mission statement occurs in the setting of a program or departmental retreat. Usually such a retreat is a daylong event, held off-site from the everyday work environment, utilizing methods such as brainstorming and nominal group technique, often with the assistance of an outside facilitator.

The organizational mission statement should reflect the underlying purpose of the program, with enough specificity to be meaningful, and enough latitude to accommodate change over a period of years. The mission then defines the nature and number of residents selected for training, the content of the curriculum, the sites and services used in the program, the dimensions of resident evaluation, and all the other aspects of implementation. These factors are the objects of the governance of residency training; they are the products of the decision making, or problem-solving process.

Where strategic planning reflects constancy, decision making embodies the change that is required to maintain the survival of the mission. Both individuals and organizations are inherently resistant to change, and the effective leader is one who facilitates change with the least disruption and conflict. The most important dimension of organizational decision making is that it is participatory; voices of all relevant constituencies are heard. Although the chair may delegate authority to the residency training director, the power to implement policy requires the participation and collaboration of all parties.

Certainly, there are disadvantages to participatory decision making. It is time-consuming, and not useful for response to immediate crises. With the diffusion of responsibility, it becomes difficult to assign either credit or blame for the outcomes. The process may lead to the leader's being viewed as weak. It requires special leadership skills to attain consensus, if not unanimity.

Nonetheless, the advantages clearly outweigh the disadvantages. According to Floyd (1985), participatory decision making provides the following:

- Greater understanding and acceptance of decisions by the involved parties
- Greater identification with the decisions and more commitment to them
- Better morale within the program
- Consistency with the needs of mature faculty and residents for autonomy and achievement
- Group pressure on dissenters to comply
- Cooperation and team identification
- Availability of the particular skills of individuals to the entire organization.

The Interrelated Objects

The contingency theory of management maintains that there is no single best way to organize. The organizational structure must relate to both the purpose and the environment (Lawrence and Lorsch 1969). The participatory processes of strategic planning and decision making require an organizational structure that represents its constituencies, yet maintains the centrality and continuity of the program's mission.

Residency training directors function as both leaders and managers. They "carry the flag" of the educational mission and serve as its most consistent advocates, and they also coordinate the individuals and committees, the faculty and the residents, in making the daily work of teaching and learning possible.

Program coordinators (or administrative assistants) are responsible for implementation of the actions and decisions of the training director and the residency training committee. Much more than secretaries, coordinators maintain resident files and contracts, arrange applicant interviews, schedule special activities such as oral examinations and graduation, facilitate curriculum scheduling, compile material for communication to such agencies as the State Medical Board and the American Board of Psychiatry and Neurology, and solicit timely evaluations, among a host of other duties. The training director and program coordinator should ideally maintain a calendar of repeating events to allow for sufficient preparation (Table 17–1).

The program coordinator's role is vital to the success of the program. Coordinators are the first contact with applicants, and with residents within the program who have issues for the training director. In practice, the administrative coordinator provides a nurturing and sustaining role that far transcends the administrative job description.

The *associate (or assistant) training director* has a role more idiosyncratically defined in each program. In smaller programs, there may be none at all. In others, there may be one assistant director for the entire program; or there may be several, with each associate director responsible for education at one affiliate institution.

The *residency training committee*, also called the educational policy committee, serves as the major collaborative planning and decision-making body in the training program. Its composition should reflect those with the greatest investment in the educational process. Typically, membership will include the residency training director as chair, the associate training

Table 17–1. Annual calendar—residency training

Month	Program Coordinator	Residency Training Director
July	New residents begin.	New residents begin.
August	Schedule semiannual reviews; send reminder to each resident about 3 weeks ahead. Schedule live patient oral examinations. Send each resident reminder plus description/instruction sheet. Resident picnic. Review recruitment materials.	Begin receiving and screening applications for residency.
September	Schedule PRITE. Clear with clinical sites; get room and preceptors. Schedule Residency Selection Committee meetings. Begin scheduling applicant interviews. Send evaluation forms for July–September.	Fall Components Meeting, APA.
October	PRITE.	PRITE. Begin interviews with resident applicants.
November		Deans' letters released.
December	Holiday party. Send evaluation forms for October–December.	Holiday party.
January	Request ABPN results of graduates.	
February	Recruiting dinner for local applicants. NRMP Match list due (fourth Wednesday).	NRMP Match list due.
March	Send appointment letters to newly matched residents. Start scheduling audiovisual oral exams for April: recruit examiners, notify sites and residents. Send evaluation forms for January–March. Send post-Match questionnaires to applicants who matched elsewhere.	AADPRT annual meeting NRMP results announced. After-Match recruiting, if necessary.

(continued)

Table 17–1. Continued

Month	Program Coordinator	Residency Training Director
April	Audiovisual oral exams. Mailings to incoming residents.	Prepare rotation and seminar schedules for July–June. Assign psychotherapy supervisors. Submit budget requests to hospitals. Chief residents selected.
May	Graduation plans.	APA annual meeting. Review and revise orientation manual.
June	Prepare certificates of completion of PGY-I and residency for graduating residents, for ABPN. Send evaluation forms for April–June. Prepare contracts for new residents. Graduation. Orient new residents.	Chief residents' national conference. Graduation. Orient new residents.

director(s), chiefs of relevant divisions or services (such as consultation-liaison and child psychiatry), other faculty integral to the curriculum, and resident representatives. The training committee is responsible for designing, evaluating, and refining the curriculum; determining policy; allocating resident workforce; disseminating information; and evaluating residents in academic difficulty.

Task forces and *work groups* may be delegated by the training director or the residency training committee to accomplish specific tasks that are of limited duration or require special expertise. Such tasks may include proposing specific didactic curricula, designing evaluation instruments, researching solutions adopted at other programs to a particular problem, or organizing a PGY-I mentorship program.

Input

The ingredients that ultimately yield classes of educated and trained psychiatrists are the residents themselves, the faculty, and the resources available to both. Other chapters of this book deal specifically with resident recruitment and faculty development. Our focus here is on the administrative integration of these elements into the training program.

Once the National Resident Matching Program results are announced, or once a resident and training program have otherwise committed to each other, a contract must be finalized. The elements of the contract will vary across institutions but should always include the identities of the parties, the exact nature of the position, the salary and benefits, the duration of the contract and terms of its renewal and cancellation, and the obligations and responsibilities of the parties (Table 17–2). There must be a "due process" policy in place at the institutional and/or program level to clarify procedures and alternatives when a resident has academic or professional difficulties. Most commonly, this policy is contained in a resident policy manual, to which reference may be made in the contract (see also Chapter 21).

The resources used by the training program include clinical facilities, clerical and administrative services, and, of course, money. Clarification of the nature of these commitments allows for optimum strategic planning. Although contracts and agreements with clinical facilities are generally conducted at the department level or higher, the residency training director should have familiarity with their content and, ideally, input into their provisions (Wilson and McLaughlin 1984). Such agreements should specify the following:

- Clinical facilities and services committed
- Staff and personnel committed
- Terms of financial exchange
- Lines of authority and responsibility
- Individual and institutional liability coverage
- Mechanisms of quality review and quality control

Contracts with faculty generally cover their obligations and commitments to the educational program, which are discussed elsewhere in this book.

The Environment

Thus far, we have considered primarily the *participants* in the educational program: the training director, his or her committees, the program coordinator, the faculty, and the residents. These figures operate in a complicated

Table 17–2. Elements of the resident contract

   I. Parties to the contract
      A. Hospital, University, School of Medicine
      B. Resident
  II. Duration of contract: beginning and ending dates
 III. Title or name of position
  IV. Salary
      A. Amount
      B. Payment schedule
   V. Benefits
      A. Insurance
         1. Health
         2. Life
         3. Disability
      B. Perquisites
         1. Travel funds
         2. Book funds
         3. Moving expenses
         4. Uniforms, laundry
         5. Meals
  VI. Professional liability insurance
 VII. Work and duty parameters
      A. Normal duty hours
      B. Vacation
      C. Sick leave
      D. Parental leave
      E. Educational leave
VIII. Employer obligations
      A. Provision of suitable educational environment
      B. Training program that meets standards of accreditation
  IX. Resident obligations
      A. Satisfactory academic and clinical performance
      B. Conformance to applicable procedures and bylaws
      C. Ethical and professional behavior
   X. Conditions and procedures for termination of contract

---

context, and their choices and behavior are shaped powerfully by nonparticipant *stakeholders*. Stakeholders are the individuals, groups and institutions that affect and are affected by the policies and products of the training program (Srivastva 1983). The missions of the department, the school of medicine, the affiliated hospitals, and the university must all be accommodated in training program decisions. Political, social, and economic elements of the community and the society at large have a powerful influence. Decisions in organizations are reached as often on the basis of environmental exigencies as on internal logic and desirability (Griffith 1979).

Training directors often operate at the boundaries of the program and its environment. They are the chief spokespeople for the training program. In this position, it is advisable that the training director reach consensus with the stakeholder about goals and missions. The position rarely carries enough authority for the training director to be a parochial advocate for the program's interests in opposition to those of the department, the college, or the hospital (Wilson and McLaughlin 1984). Cultivation of relationships with stakeholders is part of the ongoing maintenance of the program's effectiveness.

Outside the local environment, a host of entities operate to influence the function of each residency training program. This jumble of acronyms is decoded in Table 17–3 (Strauss and Preven 1991).

Feedback

Maintaining and improving quality education requires "closing the loop," constantly assessing the process and the product. The principles and practice of evaluating individuals are discussed elsewhere in this book. The evaluation of program quality may use some of the same measures but constitutes a separate process.

The Residency Review Committee (RRC) for Psychiatry of the Accreditation Council on Graduate Medical Education (ACGME) undertakes regular evaluations of training programs for the purpose of certification. This ACGME accreditation, however, certifies only that minimum standards have been met and does not comprise a true measure of quality. By the time RRC certification is in danger, there have generally already been serious deficits in program quality.

Success at recruiting new residents is a measure of the program's quality as perceived by applicants. Group mean scores on the Psychiatry Resident In-Training Examination (PRITE) allow cognitive gains to be followed from year to year. The American Board of Psychiatry and Neurology (ABPN) provides records of the test results of a program's graduates. More direct, but more difficult to obtain, are evaluations of graduates' performance by their employers or colleagues. Similarly, recent graduates can be

Table 17–3. Organizations influencing functions of the training program

AADPRT—American Association of Directors of Psychiatric Residency Education. Includes the training directors of nearly all training programs in the United States. Also includes associate directors and fellowship directors. Provides education and advocacy for training directors.

AAP—Association for Academic Psychiatry. An organization of psychiatric educators providing education and camaraderie for teachers of students and residents.

ABPN—American Board of Psychiatry and Neurology. The organization that administers written and oral examinations to postgraduate physicians and certifies their safety and competence.

ACGME—Accreditation Council for Graduate Medical Education. Sponsored by the American Board of Medical Specialties, the American Hospital Association, the American Medical Association, the AAMC, and the Council of Medical Specialties. Certifies that institutions have met standards for accreditation of their residency training programs. See also **RRC**.

APA—American Psychiatric Association. The chief professional organization of American psychiatry. Represents the political, economic, and educational interests of its 40,000 members. APA's Office of Education provides information, consultation, assistance, and liaison with other wings of the APA. Within the Component structure of the APA, the Committee on Graduate Education deals specifically with residency issues, and reports to the Council on Medical Education and Career Development.

ECFMG—Educational Commission for Foreign Medical Graduates. Provides certification of graduation from non-U.S. medical schools and administers examinations of readiness of international medical graduates to enter residency training in the United States.

HCFA—Health Care Finance Administration. The regulatory agency that sets and administers policy for distribution of Medicare funds, the largest single source of residency stipend money.

NBME—National Board of Medical Examiners. Organization that formerly administered the examination for licensure eligibility in the United States. See also **USMLE**.

NRMP—National Resident Matching Program. The official cooperative plan for appointments to graduate medical education. NRMP operates the "Match" each spring that constitutes the primary vehicle for U.S. medical graduates to enter residency training programs.

PRITE—Psychiatry Resident In-Training Examination. Sponsored by the American College of Psychiatrists, this 5-hour written examination is administered each fall. Results are for internal use only.

RRC—Residency Review Committee. A subgroup of the ACGME that reviews programs in each respective specialty. The RRC for Psychiatry certifies psychiatric training programs.

USMLE—United States Medical Licensing Examination. The three-step examination required for licensure eligibility in the United States. Replaces the former FLEX and NBME examinations. Non-U.S. medical graduates must first pass an examination of English proficiency.

surveyed or interviewed about the relevance of their training to the needs of their careers (Langsley 1986).

Within the program, evaluations of rotations, seminars, and teachers by the residents can provide a picture of their perceived value. Such evaluations must be tempered by the realization that popularity and quality are separate dimensions; an unpopular rotation or an uncharismatic teacher may wind up providing the knowledge and skills that will ultimately prove most useful to the graduate physician.

In the end, evaluation is an ongoing process. It is among the most important functions of the residency training committee. Determining the desired outcomes allows the committee to have in mind its benchmarks as it assesses the quality of the training program.

References

Floyd CE: Faculty Participation in Decision Making: Necessity or Luxury? Washington DC, Association for the Study of Higher Education, 1985, pp 1–10

Griffith F: Decision-making, in Administrative Theory in Education: Text and Readings. Midland, MI, Pendell, 1979, pp 233–244

Langsley DG: Evaluation during residency, in How to Evaluate Residents. Edited by Lloyd JS, Langsley DG. Chicago, IL, American Board of Medical Specialties, 1986, pp 11–30

Lawrence PR, Lorsch JW: Organization and Environment: Managing Differences and Integration. New York, Irwin, 1969

Mann D: Problems of organizational calculation, in Policy Decision-Making in Education: An Introduction to Calculation and Control. New York, Teachers College Press, 1975, pp 53–83

Srivastva S: Common themes in executive thought and action, in The Executive Mind: New Insights on Managerial Thought and Action. Edited by Srivastva S. San Francisco, CA, Jossey-Bass, 1983, pp 1–14

Strauss GD, Preven DW: Administering the residency program, in Handbook of Psychiatry Residency Training. Edited by Kay J. Washington, DC, American Psychiatric Association, 1991, pp 1–16

Wilson MP, McLaughlin CP: Organizational relationships and leadership roles, Leadership and Management in Academic Medicine. San Francisco, CA, Jossey-Bass, 1984, pp 78–114

18

Developing and Monitoring the Curriculum

Linda Andrews, M.D., and James W. Lomax, M.D.

In the first edition of this *Handbook*, Yager et al. (1991) asserted that the identity of the training director as a department expert in education was "forged and reaffirmed on a daily basis through the development and monitoring of the curriculum" (p. 17). We agree with this assertion and add that, in contrast to some other aspects of residency administration (particularly management of "troubling or troubled residents"), the tasks related to curriculum development are extremely gratifying and substantially contribute to job satisfaction in residency education.

This is not to say that curriculum development is without significant tensions and conflict. In fact, such tensions are inherent and range from conceptual and philosophical differences to the most mundane financial and logistical considerations. Each program must consider the core elements of a psychiatrist's professional identity and how these are formed from clinical and didactic educational experiences. And, within each program, sharp philosophical differences may exist about the relative emphasis on "biological," "psychological," and "sociocultural" perspectives represented in the curriculum (Mohl 1995).

At no other time in the history of American medical education has there been more tension around the economics of the current educational enterprise and the future practice of psychiatry. Is the residency director helping or hurting residents by emphasizing "education for managed care"?

This is an important question for programs to discuss. What is perhaps most clear is that new educational partnerships must be forged to support the educational enterprise. Difficult decisions may have to be made regarding whether traditional educational sites can continue to be used when they are being transformed to meet the needs and expectations of cost containment. Of course, these theoretical and practical considerations must also fit with local resources.

It is impossible for any residency program, even within the most prestigious and largest departments, to provide experiences in all treatment modalities with all types of patient problems. The residency director, with input from the educational committees of the department, must forge a curriculum that provides "broad" enough didactic and clinical exposure to enable graduates to choose many posttraining practice options, yet also "deep" enough to allow graduates to perform at a specialist level of competency.

The criteria for required didactic and clinical experiences are covered in other sections of this text and are delineated in the Residency Review Committee's Essentials for Psychiatry. However, the specifics of "content" and "timing" of didactic and clinical experiences remain the residency director's decision.

The educational principle of "first things first" is germane and helpful in making "content" and "timing" curriculum decisions. Teach first in the most-supervised settings with expansion to less-structured and less-supervised settings as trainees gain experience. Teach first the easiest material and concepts, followed by more difficult and complex material and tasks (i.e., memorization of drug doses may be easier than understanding and experiencing transference and countertransference phenomena). Teach first what residents need to know immediately or material and concepts that will get residents in the most trouble if they don't know them. Teaching what residents will likely see while on call, or teaching about common psychiatric emergencies, will be quickly absorbed and retained, whereas teaching about gender differences in psychological development may seem esoteric and irrelevant during the first 6 months of residency. Of course, residents will feel that they need to learn everything at the beginning, but residency education is a process and one of the first curriculum struggles will occur around what should be taught first.

Another guiding principle for curriculum development is that the more people you involve in planning and the more people who agree before implementation is attempted, the more successful you will be in developing, changing, or monitoring that curriculum. We recommend a two-tier planning approach. First a "core planning group," consisting of the training director, associate/assistant training director, chief resident, and possibly service chiefs, should initiate the curriculum review process, and the core group should know the rules and requirements of training, the financial resources, and idiosyncratic scheduling issues. A larger "consulting" group should consist of greater numbers of faculty and residents, including teaching faculty, clinical and supervising faculty, and resident representatives from all training levels. Many programs have a Residency Program Committee (RPC), which essentially equals this "consulting" group or might serve as the initial core on which to add additional faculty and residents. In a new program, the consulting group could develop suggestions for the curriculum. For existing programs, the consulting group could (a) review current didactic and clinical curricula, (b) provide suggestions for change in existing experiences, and (c) provide suggestions for how to implement any changes. The larger consulting group should also be involved in the ongoing assessment and evaluation of various curricular elements. This may be best accomplished by assigning subcommittees of the larger consulting group the task to review specific curricular elements. The larger consulting group can also serve to assist the core planning group when site visits are expected from the Residency Review Committee.

A suggested timetable for curriculum development is as follows: (1) fine-tuning should occur monthly (via RPC meetings) with annual implementation of suggested changes, (2) all new curricular elements should be thoroughly reviewed during their first year of implementation and then as part of subsequent routine reviews if no special problems arise, and (3) the entire curriculum should be reviewed every 4 to 5 years. This more extensive review should include solicitation of feedback and suggestions from 5 to 10 years of recent program graduates, and solicitation of feedback from outstanding residency programs in the country regarding their curricular development. Obtaining such feedback allows one to assess the program's past performance and plan for its future, building on old strengths or creating new strengths when necessary. The entire faculty should be notified annually of significant curricular changes. The training director and associate/ assistant training director should begin by April or May to plan all curricular elements to be implemented that next July 1. The larger review, occurring every 4 to 5 years, should occur either in the late fall or early spring so that major changes can be organized for implementation the following July 1.

Evaluation of the resident, faculty, and the educational experience itself should occur in both verbal and written forms at the end of each didactic experience and clinical rotation and via formal semiannual evaluations with each resident. We also suggest regular monthly resident forums to discuss training experiences and a mechanism whereby this feedback can be transmitted by the chief resident to the training director. A monthly "resident business meeting" or "residents' association" chaired by the chief resident with faculty present only by specific invitation is a particularly useful vehicle to obtain candid feedback. An annual resident retreat or some similar mechanism for a structured review of the curriculum by residents should take place in the early spring, to leave time to plan for July 1 implementation of suggestions (Claman et al. 1995). For new curricular elements, special attention should be paid to evaluation of the faculty teachers and of the new elements themselves.

The following is a general outline of goals for and models of didactic curriculum, clinical curriculum, and supervision. For didactic, clinical, and supervision curricula, each experience must have written goals and objectives. Although initially labor-intensive, creating goals and objectives ultimately makes easier reviews of minor or new elements as well as large program reviews. In the appendixes at the end of this chapter, you will find graphic templates of specific models for the didactic and clinical curricula. We will close this chapter with some comments about special curricular elements, collaborating with other departments, and faculty as teachers.

Models for Didactic Curriculum

As mentioned in the introduction, the tension about a relative balance among biologic, psychologic, and sociocultural aspects of psychiatry will be played out when developing the didactic curriculum. Baylor recently developed a system using "tracks," representing six core content areas, as a strategy for structuring didactics. The tracks include: (1) Psychotherapy, (2) Psychopharmacology, (3) Research, (4) Ethics, (5) Neuroscience, and (6) Descriptive Psychiatry, which encompasses psychopathology, phenomenology, and specialty areas such as child psychiatry, geriatric psychiatry, consultation-liaison psychiatry, and addiction psychiatry. All six of these tracks are taught during all four residency training years. The complexity and sophistication of content within a given track builds over the 4 years, focusing on learning the basics first, then special situations, then advanced concepts, and, last, integration. A faculty member and resident serve as track coordinators to oversee the content across all 4 years and to monitor for planned and unplanned redundancy (see Appendixes 18–A to 18–F). This *Handbook*, the expansion of computer learning, and nationally developed model didactic curricula should make curricular design easier for new programs, for training programs undergoing curriculum revisions, or for training programs combining with other programs (Burt et al. 1995; Garza-Trevino et al. 1997; Klein and Glick 1996; Lambert and Fowler 1996; Marin et al. 1988; Scully 1996; Spielvogal et al. 1995; Thompson 1996; Yager et al. 1988).

Models for Clinical Curriculum

Similar questions about balance occur when planning the clinical curriculum. The conceptual framework that residents be taught the basics first, then special situations, then advanced concepts, and conclude with integration, can apply to the clinical curriculum as well. Clearly, site availability and clinical supervisor availability will dictate some of the specifics. However, the following general structure is followed by most programs. Inpatient psychiatry, emergency psychiatry, and consultation-liaison psychiatry with adult patients tend to precede outpatient experiences or experiences with subspecialty populations, such as children or geriatric patients (see appendixes). The level of clinical supervision should progress from most intense to least intense, with almost independent practice occurring in PGY-IV. Elective and selective rotations usually appear later in training, as residents have greater levels of expertise, confidence, and notions of the type of psychiatry they aspire to practice.

A residency documentation system can be helpful for monitoring gaps in residency education. These documentation systems are becoming more useful and necessary as residents apply for jobs in controlled-care settings where they must prove their level of expertise and training experience for treating various patient populations. Therefore, quality monitoring/documenting should be discussed and formalized for both the didactic and clinical curriculum. At Baylor and an increasing number of other programs, a computerized scanner read log of clinical experiences greatly facilitates this documentation process.

Models for Supervision

Providing supervision is clearly program-specific since resources vary widely across programs. However, the same conceptual framework can be used to educate supervisors about expectations of supervision varying by residency level, that is, basics, special situations, advanced concepts, and integration. Questions about attendance and evaluation must be carefully discussed, because this curricular element's success depends highly on the individual supervisor and implementation can more easily "fall through the cracks." The residency director must know the financial arrangements that the department makes with its supervisors and the departmental requirements for voluntary faculty participation. Supervision is frequently a popular way for voluntary faculty to maintain a faculty appointment.

Supervisory Interventions (Jacobs et al. 1995)

1. Modeling—demonstrate how supervisor thinks, reasons, and arrives at decisions by discussing this process with supervisee.
2. Didactic instruction—directly explain specific content areas (i.e., DSM-IV [American Psychiatric Association 1994] criteria, defense mechanisms, differential diagnosis, etc.).
3. Socratic questioning—use questions to increase supervisee's active exploration of issue/content.
4. Encouragement and permission—help supervisee discuss countertransference, try new therapeutic techniques, and develop his or her own style.
5. Clarification—comment on aspects of the supervisee's attitude or behavior to encourage self-reflective thinking (slight shift from "focus on patient" to "focus on resident")
6. Interpretation—(riskiest of techniques) interpret "parallel process," comment on supervisee's affect, dynamics and defenses of which resident seems unaware.

Qualities of Good Supervision (Kline et al. 1997)

1. Supervisor is *active* and *aggressive* in teaching.
   a. Stimulates resident to conceptualize a theoretical understanding
   b. Pushes resident to limits of capacity
   c. Shows unambiguous communication

    d. Is in touch with therapeutic problem

    e. Communicates emotional involvement

2. Supervisor is *focused on the patient* and cases' details.

    a. Discusses the transference

    b. Understands patient's dynamics or the content

    c. Understands the process between the patient and therapist

    d. Uses extrapolation

Special Curricular Elements

There are several areas within a residency program that do not clearly fall under the rubric of either the didactic or clinical curriculum. These elements tend to be monitored more directly by either the clinical site supervisors or the residency training directors. Examples include site-based clinical case conferences, teaching rounds, journal clubs, and grand rounds. The training director must be aware of the goals, objectives, and content of each didactic and clinical element in the program to guide clinical site supervisors about teaching emphasis. Most typically, these special curricular components are used to either supplement material already taught in the core didactic and clinical elements or to be sure that concepts taught in the didactic curriculum can be implemented in actual clinical situations.

Chapter 16 discusses collaboration with other departments in greater detail. We would only like to comment that in these financially challenging and constraining times and during the current emphasis on primary care, it may become fiscally necessary and clinically relevant to teach psychiatry in nonpsychiatric settings and to collaborate across departments for seminars, grand rounds, journal clubs, and board reviews. The current academic climate makes such collaboration significantly more possible than in past times. As requirements for psychiatric experiences increase for nonpsychiatry residency training programs, and as the cost of training increases for everyone, collaboration may allow programs within a school to share the ever-expanding educational burden and create even more useful training experiences for psychiatry and nonpsychiatry residents alike.

The availability of faculty to teach formally in the didactic curriculum and less formally in the clinical curriculum and the ratio of full-time to voluntary faculty is variable across training programs. As mentioned in the introduction, programs with large faculty pools will have the most resources upon which to draw. However, potential disadvantages exist as programs get larger. As program size increases, it is more difficult to check feedback mechanisms, monitor resident and faculty participation, and ensure consistency across experiences. The training director, in concert with the department chair, ought to know the faculty pool and who is available to teach in various capacities. Some of the special curricular elements provide the easiest and optimal ways to involve voluntary faculty. Other tasks that allow faculty involvement include mock board exams, student oral exams, and research mentoring. It is useful to poll your entire faculty for any suggestions of innovative teaching techniques. This helps keep the curriculum from becoming stagnant or routine. Finally, do not hesitate to use teaching resources that have been developed by other departments of your school or hospitals.

References

American Psychiatric Association: Diagnostic and Statistical Manual of Mental Disorders, 4th Edition. Washington, DC, American Psychiatric Association, 1994

Burt VK, Yager J, Lundgren J: Providing residents with a comprehensive educational program in outpatient psychiatry: integrating an outpatient curriculum into outpatient management teams. Academic Psychiatry 19(1):22–29, 1995

Claman L, Miller DA, Altshuler KZ: Psychiatry department retreats: uses and benefits. Academic Psychiatry 19(12):45–47, 1995

Garza-Trevino ES, Ruiz P, Venegas-Samuels K: A psychiatric curriculum directed to the care of the Hispanic patient. Academic Psychiatry 21(1):1–10, 1997

Jacobs D, David P, Meyer DJ: Supervisory interventions, in The Supervisory Encounter. Edited by Jacobs D, David P, Meyer DJ. New Haven, CT, Yale University Press, 1995, pp 179–206

Klein DF, Glick ID: Curriculum for Residency Training Directors and Teachers of Psychopharmacology. New York, American Society of Clinical Psychopharmacology, 1996

Kline F, Goin MK, Zimmerman W: You can be a better supervisor! J Psychiatr Educ 1(2): 174–179, 1977

Lambert MT, Fowler DR: Psychiatric education at a veteran affairs medical center. Academic Psychiatry 20(1):56–63, 1996

Marin RS, Foster JR, Ford CV, et al: A curriculum for education in geriatric psychiatry. Am J Psychiatry 145:836–843, 1988

Mohl PD: What is a balanced program? Academic Psychiatry 19(2):94–100, 1995

Scully JH: A basic model ethics curriculum for psychiatric residents. APA Taskforce to Develop Model Curricular Material on Medical Psychiatry Ethics, APA Office of Education, Washington, DC, January 1996

Spielvogal AM, Dichstein LJ, Robinson GE: A psychiatric residency curriculum about gender and women's issues. Academic Psychiatry 19(4):187–198, 1995

Thompson JW: Curriculum for learning about American Indian and Alaskan natives in psychiatric residency training. Academic Psychiatry 20(1):5–12, 1996

Yager, J, Borus JF, Robinowitz CB, et al: Developing minimal national standards for clinical experience in psychiatric training. Am J Psychiatry 145:1409–1413, 1988

Yager J, Kay J, Winstead DK: Developing and monitoring the curriculum, in Handbook of Psychiatry Residency Training. Edited by Kay G. Washington, DC, American Psychiatric Association, 1991, pp 17–47

Goals

Didactic Curriculum

1. Meet RRC requirements.
2. Follow a logical, systematic, and organized sequence through all 4 years of training.
3. Be appropriate in content and process to the level of residency training.
4. Be reasonably temporally "paired" or parallel to related clinical curricular elements.
5. Use textbooks to organize seminars whenever possible. Current journal articles to be used PRN.
6. Use active teaching/clinical demonstrations whenever possible.*
7. Didactic experiences should be supported by the chairman and residency director so that attendance is encouraged, expected, monitored, and rewarded.
8. Involve as many faculty, clinical and voluntary, as possible to maximize resources to produce optimal didactic experiences.

Clinical Curriculum

1. Meet RRC requirements.
2. Follow a logical, systematic, and organized sequence across all 4 years of training.
3. Be appropriate in content and experience to the level of residency training, especially with respect to the level of supervision needed for the appropriate level of training.
4. Be reasonably temporally "paired" or parallel to related didactic curricular elements.
5. Consider clinical site availability for the individual program and adjust clinical curriculum content and process accordingly.
6. Allow flexibility to maximize strengths and minimize weaknesses of the individual program.

Supervision

1. Meet RRC requirements.
2. Use supervisors who are aware of cognitive and experiential skill levels for

---

* This may require lecturers to update their teaching styles, and, therefore, teaching skill development should be included in overall faculty development.

various residency training levels and use supervisors' experience appropriately (i.e., ask the voluntary faculty members to request the level of trainee that they wish to supervise, given their own abilities to teach "novices" or "experts").

3. Involve as many faculty, clinical and voluntary, as possible to maximize resources to produce optimal supervisory experiences.

4. Provide supervisors with expectations and goals and objectives of supervision and education of what constitutes "good supervision." Provide feedback to supervisors, especially for new supervisors, to help model good supervision and mold the supervisory practices.

Baylor College of Medicine Department of Psychiatry Four-Year Rotational Outline

| PGY-I | Medicine 4 mo. or Pediatrics & Medicine 2 mo. each | | Neurology 2 mo. | Harris County Hospital District Hospital Psychiatry 6 mo. | | |

| PGY-II | Methodist Inpatient 3 mo. | Consultation and Liaison 3 mo. | Child and Adolescent 2 mo. | VA Inpatient 2 mo. | Emergency Psych 1 mo. | Gero-Psych 1 mo. |

PGY-III	Outpatient Treatment of Special Populations—1/3 time, 12 mo.
	Community Treatment of Severe Mental Illness—1/3 time, 12 mo.
	Baylor Psychiatry Clinic—1/3 time, 12 mo.

PGY-IV	Teaching and Administrative Psychiatry 3/4 time, 3 mo.	Electives 3/4 time, 3 mo.	Selectives: St. Luke's Hospital C/L, Advanced Psychopharmacology, Women's Home Halfway House, Jewish Family Services, etc. 3/4 time, 6 mo.
	Baylor Psychiatry Clinic—1/4 time, 12 mo.		

During PGY-I, the Harris County Hospital District psychiatry rotation is divided between the inpatient service at Quentin Mease Community Hospital (appropriately 4 months), the Emergency Psychiatry Service at Ben Taub (4–6 weeks) and the Consultation and Liaison Service at Ben Taub (4–6 weeks).

During PGY-II, the Geropsychiatry month may be replaced by a rotation with a research mentor if a resident is interested in the research tract or by an "away" elective. The program does not provide any funds for away electives. These substitute rotations are negotiated during March of the resident's PGY-I year.

During PGY-III, the "special populations" rotation includes outpatient assignments in geriatrics and substance abuse for all residents and elective assignments with a variety of other special patient populations (HIV +, abused women, high-risk pregnancies, etc.) or treatment techniques (group therapy, family therapy, etc.). Each year up to four residents may apply for a research track. These residents divide their time between research with an approved departmental mentor and their assignments to the community-based treatment of severe mental illness, the Baylor Psychiatry Clinic (the rotation dedicated to the learning of psychotherapeutic treatments) and the outpatient treatment of special populations and reduced in quantity. Research track assignments are individually negotiated and approved during March of the PGY-II year.

In PGY-IV, the only required new assignment for all residents is the administrative psychiatry rotation with teaching and administrative responsibility for medical students and more junior residents on the inpatient units at the VA or Hospital District. Most residents continue their Baylor Clinic patients as a quarter-time assignment throughout the year. A wide variety of electives are available.

Sample of PGY-I Didactic
Curriculum Outline
(6 months: July–December/January–June)

Month	1	2	3	4	5	6

| Psychopharmacology (16) | | | | | | |

| Descriptive Psychiatry (13) | | | | Psych Testing (5) † | Intro to Research (4) | |

| Emergency Psychiatry (8) | | Interviewing (8) ‡ | | Intro to Psychotherapy (6) | | |

| | Forensics and Ethics (11) | | | Intro to Neurosciences (9) | | |

Psychopharmacology	16
Psychotherapy	19
Descriptive Psychiatry	21
Neurosciences	9
Ethics	11
Research	4
	80

---

† case examples to demonstrate testing
‡ resident videotapes
All other seminars are lecture with assigned reading format.

Sample of PGY-II Didactic Curriculum Outline (12 months)

Advanced Psychopharmacology (20)

Psychotherapy (85)

Descriptive (65)

Neurosciences (10)

Ethics (8)

Research (8)

Psychotherapy (85)—Includes courses:

Empathy Seminar	Movies & audio/videotaped examples &
Introduction to Psychotherapy	resident videotapes
Basic Principles of Human Behavior	Videotaped examples
Cognitive Therapy	Lecture and readings
Behavioral Therapy	Audio/videotaped examples
Process Group	Demonstration of techniques
Introduction to Baylor Clinic	Experiential group
	Lecture & charting demonstration

Descriptive Psychiatry (65)—Includes courses:

Consultation/Liaison Psychiatry, Cultural Psychiatry, Geriatrics, Hypnosis, Sleep Disorders, Psychopathology, Child Psychiatry

Total Hours: 175

APPENDIX 18-E

Sample of PG-III
Didactic Curriculum Outline

July	Aug	Sept	Oct	Nov	Dec	Jan	Feb	Mar	Apr	May	June
Community Psych (6)		Marital Therapy (7)†	Psych & Religion (6)	Human Development (23)							
		Adv. Research (5)		Adv. Psychopharm II (10)		Advanced Ethics (12)			Teaching Res to Teach (4)‡		
Family Therapy (4)		Adv. Ind. Psychotherapy (16)§				Brain & Behavior (24)					

Psychopharmacology	10
Psychotherapy	50
Descriptive	16
Neurosciences	24
Ethics	12
Research	5
	117

There are also two case conferences in PGY-III: one Psychotherapy and one Psychopharmacology.

† lecture and case examples; ‡ demonstration of techniques; § case examples to illustrate principles. All other seminars are lecture with assigned reading format.

379

Sample of PGY-IV
Didactic Curriculum Outline

July	Aug	Sept	Oct	Nov	Dec	Jan	Feb	Mar	Apr	May	June

Board Review Course (29) — Resident organized   Integrated Patient Mgmt (8)[†]

Brief Psychotherapy (15)[†]

Transition to Practice (8)[§] | Advanced Ind.[‡] Psychotherapy (10) | Adv (5) Forensics

Psych Issues of Men/Women (14)   Sex Dysf. (4)

Psychopharmacology	37 integrated
Psychotherapy	39 + 37 integrated
Descriptive	12 + 37 integrated
Neurosciences	37 integrated
Ethics	5 + 37 integrated
Research	37 integrated
	93 total hours

[†] case examples to illustrate principles
[‡] open discussion of problems
[§] guest speakers discussing practice options
All other seminars are lecture with assigned reading format.

19

Fulfilling the Special Requirements

Stefan Stein, M.D.

We Know How Difficult Accreditation Can Be— So What's Good About It?

Accreditation is a critical element in maintaining the quality of graduate medical education in the United States. It establishes uniform minimal standards for residency programs responsible for preparing physicians for independent practice and ensures that residents are not exploited or carelessly trained. And, particularly in a climate of economic scarcity, it provides program directors with powerful weapons to use in dealing with administrators who would prefer residency programs that cost little and supply much service. Finally, it ensures that sponsoring institutions provide the administrative support necessary for educationally sound residency programs.

The Accreditation Process—An Overview

All U.S. graduate medical education programs are accredited by the Accreditation Council for Graduate Medical Education (ACGME), which is jointly sponsored by the American Board of Medical Specialties, the American Hospital Association, the American Medical Association, the Association of American Medical Colleges, and the Council of Medical Specialty Societies. In psychiatry the ACGME accredits programs in general psychiatry, and in the specialties of addiction psychiatry, child and adolescent psychiatry, forensic psychiatry, and geriatric psychiatry.

The ACGME delegates responsibility for the accreditation process for all psychiatry programs to the Residency Review Committee for Psychiatry (RRC). The RRC is composed of representatives nominated by its "parents," the American Board of Psychiatry and Neurology, the AMA Council on Medical Education, and the American Psychiatric Association.

The ACGME itself reviews all institutions in which residency programs are cited using the standards of the institutional requirements (American Medical Association 1995, pp. 14–16). This component of the accreditation process ensures that the institution (usually a hospital) provides the support and resources necessary for residents to function in an educationally sound manner.

The institution is required by the ACGME, for example, to maintain a graduate medical education committee that regularly reviews and oversees the educational programs in the hospital. It must also guarantee that financial support for resident stipends and benefits is available. It is charged with the responsibility of ensuring that applicants to residencies are informed about sickness and parental leave policies, liability insurance as well as health insurance, and other benefits. It requires that on call responsibilities be specified and that residents not be required to perform hospital duties appropriate to other staff. In summary, the ACGME institutional requirements specify the conditions that the hospital must meet to provide a setting where graduate medical education can take place with a minimum of interference by institutional problems and demands.

The RRC has two major functions: (1) It prepares and publishes the Program Requirements (often referred to as "the Essentials") for each specialty and subspecialty (American Medical Association 1995, pp. 218–238) program for which it has responsibility, and (2) it conducts reviews of individual programs. The Program Requirements are the written standards against which the programs are measured for accreditation purposes.

The Process of Review of Individual Programs

Documentation

Each program seeking accreditation or reaccreditation must prepare and submit a Program Information Form (referred to as the PIF and available on computer disk) provided by the RRC. This lengthy document provides the program's description of itself, and is used by the site visitor and the

RRC to evaluate the program. In addition to asking for specific information about the program's facilities, residents, and faculty, the PIF asks a series of questions linked to the requirements in the Essentials.

The following suggestions may be useful to new training directors:

1. Notification that the RRC is to review a program should trigger a two-stage process, the first being a self-study review carried out by the faculty of the program, to be followed by the official RRC review.
2. The form is long and requires much detailed information. Begin the process necessary to prepare a draft as soon as you learn that you are to be reviewed. It is not a weekend project.
3. Speak with an experienced program director about completing the form. You will need information from your administration about affiliations, from the office in your institution that maintains faculty records, from the house staff office, and from your faculty.
4. The pages of questions after the sections listing faculty and residents that refer to the curricula and clinical rotations should be distributed to the responsible faculty for completion. The responsibility for the review (and the completion of the form) should be shared. Although the program director has ultimate responsibility for the program, the faculty should actively participate in the preparations for the site visit and the entire accreditation process

The Site Visit

1. You will be notified of the site visit by letter from the ACGME. The site visitor will be either a field surveyor (FS) from the ACGME pool of individuals who do routine surveys of programs in all specialties, or a specialist site visitor (SSV) selected by the RRC, if it believes the visit would better be carried out by a psychiatrist. New programs and programs on probation or whose last review raised major questions about compliance are routinely surveyed by SSVs. You will be asked to contact the surveyor to schedule the visit. After you agree on a mutually convenient date, the surveyor will work out a schedule for the visit. Be sure to arrange the visit on a day when your senior administrators and faculty are available. Surveyors want to at least meet briefly with the chair of the department, or the director of the hospital in which the program is located.

The visit will also include meetings with all key faculty, both didactic and clinical, who have major responsibility for the program. The director of the inpatient service to which residents rotate, the chief of the outpatient service, and the major coordinators of the curriculum will, for example, be scheduled for meetings. Some surveyors prefer to meet with groups of faculty; others prefer individual meetings. In addition, the surveyor will review resident files (current and past), patient charts, and program files, including minutes of the residency education committee. If a program uses more than one facility, faculty and possibly administrative personnel from the other facilities may be asked to meet with the surveyor. The surveyor will meet with residents without faculty present, in order to verify the information with them. Residents should be familiar with the process of accreditation and, of course, will have copies of the Essentials (as required by the Essentials!). They should not be programmed for the meeting. Surveyors quickly recognize gagged or programmed residents and react negatively.

In addition, the surveyor will tour the facilities and will inspect resident offices as well as clinical service areas. Surveyors vary in their preferences, and it is important to establish what your surveyor wishes to see so that you can arrange the visit in an efficient manner.

2. Involve your senior faculty in the preparation for the survey. Distribute copies of the complete PIF as submitted to the RRC, and ask faculty members to review sections of the document that refer to the areas in which they work and identify any inconsistencies or problems that relate to the PIF. The site visitor's job is to verify the information in the PIF, so it is important that it be accurate and correspond to what is actually happening. In addition, it is useful to involve a few senior residents in the process. Since residents will be interviewed by the site visitor on the day of the survey, their familiarity with the process is helpful. Residents should know about the PIF and what it contains.

3. The site visit is not an educational experience for the program. *The surveyor will offer no feedback at the end of the day.*

The Committee Review and Notification Process

1. After the visit, the site visitor will prepare a report and send it to the RRC. The executive director then distributes it to two members of the

RRC, along with the program's file. The committee meets twice a year, once in the fall and once in the spring. It will review the program at the next meeting using the reports prepared by the two committee members who have studied the site visit report, and all other program documents.

2. The RRC will either defer a decision for more information or will reach a decision about the program's status. Table 19–1 summarizes the possible decisions for an initial application. Table 19–2 summarizes the decisions for a renewal application.

3. The RRC then prepares a letter informing you of the decision. Because of the twice yearly meeting schedule, there may be a wait of several months after the site visit before you receive the notification letter. The RRC executive director may be able to inform you of the decision by telephone approximately 2 weeks after the committee meeting.

4. If the RRC wishes to take an adverse action, it will so inform you, and you may then write a rebuttal. The program will remain in its current accreditation status. You may include only information that reflects what was in place at the time of the site visit. The rebuttal will be considered at the next meeting of the committee, delaying the action for at least an additional 6 months.

5. The RRC will often grant approval but will also ask for a progress report from the program director, a mechanism designed to provide the committee with information about compliance without the necessity of an additional full survey.

6. If you have questions about the decision, you should call the executive director of the RRC. He or she may be able to clarify the language (sometimes arcane and technical) and explain the decision.

Table 19–1. Actions regarding accreditation for new programs

Withhold Accreditation—This action reflects the RRC's view that the program is not in substantial compliance with the Essentials.

Provisional Accreditation—This is the only initial accreditation possible for a new program, or for a program reapplying after its accreditation had been withdrawn. There is usually a 2-year interval until the next review. The maximum permissible period of provisional accreditation for a general psychiatry residency is 5 years.

Table 19–2. Actions regarding accreditation for existing programs

---

Full Accreditation—This action is used for programs that have "graduated" from provisional accreditation, for programs holding full accreditation judged to be in continued substantial compliance, and when programs on probationary accreditation are judged to have returned to substantial compliance.

Probationary Accreditation—This adverse action is conveyed to the program director in a letter of intention to grant probationary accreditation in which the specific citations are specified. The program director then may respond to the letter and rebut the citations. The response will be considered at the next scheduled RRC meeting.

Probationary status reflects the RRC's view that a program is no longer in substantial compliance.

Withdrawal of Accreditation—This status reflects that view that the program is out of compliance and must be closed. It can follow:

- Provisional Accreditation
- Probationary Accreditation
- Institutional Noncompliance with the Essentials
- Request of Program (Voluntary Withdrawal)
- Other Administrative Factors including non-payment, program inactivity, etc.

Warning—If the RRC has grave concerns about a program's compliance, it may continue full accreditation, but also warn the program that unless it improves its compliance a further negative action will follow, i.e. probationary accreditation or withdrawal of accreditation.

Deferral of Action—If the RRC does not have adequate information for the accreditation decision, it may defer, and ask the program director for additional information.

The Essentials and Program Design

The starting point for planning or revising a residency program is the Essentials. It is thus critical to be familiar with the Essentials; every training director should have a working knowledge of this document. Although they are lengthy and quite detailed, the Essentials has relatively few numbers. Specifically, the inpatient, outpatient, consultation-liaison, and child and adolescent experiences have minimum time requirements. There are many requirements for experiences that do not specify lengths of rotations, leaving the specific shaping of the program up to the discretion of the program director. The Essentials are periodically revised, so it is important to be certain you are using the current version. The current *Graduate Medical*

Education Directory, published by the American Medical Association (the *"Green Book"*) will contain the most recent version. The *Green Book* is distributed widely and contains information about residency programs, the Essentials and board requirements for certification. Every residency director should have a copy of this reference volume. Be sure to check your own program listing for accuracy.

Many program directors fail to recognize that the Essentials are written so that there is room for considerable latitude in program design. You should be prepared to defend your programmatic decisions on the basis of their educational merit, but you need not slavishly repeat what others have done. Although the RRC measures programs against the standard of the Essentials, it recognizes that all programs have strengths and weaknesses. It is not, however, acceptable to omit a required experience for any reason.

Program directors are often unsure of the specific requirements for a rotation. Such concerns may focus on whether consultation liaison may include ambulatory experience (it may), whether child and adolescent psychiatry may include both inpatient and outpatient experience (it may), and whether substance abuse experience must be fully inpatient (it may include ambulatory placements). The RRC will examine these rotations from the viewpoint of their educational soundness. Is there a suitable patient base for learning? Is the supervision of the experience carried out by adequately qualified specialists? and so on. Discussions with fellow training directors can be helpful in providing information about other programs' rotations that will inform a new training director about the range of possibilities for planning.

Major changes in the program require advance approval by the RRC. The biannual meeting schedule requires that you submit the proposed change by October of the year preceding the anticipated (July) implementation date to receive approval so that you will be notified with sufficient time to make a complicated change.

How to Manage an Accreditation Site Visit Without Losing Your Sanity

First and foremost—*be prepared.*

The key person in your office in preparing for a site visit is the administrative assistant in charge of the residency files, appointments, schedules, and so on. The administrative assistant's full cooperation is an absolutely essential starting point. As already noted, records of present and past residents, of patient logs, of supervisory schedules, of resident and faculty evaluations, of minutes of meetings . . . all these and more will be needed for the site visit. In addition, the administrative assistant will be a key person for scheduling special meetings, including a rehearsal site visit, and the survey day itself.

Accreditation site visits are not surprise events. Every notification letter includes the date of the anticipated resurvey, so that you are always informed of the approximate date of your next survey.

Ideally, you should begin a self-study process leading to the preparation of the PIF *1 year* before the date of the anticipated survey, to allow time to correct problems you identify. The responsibility for the self-study should be shared by the faculty; it is not yours alone. It is useful to empower a subcommittee of the residency education committee to coordinate this effort. In the current era of rapid change, a self-study process in anticipation of a survey has become even more important, since it is almost inevitable that significant changes will have taken place since the last site visit.

Some important steps to be taken are as follows:

1. Inform all faculty and residents of the visit as soon as it is scheduled. They should understand that they will be expected to be available on that day, should their participation be required.
2. Confirm the date with the chair and/or other senior administrators who may be involved.
3. As mentioned, be certain that the PIF preparation is proceeding rapidly.
4. After you have scheduled the visit with the surveyor, work toward completion of all preparation by an earlier date, when you will schedule a mock site visit. The mock site visitor can be another training director from a department in your hospital who is experienced in managing site visits, a fellow psychiatry training director from another program (which some find uncomfortable), or one of your faculty who is experienced in participating in surveys.

A full run-through will be most helpful, including review of resident files, evaluations, logs, and so on, to ensure that the files are orderly and complete. Table 19–3 highlights critical issues in preparing for an accreditation survey:

Table 19–3. Some accreditation do's and don'ts

Do's

1. Start the preparation early, i.e., as soon as you know there is a survey scheduled. Even better, review your last RRC letter and begin to prepare 1 year before the anticipated revisit. The RRC does not forget about programs!
2. Become familiar with the Essentials. The outline headings are useful as a guide to a self-study program review, as noted.
3. Spread the work widely among your faculty. You should delegate the preparation in a manner similar to the delegation of the program responsibilities.
4. Again, early self-study reviews allow for identification of problems with time to make necessary changes in a calm and planned way. The realization that there is a problem at the last minute leads to frantic and often inadequate changes. Self-study should be built into your residency education committee agenda.
5. Tell the truth on the PIF and in meetings with the surveyor. If you do not know the answer to a question, be direct in informing the surveyor, and arrange to get the required information. If the surveyor realizes that you are "fudging" answers, all the data of the survey and PIF will be thrown into doubt.
6. Inform the residents but do not program them for their meeting with the site visitor. Surveyors are sensitive to residents who have been tutored on what to say.
7. Call the RRC if you believe a surveyor selected for your program has a conflict of interest.

Don'ts

1. Do not "fudge," lie, or otherwise dissemble. The site visit is designed to verify information about the program, and inconsistencies and deceptions will emerge.
2. Do not argue with the surveyor. If you believe you have not been treated fairly, notify the RRC at once in writing. Call if you are having problems in setting up a survey.
3. Do not ask the surveyor for his/her opinion. Surveyors are instructed not to give any feedback to program directors.
4. Do not ask the RRC about individual resident's training. It is your responsibililty to develop a complete experience for each resident. The ABPN is responsible for certification of individuals and should be consulted if there is a specific question about eligibility for admission to the certification process.
5. Do not "go it alone." Ask for help from other training directors, from the AADPRT (regional caucus leaders) or the consultation service of the Office of Education of the APA.

How to Get Help

Help is available from several sources. Your first resource is other training directors. The American Association of Directors of Psychiatric Residency Education (AADPRE) regional caucuses can be helpful in identifying program directors in your area, if you are new and have not met them. In addition, the leadership of the AADPRT will connect you to training directors who may have particular expertise or experience in the area about which you are concerned.

The executive director of the RRC is an additional resource. Although not able to give official approval to anything, the executive director may be extremely helpful in clarifying the Essentials and helping you with "interpretations" of the written rules.

It is important to remember that the RRC can never answer a question about an individual resident's program. The RRC is only able to consider matters related to program accreditation. The American Board of Psychiatry and Neurology (ABPN) is responsible for certification of individual residents, and questions about an individual resident's training pattern should be directed to the ABPN.

Finally, programs that feel themselves to be in trouble and in need of external consultation may use the consultation service of the Office of Education of the American Psychiatric Association. The confidential review conducted by an experienced, senior educator includes a site visit, and a report with feedback and the possibility of an ongoing consultation process.

A Few Words About the Essentials

To the relative newcomer, the Essentials seems like a morass of fine print details. The Essentials is best used by following the outline of its Roman numeral and capital letter headings. That outline can serve as an excellent guide for an internal review in preparation for a site visit. This allows the internal review to examine the major areas of the program using the RRC's own review plan, the same one used during the official survey. This approach is most likely to catch details easily missed in a casual hunt for problems using the document as a whole.

There are many ways of assigning faculty responsibilities in the review process. The Essentials lend themselves to being used for this purpose, as just noted, in following the major headings in the outline. Many program directors have found it useful to assign one faculty member as coordinator for each year of the residency. This helps in the overall coordination of the didactic and clinical elements of the program and provides a resource for the residents to use if they find that the integration of their program as a whole is not working well.

Accreditation Actions for Subspecialty Programs

The RRC reviews and accredits subspecialty programs, similarly, with one major additional factor, the accreditation status of the general program. In psychiatry, the accreditation status of subspecialty programs *except child and adolescent psychiatry* depends on the general program having full accreditation. If the general program is on probation, or is appealing from a negative action, these subspecialty program cannot be accredited. If the parent program has its accreditation withdrawn, the RRC will administratively withdraw the accreditation of the subspecialty program. At present, as noted, accreditation of 1-year residencies leading to eligibility for a subspecialty certificate (by examination of the ABPN) is offered for addiction psychiatry, forensic psychiatry, and geriatric psychiatry. The child and adolescent psychiatry residency remains a 2-year program, which may begin in the PGY-4 year, leading to eligibility for a subspecialty certificate of the ABPN after examination.

The overall accreditation procedure is identical to that for general psychiatry, except that the "special essentials" for the particular program are used as the standard for the review and decision. The accreditation actions for subspecialty programs except child and adolescent (which is accredited with the same actions as the general program) are as follows:

1. Accreditation
2. Withhold accreditation
3. Accreditation with warning, administrative (action taken when parent program has accreditation changed to probation)
4. Accreditation with warning
5. Withdraw accreditation
6. Withhold accreditation, administrative (action taken when parent program has accreditation withdrawn)

Adverse Actions and the Right of Appeal

As mentioned, if the RRC decides to take an adverse action, they will notify the program with a detailed letter specifying the citations and "proposing" to take that action. The program then has an opportunity to rebut by letter, and the committee will reconsider the proposed adverse action. If the committee decides to take the adverse action, the program has the right of appeal after this reconsideration and final notification.

Appeals are conducted by the ACGME itself, rather then the RRC. The members of an appeals panel are selected from a list prepared by the committee, and the program director has some role in selecting the final membership of the panel. A hearing is convened at which the program may present arguments related to the issues of compliance, but it must limit its presentation to the program as it existed at the time of the RRC review. The decision of the appeals panel is final.

Summary and Conclusions

The notification of a site visit is often received by a program director (particularly a newly appointed one), with all the enthusiasm that greets a letter from the IRS informing someone of an audit! A site visit need not be an ordeal if the program director prepares adequately. The worst enemy of a successful survey is the inclination to delay preparation until shortly before the visit.

Program directors are responsible for the accreditation process and for site visits, but they should not prepare for them on their own. Involve the faculty and the residents. Be certain the administration of the facility that sponsors the program is informed and involved. And ask for help, from other program directors, from the leadership of the AADPRT, who can help direct a question to someone likely to know the answer, or from the RRC, if the question refers to a procedural question or confusion about the interpretation about the Essentials.

Accreditation is ultimately designed to maintain quality in graduate education. One can argue about the specifics, but the overall process ensures national minimum standards for education. It also provides an opportunity for every program to periodically examine itself. In situations where hospital administration is reluctant to provide needed resources for the program, the Essentials and notification letters can be powerful tools. The usefulness of the accreditation process to a program is contingent upon the training directors' use of the process to assist in achieving the best educational program possible.

References

American Medical Association: Graduate Medical Education Directory, 1995–96. Chicago, IL, American Medical Association, 1995

20

Evaluations of Residents

Carl Greiner, M.D.

Goals and Principles of Evaluation

Resident evaluation is important for at least three central reasons: (1) It assesses individual performance in a timely manner, (2) it is an opportunity to determine whether the training program is meeting its clinical and educational goals, and (3) it provides required documentation for site reviews. The evaluation process plays an integral role in resident development and the ongoing revision of a residency training program. Developing an evaluation style that anticipates fine performance yet acknowledges genuine deficiencies when necessary is an essential task of the residency training director (RTD).

The Accreditation Council for Graduate Medical Education (ACGME) offers a specific outline for the requirements of evaluation in the New Special Requirements (Accreditation Council for Graduate Medical Education 1994). Sections III.B and VI provide the guidelines for the RTD. It is noteworthy that the word *must* is included in describing the evaluation requirements. The guidelines provide a template to which the RTD can refer in discussions with the chair, faculty, and residents.

The primary goal of evaluation is to assess the resident's competency. The components of a complete evaluation are as follows:

1. Accuracy
2. Completeness
3. Timeliness
4. Appropriate process
5. Communication

A good evaluation combines all of these elements in an artful way. Residents deserve a fair and accurate appraisal of their work. The attending should provide tactful and specific comments in the areas of attitude, skill, and knowledge. If the resident receives a failing grade, the individual needs to know what portion of the experience was failed and what would constitute remediation. Completeness calls for an appraisal of both strengths and weaknesses with specific examples to corroborate the assessment. Timeliness requires that the evaluation occurs in such a way that the resident has the opportunity to remediate deficiencies or consider fellowships or local/national awards. The Residency Review Committee (RRC) requires semiannual reviews; a set schedule such as October-November and April-May allows the resident to plan for the event. Additionally, such scheduling avoids other busy times such as recruiting season and the beginning of the academic year. The resident can anticipate and prepare personal goals and objectives, and faculty can finish "late" paperwork. Appropriate process requires that the RTD follows contractual and institutional guidelines if there are deficiencies, potential probationary status, or suspension. The wise RTD must be aware of the possibilities of litigation if there is a negative assessment. Communication dictates that residents be fully aware of the implications of a negative evaluation and what avenues they have to remediate the problem. The new director may find the range of evaluation expectations bewildering; maintaining contact with a senior colleague at another institution or asking for a basic review by the Graduate Medical Education committee in your home institution will greatly aid the first series of evaluations.

Obstacles to Evaluation

There are many obstacles that may impede giving and receiving a good evaluation. Some of these obstacles are attitudinal. Rosenthal (1995) noted overarching themes that impair a physician's abilities to define impaired performance in colleagues; a partial list includes the following topics with my commentary:

1. Permanent uncertainty exists in clinical evaluation, which indicates that no physician has all the relevant information to make a decision. Clinical care is delivered in the context of incomplete information. What are the levels of information collection that we consider to be competent?
2. Necessary fallibility is a concept derived from comparing premortem

and postmortem diagnosis. From an extension of this analysis, a current hypothesis is that there is an irreducible error rate in the diagnostic process.

3. Shared personal vulnerability in facing uncertainty is intrinsic to clinical practice. Both the supervisor and the resident are in the same boat with regard to an irreducible error rate. Knowing the ever-present possibility of error, the supervisor may be more hesitant to identify error in the resident's work.

Minor themes include faculty hesitance that their evaluations will result in unfavorable assessments by residents, and they may be tempted to give a bland or stereotypic review of a resident's performance. Such a review, however, is an avoidance of the RTD's or attending's duty to expect and monitor change. Although the faculty may be well trained regarding collusion in psychotherapy, less attention may be paid to this factor when reviewing one's residents.

Time limitations present further obstacles. In a busy clinical setting, evaluation may appear to be a peripheral and unwanted exercise. A thorough evaluation requires a commitment of time. Thoughtful consideration must be given to place the resident's performance in a relative context of experience (i.e., being at R-1), difficulty of assignment (i.e., transplant service consultation), and training contingencies (i.e., the loss of a beloved teacher on the unit). With increased clinical demands on faculty, one is more likely to hear the claim "I am too busy" to provide a thorough evaluation. Faculty who are "too busy" must understand that unless they participate fully in the evaluation process, further resident assignments to their service may not be possible.

Organizational obstacles exist as well. The RTD must ensure adequate department financial support for staffing the residency training office. In addition, a close working alliance with the chairman is critical to the RTD's success. The emerging new patterns in psychiatric practice make it a confusing time to clearly articulate a model of the excellent psychiatrist. The chair and RTD can help define and model the expectations for competency in their particular program.

Finally, the lack of a consensus on the moral and professional issues that are part of the evaluation process presents a unique obstacle. Wagner (1993) highlighted this issue in his discussion of medical student cheating and the controversy surrounding what the outcomes should be. Although lack of consensus can provide the springboard for a more comprehensive understanding, the RTD and training committees have a more complex task in formulating and presenting a credible evaluation process.

Development of a departmental committee for evaluation of misconduct that focuses on whether the administrative action is consistent with published professional codes, such as the American Medical Association (AMA) and American Psychiatric Association (APA) Ethics Guidelines, and/or mission statements of the home institution would be a potential way to address this problem.

Types of Evaluations

Residency training directors have a wide variety of evaluation tools at their disposal, including the following:

1. Resident self-evaluation
2. Faculty evaluation of clinical performance
3. Faculty evaluation of didactic participation
4. Chief resident evaluation of trainee's interpersonal skills, knowledge, and attitude
5. Psychiatry Residents In-Training Examination (PRITE) score
6. Performance-based assessment

Not all programs may use all the preceding tools, but the list suggests the broad perspectives available to provide an interconnected view of the resident's attitudes, skills, and knowledge.

The semiannual review is an ideal place to synthesize the different sources of resident evaluation. The resident self-evaluation can be one of the most valuable insights into the resident's development. Providing written, personal goals allows residents to put their "best foot forward" and provides a background for ongoing review. Knowledge of these personal goals enables the RTD to recommend appropriate mentors who could facilitate the resident's growth. This recommendation is particularly important for the junior residents who may not have a clear idea about the range and depth of the faculty.

The chief resident's insights can be invaluableand are often distinctive evaluations of attitude and willingness to work with others (Reuben and

Noble 1990). The critical material that is often absent from faculty evaluations may be present with a near peer review.

Essay-type examinations developed by individual programs have particular usefulness in testing core material mastery. The knowledge base is often not as clearly distinguished on a busy clinical service except at the levels of "very good" and "very poor." Additionally, "morning report" or its equivalent may be used for evaluation of on call capability; this assessment can be one of the best indicators of knowledge base, confidence, and ability to work with others. Persistent difficulties on call can be one of the earliest warning signs of a resident who has problematic performance. The mock boards are informative about how the resident actually interviews. Unfortunately, as the clinical world becomes busier, there are fewer opportunities for the faculty to participate in a resident's complete interview of a patient. The mock board provides an important glimpse on the establishment of rapport, capacity for empathy, and ability to do a focused interview.

If the RTD reviews this range of material about the resident prior to the semiannual review, the RTD will have the opportunity to provide succinct and reasoned assessments of strengths and weaknesses. Common patterns will appear such as the resident with strong descriptive skills but with a great hesitancy to examine intra/interpersonal issues, the bright resident with limited confidence, the relationally skilled resident with a minimal knowledge base, and the resident who has excellent skills in one domain but has limited ability to connect with patients of other groups. The RTD can make specific recommendations about ways to broaden and deepen the resident's capacity to work with a wide variety of patients.

An important educational development is the incorporation of performance-based examination, which can aid the RTD in evaluating how the resident handles complex problem solving. Swanson reviewed four important performance-based assessments: patient management problems, computer-based clinical stimulations, oral examinations, and standardized patients (Swanson et al. 1995; abstracted in Juul 1995). These newer techniques are to be used in combination with multiple-choice tests.

An excellent description of the Objective Structured Clinical Examination (OSCE) was provided by Loschen (1993). He noted that "mock boards" have the usual limitation of examining only one or two patients. In distinction, Loschen described the OSCE as using examination "stations" to test discrete clinical skills in short sessions (5–15 minutes). For practical considerations, a group of six stations has typically been used. A variety of materials could be used such as clinical data, an emergency scenario, or standardized patients. Faculty are discouraged from using rare or unusual case material. Standards for performance are specified prior to the examination. The resident could receive feedback from the standardized patient. The virtue of this type of examination is its comprehensiveness, fairness, and objectivity, which may be lacking in supervisory commentary. As we face increasing demands to certify residents' competence, the performance-based exams will become more important.

The Resident With Disabilities or Special Needs

The RTD is expected to provide training to residents within a broad spectrum of ages and physical health status. For example, a beginning resident may have completed a successful career in another area of medicine and be starting a new career in her 50s. A resident may have a chronic illness that can require periods of time away from the residency.

The 1990 Americans with Disability Act provides that "no qualified individual with a disability shall, by reason of such disability, be excluded from participation in or be denied the benefits of the services, programs, or activities of a public entity, or be subjected to discrimination by any such entity." (42 USC §2132). The booklet *Disabled Students in Medical School* is essential reading (Association of American Medical Colleges 1993). An abbreviated list of the summary recommendations is as follows:

1. Schools should judge persons on the basis of their ability to complete the educational program rather than on their status as disabled persons.
2. "Reasonable accommodations" or "modifications" may be needed and, if so, must be provided.
3. Each school must determine the "essential functions" or "essential eligibility" requirements of its program.

Amy Longo, R.N., J.D., a hospital attorney, provided an important insight when she noted that the "essential functions" remain constant but the way they are accomplished may be flexible. The institution must demonstrate that reasonable attempts have been made to accommodate the resident's needs. The potential resident has the responsibility to describe what needs are to be addressed. For example, a potential resident may request a limited call schedule due to auditory impairments and vertigo. A potential resident in his 70s may require a physical assessment to determine whether he has adequate stamina to participate in the residency. It is important to remember that special needs are usually a *prospective* matter of identifying an issue and working toward an accommodation; a resident's statement of special needs *after* academic failure should be viewed with caution. The hospital attorney can be helpful in reviewing recent case law on what types of conditions have been considered disabilities.

Record Keeping

"God is in the details" is a widely quoted aphorism. New RTDs will quickly confront the reality that they have inherited the job of being a record keeper. They face the same range of challenges as the medical records department and must employ their ingenuity (from gentle reminders to threats of withholding paychecks or vacation) in trying to keep records up-to-date. How one maintains sanity during these experiences is an early test of the RTD's adaptive capacity. Some thoughts on surviving this task include the following:

1. Hire or develop a responsible executive secretary who has a strong sense of joint ownership in the residency. The RTD must actively participate in the record keeping. It will usually require that the RTD have institutional authority to "encourage" wayward faculty to provide required documentation. The executive secretary *can* provide a list of delinquent evaluations, missing residents' patient lists, and up-to-date management of correspondence; what the secretary *cannot* do is generate a departmental atmosphere for the importance of records. This is a task for the RTD and chairman. An ongoing negotiation for the RTD is to acquire adequate space and resources to maintain the residency program.
2. Regular attention to records gives the RTD the advantage of access to a full range of materials for the semiannual reviews. It is in your own best interest to have a system that works.
3. Who were all those past residents, and what was the final assessment of their performance? HMOs and hospital medical staff services ask for detailed training assessments to use for credentialing. Providing such assessments for a resident who graduated a decade or more ago can be a challenge. Older files prepared with different expectations are

oftentimes inadequate. One can do very little about the shape of past records. However, the RTD can improve his or her life and that of a successor if a final, summary assessment of each resident is made. This approach avoids the problem of commenting on a former resident's probation when there is no clear record about the specific issue or its resolution. Without further information, the RTD is left with the unpleasant task of simply noting that the resident had been subject to disciplinary action.

4. A good record-keeping system means that the preparation for the RRC visit is only a minor task rather than a monumental one. If the documentation is organized, the RTD is not in the unenviable situation of asking faculty to provide evaluations that are "reconstructed from memory."

5. Develop computer-based record keeping to minimize the paper avalanche. E-mail simplifies communication regarding management issues. Some evaluations, such as the semiannual review, should be kept on paper unless there is a foolproof backup system. Keeping residents' patient logs on a computer system allows a better assessment of the range of patient contacts and categories of treatment as well as a more rational review of what types of training experiences need to be improved.

Due Process Procedures and the "Problem Resident"

It is important for the RTD to be thoroughly familiar with both the departmental and institutional requirements for a resident who is facing academic sanctions. Not surprisingly, most litigation occurs when dismissal from medical school becomes necessary (Helms and Helms 1991). By extension, however, one can consider the parallel situation that could occur in a resident dismissal issue. Departmental and institutional guidelines must be followed explicitly. A meeting with the associate dean for graduate medical education and a review of the institution's academic sanctions and dismissal process would be recommended for a new director or anyone who has had a change in deans. The RTD is responsible for advising the resident in a timely fashion about the action being contemplated and avenues for redress, and for notification of the appropriate institutional committees. In our institution, a formal warning is usually a precursor to a formal probation, which is organized with the graduate medical education committee. The specific requirements include an identification of the problem, a recommended solution, and the organized supervision that will monitor compliance. Many issues overlap with the "problem resident"; however, most residents find themselves facing warnings or sanctions due to being disorganized or unskilled rather than because they suffer from a major illness or personality disorder.

In many ways, the "problem resident" has been a leitmotiv in discussion of the arduous aspects of evaluation. It is helpful to consider the duration, intensity, and gravity of impairment. Since the early 1970s the AMA has provided important readings on physician impairment; Tokarz's assessment of resident vulnerability is an impressive work; he noted that 9% of physician addicts die by suicide (Tokarz et al. 1979). The AMA's 1995 report on substance abuse among physicians provided a critical review of the literature and offered an international perspective on drug/alcohol abuse and dependence; the claims of drug dependence at 30- to 100-fold greater than the national average is not supported by data. However, the United Kingdom has provided several thought-provoking articles. Brooke et al. (1991) clearly identified a central problem in effectively evaluating the substance impaired physician:

> Awkward moral overtones intrude; we are embarrassed to confront a colleague and uncertain what course to follow. The afflicted doctor continues in misery while colleagues turn away, having furtive meetings, but failing to get to grips with the problem. (p. 1011)

Firth-Cozens (1987) reported that residents have a higher level of emotional distress than other occupational groups, with 50% reporting emotional distress, 28% having evidence of depression, and approximately 20% having frequent bouts of heavy drinking. Although RTDs need to be familiar with common illnesses among trainees, they should focus their concerns in terms of competency to do the work.

A helpful checklist for more common problems would include the following:

1. Is the resident a frequent name listed for late dictations and mismanaged discharges?
2. Is the resident in an unusual number of conflicts with students, fellow

staff, and faculty? Unwillingness of other residents to cover call for a particular resident is an important marker.

3. Are there indications of gradually increasing absenteeism and decreasing job performance? The RTD needs to maintain an index of concern for drug/alcohol abuse. Unfortunately, it may require an extended period before residents/faculty identify the issues, usually after resident and faculty "forgiveness" has been exhausted.

4. Is the resident withdrawing from usual activities and failing to participate in social events? The resident's decreased availability may come as a late report to the RTD from other residents or faculty.

5. Is the resident having repeated difficulty with diagnosing and treating patients while on call? The challenge of call reveals confidence, knowledge base, and ability to manage a wide range of disorders. Problems on call should be reviewed quickly by the RTD.

6. Are there indications of a resident having problems with maintaining appropriate boundaries with patients? Are patients being seen at inappropriate times or circumstances? Is the therapeutic situation being transformed into a social one? Defining the issues for the resident in a straightforward and useful manner is perhaps the single, most complex challenge to the RTD. Defining what would be required in remediation is the administrative task.

Three cases will illustrate the range of issues and the types of problems the RTD might face. These are composite cases and other RTDs would have "variations on a theme." It is important to remember when discussing difficulties that they should be described in behavioral terms with specific examples and appropriate and observable remediation.

Case I. A junior resident had persistent difficulties in completing both inpatient and outpatient records. The medical records committee issued a series of warnings about incomplete records. Clinical care was compromised in that the discharge summary was unavailable when a patient returned to the emergency room. The resident was given a verbal warning to have all charting completed within 72 hours, and the medical records department agreed to track this performance. If the resident did not comply with the requirement, he would be placed on written probation with a copy sent to the graduate medical education committee. A typical probation would include a 3-month monitoring period for compliance to determine if the requirements were met. If after the probationary period the requirement were still not met, the resident could be discharged from the program. If the resident complied with the expectations, the probation would be dropped. Again, plans for remediation require specific actions by both the resident and the RTD.

Case II. A senior resident arrived for an emergency room call and was obviously intoxicated and belligerent. The resident refused to acknowledge any impairment, noting that residency was stressful and that he had "just been relaxing prior to the call." In discussion with the chief resident, the RTD learned that there had been growing concern about the resident's performance. In such a circumstance, the most appropriate step would be an immediate suspension until a full evaluation could be made. Full and tactful assessment of the resident should be made by a respected chemical dependency program.

Case III. A senior resident prided herself on being "warm and sharing with a flair for innovation." She had the style of taking action and then, if questioned, would discuss the case with her supervisors. After the fact, she informed her fellow residents that she had taken a patient out shopping and purchased a present for him in an attempt to "break down" the artificiality of meeting in the clinic. Prior attempts by faculty who offered suggestions were quickly met with disbelief and denial of responsibility. Significantly, she had thus avoided a serious discussion of her performance. In taking the patient shopping, she had "crossed the line," and the RTD met with her to review doctor-patient boundaries, the expectation that no sessions would occur outside the clinic building, and the necessity for faculty involvement in treatment planning. The resident argued that "a warm heart is always the best medicine." No significant change was seen as necessary by the resident. An official warning letter was sent with specific requirements about the needs for faculty supervision and references about "boundary crossings" in the standard literature.

It is a great temptation for the RTD to attempt a full evaluation of a problem resident. However, an assessment of the gravity or degree of impairment is all that should be done. A full evaluation, including identifying diagnostic issues, is best left to the employee assistance program, an outside consultant, or a chemical dependency program. Dr. Anne Marie Riether (1996) noted that an outside evaluation program can provide a diagnosis and a four-point assessment recommendation ranging from immediate return to work to no return to work. Such an outside assessment would allow the RTD and the evaluation committee to make a responsible decision about the resident's future in the program. Resources for follow-up such as the impaired physician committee and special AA groups for chemically dependent physicians could be identified if the resident returns to service. The graduate medical education committee must be informed of the circumstance, and the impaired physician committee can be helpful in offering guidelines for compliance.

One of the most problematic issues facing the RTD is responding to boundary violations. As has been noted by some scholars, the decline of psychoanalytic teaching has resulted in less understanding of the therapeutic relationship and has diminished our capacity to discuss both subtle and pronounced violations. Gutheil and Gabbard (1993) reviewed this topic and offered the valuable distinction of harmful versus nonharmful boundary crossings. All residents need to be informed regarding issues of touching, money, gifts, and special requests. The power issues involved in dating and socializing with patients need to be overtly discussed and reviewed with incoming residents. In reviewing sexual misconduct cases, Gutheil and Gabbard noted there can be a "slippery slope" from minor violations of boundaries (such as treatment at unusual hours and increased familiarity) to touching and intercourse.

Some aspects of "border shifts" are difficult to anticipate. A resident from a primary care service was rotating on a inpatient psychiatric unit to meet a training requirement. A patient with borderline personality disorder and a surgical condition wished to attend her appointment. At discharge, she convinced the resident to drive her to her appointment at a distant clinic. After being dissuaded by senior psychiatric nurses in the parking lot, he relented. A phone call was placed with his training director in primary care who indicated in such a situation he would have driven the patient to the appointment as a friendly gesture! The complexities of trainees from other clinical traditions and varied personal backgrounds encourages the RTD to find the fine balance of respect for the resident, the patient's care, and professional norms.

Standardized Written and Clinical Examinations

The PRITE examination, a 300-item exam, provides an important quantitative measure of performance that compares the resident to all general residents as well as residents at their own level of training. PRITE helps to identify strengths and weaknesses in performance and is a useful tool for providing specific feedback. The PRITE scores allow the RTD to address current performance and to review possible areas for improvement prior to taking the American Board of Psychiatry and Neurology examinations. Although the PRITE exam cannot be used for decisions regarding advancement, it does help the RTD to scrutinize curriculum content and educational effectiveness. For example, if a single resident had strong scores in pharmacology but weak scores in child-adolescent, the recommendation would be increased reading in that area. However, if a significant number of residents were not doing well in child-adolescent, a review of the curriculum would be in order. Importantly, because there is diversity among training programs and varying opinions about what specific knowledge and skills should be acquired during a psychiatric residency, the test policies and content are developed in consultation and collaboration with many different groups.

As a general rule, the RTD should establish a minimal recommended score level for discussion in the semiannual reviews. Given candidates' failure rates at the American Board of Psychiatry and Neurology, the residents should be encouraged to maintain performance levels above a specific level such as the 50% percentile. The RTD must maintain the confidentiality of the scores; however, residents who have done well may take the opportunity to share their successes.

Despite its value, several problems have occurred with using the PRITE. The expectation that *all* residents take the PRITE has been ill-received by residents on maternity leave. In addition, the RTD is in the awkward situation of possessing knowledge that cannot be shared. We are in the unusual position of having a responsibility both for the resident and for the general standards of performance in the program. With "high grading" being typical of many academic centers, the PRITE may be one of the most reliable instruments for the RTD to use to assess competence. There is, however, an inherent ethical conflict between protecting the resident and protecting the public. If a resident's scores indicate a serious knowledge base competency issue, the RTD currently may not breach confidentiality to address those competency concerns. I would recommend that the confidentiality issues would not be regarded as absolute and that guidelines for breaking confidentiality be established.

Departments should have "uniform" semiannual review forms so that all residents will be reviewed for similar performance parameters. Some institutions have the same form for residents in all training programs. Likewise, a uniform review for mock boards is recommended.

Summary

The ACGME mandates much of what is to be evaluated. The issue that distinguishes the particular program and RTD is how the evaluation is conducted. As this review has demonstrated, the RTD is walking a tightrope between providing empathic and growth-oriented information and providing suitable documentation for potential litigation. I would recommend finding a style that places more emphasis on growth-oriented evaluation, with possible litigation being a background consideration.

If there is a "universal precaution" rule in administration, it would be to keep records that are accurate, timely, and comprehensive in all circumstances. If litigation occurs, the necessary documentation is available. The alert RTD will keep abreast of changes in the legal arenas of disability and common law for misconduct. A good relationship with the university/hospital attorney is helpful. Similarly, thorough familiarity with the due process requirements of your institution will encourage a reasonable and uniform approach to dealing with misconduct.

The style we develop with residents in evaluation should be focused on helping them develop their maximal level of skill. By including aspects of faculty evaluation and self-evaluation in the process, the experience of evaluation becomes more of a bilateral experience than a unilateral one. Such a format will best express regard for the colleague in training.

The institutional requirement for the RTD is to monitor if the program itself is a persistent factor in a resident's diminished performance. Overwork can be one of the major stresses in residents' lives. If the evaluation process reveals that some services are "outliers" in the expectation of residents and results in a high rate of poor performance, the RTD would need to work with the service chief to modify the experience. The RTD is in a special position to recommend changes in the training that will allow a successful educational experience.

Resources
Director of graduate education at your institution
Hospital attorney at your institution

Local AA regarding Caduceus Groups
State impaired physician office
AMA Physician Wellness Committee
Senior RTDs at AADPRT
ACGME office

Acknowledgment: I would like to thank Dr. Jay Scully for his assistance on this chapter, Amy Longo, J.D., for her commentary, Mindy McNeil for her research efforts, and the AMA for its contribution of recent work on physician impairment.

References

Accreditation Council for Graduate Medical Education: New Special Requirements for Residency Training in Psychiatry. Chicago, IL, Accreditation Council for Graduate Medical Education, 1994

Association of American Medical Colleges: The Disabled Student in Medical School: An Overview of Legal Requirements. Washington, DC, Association of American Medical Colleges, 1993

American Medical Association: Substance among physicians. Report of the Council on Scientific Affairs (CSA Report 1-A-95). Chicago, IL, American Medical Association, 1995

Brooke D, Edwards G, Taylor C: Addiction as an occupational hazard: 144 doctors with drug and alcohol problems. Br J Addict 86:1011–1016, 1991

Firth-Cozens J: Emotional distress in junior house officers. BMJ 25:533–535, 1987

Gutheil TG, Gabbard GO: The concept of boundaries in clinical practice: theoretical and risk-management-decisions. Am J Psychiatry 150:188–196, 1993

Helms LB, Helms CM: Forty years of litigation involving students and their education: I. General educational issues. Acad Med 66:1–7, 1991

Juul D: Educational abstracts. Academic Psychiatry 19:175, 1995

Loschen EL: Using the Objective Structured Clinical Examination in a psychiatric residency. Academic Psychiatry 17(2):95–104, 1993

Reuben DB, Noble S: House officer responses to impaired physicians. JAMA 263(7): 958–960, 1990

Riether AM: The substance abusing physician patient. Paper presented at the meeting of the Academy of Psychosomatic Medicine, San Antonio, TX, November 1996

Rosenthal MM: The incompetent doctor. Birmingham, England, Free University Press, 1995

Swanson DB, Norman GR, Linn RL: Performance-based assessment: lessons from the health professions. Educational Researcher 24:5–11, 35, 1995

Tokarz JP, Bremer W, Peters K: Beyond Survival. Chicago, IL, American Medical Association, 1979

Wagner RF: Medical student academic misconduct: implications of recent case law and possible institutional responses. Acad Med 12:887–889, 1993

21

Special Problems

Paul C. Mohl, M.D.

Most residency training directors (RTDs) seek their jobs out of an interest in education, supporting residents, and developing curricula. However, their success will be judged primarily by how they perform at two other functions: recruitment, and handling of problems and problem residents. This chapter addresses the latter of these two functions. Effective handling of special problems will be almost invisible to both residents and faculty, garnering little praise. Ineffective handling will be noticed by all, provoke intense criticism, erode both faculty and resident morale, and compromise efforts in other areas.

In considering various special problems it is useful to keep in mind the numerous roles of the RTD: personnel officer, mediator, evaluator, icon and caricature, role model, parent (as seen by the faculty), and curriculum developer (see Table 21–1). Difficulties encountered handling the problems enumerated in this chapter can be understood as arising from inherent conflicts in these roles. Most problems require some form of personnel officer management, something very few RTDs are prepared for. Yet the personnel officer decisions (enforcing institutional or departmental procedures, protecting the program from legal liability) must be modulated by the impact on the training of the particular resident involved and on the curriculum as a whole. Although the service impact of a particular decision is not the immediate concern of the RTD, a significant change in the service load must be seen as affecting the training of other residents and, thus, the clinical curriculum.

Table 21–1. Roles of the residency training director

Systems engineer
Personnel officer
Public relations agent
Caricature and icon
Parent surrogate
Mediator
Role model
Evaluator
Curriculum developer

Like it or not, how the RTD is seen by both the faculty and the residents is a, if not *the,* major determinant of how the program is seen. Thus, the RTD must be a public relations person as well. It is here where the roles of icon, role model, and parent must be carefully thought through in any decision. The RTD is viewed as a role model by all residents in the program. As such, how special problems and problem residents are handled will be seen as a demonstration of how all residents should handle difficult problems. But at times, being a role model slides into being a caricature or icon (either good or bad), a transference figure. The wise RTD learns when to use these projections to get things done, and when to dispel them to facilitate others getting things done.

To the faculty, the RTD is often regarded as the residents' parent, who is responsible for their behaving well or badly. All of this can conflict with the RTD's own needs, both personal and professional, but most especially with those needs that led the training director to seek the job in the first place.

In general, there are two basic models of being a training director, the *charismatic type* and the *honest broker* type. Charismatic types take advantage of all of the projections coming their way to make decisions and make them stick. Honest broker types see themselves as *systems engineers,* whose job is to make a program composed of complex pieces function smoothly and effectively to train and educate the residents optimally. Honest brokers are more concerned with how fair the system is, and is perceived to be, than with how good they are seen to be.

My opinion is that the honest broker type is far superior to the charismatic type, and the solutions to problems suggested in this chapter reflect that belief. Faculty and residents will accept many disappointments if they believe that the system of decision making is fair and has considered their points of view. The key word here is *believe*. It is important that the system not just be fair, but *be perceived as fair*. Much of what I advocate relates to this important distinction. This means constant ongoing consultation and keeping important people informed well in advance as things develop. Often the direction of a decision may be obvious, but the process of informing people and soliciting their input is crucial to the *perception* of fairness.

Residents and faculty, if they believe themselves to be part of a fair and honest system, will work hard to solve problems that arise. This means that RTDs must know not just what to do, but whether to do anything, when to do it, when not to step in (to avoid possibly interfering with others' attempts to solve a problem), and how to appear to be doing something, when in fact they are temporizing.

In the discussion of specific problems to follow, I may not always refer back to these principles, but they are the basis for the solutions suggested.

When a Resident Becomes Ill or Injured

Many of the problems listed in the following discussion fall under the general category of a resident not being available to a clinical service that was expecting the resident and depending on the presence of that resident to assist in the care of patients. Not only does this threatened absence tap into the faculty's perception that they "need" the resident and can't function without him or her, it raises the specter, if the site functions effectively without a resident for a period of time, that the RTD might conclude that the site can do without a resident during future shortages. Further, sites and faculty are often in a complicated competitive position with each other about which one is the better rotation. All of this conspires to create a "give us our body" message from the faculty. They will watch the RTD's response carefully to gain a sense of to what extent the RTD "understands" the needs of the site, how the role of the service is perceived, and how valued the faculty's educational efforts are.

Residents are exquisitely sensitive to schedule changes. Their fundamental issue in almost any conflict is the feeling of not being in control of their lives. Nothing reinforces this more than an abrupt, unexpected shifting of the schedule, even if only one resident is involved only for a brief time. At the same time, the other residents assigned to the same service as the ill or injured resident fear that they will have to carry an extra service load. This subgroup of residents becomes a group pressuring to change the schedule and a source of anger, ambivalence, and guilt among the rest of their class. Compounding this is the general reaction among the residents of "could this happen to me?" How all this is handled becomes a test case in the residents' eyes for the compassion with which they will be dealt should something untoward occur to them, how they are truly viewed by the faculty, and whose side the RTD is on.

Thus, even this routine event of life raises fundamental questions in the minds of both faculty and residents. The RTD must keep all this in mind.

If the resident's illness occurred in connection with the residency (e.g., a violent act by a patient), then the issues are compounded further. The faculty experiences some sense of guilt, and the residents see before them the lifelong risks of their chosen profession and the inability of the faculty to provide for their security, welfare, and well-being.

A number of principles should guide handling this situation. First, as an RTD I want every site to believe that it is the best, most important one in the program. Any site that doesn't believe this, is willingly accepting a second-rate position. Similarly, I also want the residents to have difficulty deciding which service is the most educational. Second, I want the residents to feel and behave, both individually and as a group, like professionals. I want them to feel professional "ownership" of the sites and to feel responsible for assisting sites, fellow residents, and faculty who are faced with some difficulty. If these values are in place, the RTD has much more latitude to respond to any problem. Instilling these values requires the systems engineer role to be implemented in a variety of verbal and nonverbal ways over a period of time.

If there is a reasonable sense of the two values just listed, *the first thing the RTD should do is . . . nothing.* Give everyone a chance to see the problem, digest it, think about it, and dialogue on-site about it. In my experience, the residents and faculty will solve it 90% of the time. Either the faculty will say, "We can survive for this short time one resident short," or the residents will say, "We need to help out." Commonly, both residents and faculty will put pressure on the RTD to make the decision quickly, to avoid processing the complicated feelings stimulated. The RTD should say things like, "Why don't we see how things go for a couple of days, first," or "Get together with the faculty up there and see what you come up with."

If it becomes clear after a few days that the problem is not moving toward a solution, the RTD's first action should be to set up meetings with everyone involved. When a problem such as this cannot be solved on-site between the residents and faculty, there is often something else going on. Through situations such as this I have discovered important issues at sites, such as changes in the service demands, structure, personnel interactions, and so on of which I was unaware. Once these are clarified and addressed, the residents and faculty will often proceed to solve the issue.

If it becomes clear, either through the failure of residents and faculty to find a site-based solution, or through consensus of both sides, that a schedule change is necessary, the implementation must be carefully handled. Within a year or two after I became an RTD, I identified in my own mind which sites could not tolerate the loss of a resident without serious damage to their educational programs, and which sites were much less resident dependent, able to function effectively in a shortage situation. That is open knowledge, with the rationale clearly explained to all attendings. This creates a sense of security among the sites and prevents a sense of surprise when a resident has to be "pulled." At times I have met with an entire resident class, explained why I thought a schedule change was necessary, and asked for volunteers. Other times I have called two or three residents and asked them to make the change. I always select the resident whose education will be most enhanced (or least damaged) by the change, and I always apologize for asking and appeal to their sense of helping out both their fellow residents and the faculty (I have yet to be turned down). When informing a service director that a resident will be pulled, I express appreciation for the service director's contribution to the overall functioning and quality maintenance of the program, and I suggest to the faculty who will get the resident that they call with gratitude to the site losing the resident.

The principle is to constantly reinforce to all parties that we are in this together, trying to maintain the best educational program in an unfortunate circumstance. It's "their" program, not mine, and we are all trying to keep it going as best we can.

The worst situation of this sort that I have encountered was when a patient struck a resident who was pregnant, precipitating premature labor, forcing her to bed rest for 4 months. Because I had established the preceding as my modus operandi, the site director called me to let me know what had happened and then said, "Let us handle this." Another inpatient unit director at the same hospital volunteered to rotate his residents into the empty slot, wisely asking his residents to "help out," first, then assigning them the task of setting up the schedule. The faculty at the site organized a resident/ faculty review committee that met at the injured resident's home for a "psychological postmortem" to assist the resident in processing her experience and to review how preventable the incident was. They tried but failed to get the patient, when he improved, to send a note to the resident.

Pregnant Residents

Of all the special situations in residency training, the issue of pregnant residents has probably received the most attention in the literature. Until around 1980, when there was a dramatic increase in women in medical schools, with a substantial proportion choosing psychiatry, a pregnant resident was a relatively rare occurrence. Now it is routine. Most residencies have more than 40% women, and it is a virtual certainty that sometime during any 1- to 2-year period, at least one of them will become pregnant.

The issues here are the same as those involved in illness and injury, with two important complicating factors. First, pregnancy is viewed by many residents and faculty as a resident's choice. Second, feelings arise about special treatment that is made available to some, but not all, residents. In terms of the shortage resulting from the pregnancy leave, compared with injury and illness, one has lead time in preparing for the absence. This is a mixed blessing. On the one hand, there is plenty of time to prepare; on the other, there is plenty of time for individuals to become very upset about things. In addition, the absence of the sense of crisis that accompanies an unexpected injury or illness reduces the shared need to find a solution.

The resident reaction to news that one of their peers is pregnant is usually mixed. There is delight and excitement, and there is resentment and envy. Interestingly, the split is rarely along gender lines. Men tend to split, with some being very supportive, even overly solicitous of the pregnant resident. Other males can be very resentful, feeling like the resident is "getting away with something," and taking advantage of her position to dump work on the rest of the resident group. Some women, especially those who are married, who have children, or who may be contemplating pregnancy, are also very supportive, even militantly so, demanding special privileges and consideration. Ironically, the most venomously resentful residents I have encountered are other women, commonly unmarried, who see any special considerations as undermining of their roles and position among their peers. Where men recognize the unique biological function of childbearing, though they may resent the timing, single women see marriage and motherhood as a choice or happenstance that excludes them.

The faculty is usually, these days, very supportive of pregnant residents, concerned simply with site coverage. However, there are still a few old guard types (which can include some senior women faculty who delayed their childbearing until after residency), who deeply resent the resident's choice to become pregnant. This small, but vocal, group can effectively stir up everyone, resulting in a totally unnecessary uproar. I have had faculty members literally say to me, "Why did you let this happen?," leaving me with the feeling that I should have been standing at the exits each night passing out birth control pills.

The stance of the pregnant resident herself becomes crucial in this situation. Some take an "I'm tough!" stance, planning to work full-time, taking their full measure of call right up to the moment of delivery, and determined to return to work 2 weeks afterward. Others engage in special pleading, demanding relief from call as soon as they learn they are pregnant, requesting easier rotations, resenting that they may have to make up some educational time if they take 6 months off before returning, and generally acting entitled. One year, I had two pregnant residents in the same class, which was already slightly smaller than most classes, who were going to deliver at approximately the same time. One was at the tougher end of the continuum, negotiating with her classmates to take extra call during her second trimester so that she could take less during the third, if necessary. The other acted much more entitled and spoke openly about the special status of pregnant women. The resident group practically fell over themselves helping out the first resident while being very resistant and resentful toward the second.

The single most important aspect of keeping this now routine part of residency training from becoming a "special problem" is to have a written policy in place. Ensure that the policy is well known and disseminated, and promote residents' and faculty acceptance of the policy as fair and humane. Such a policy is best proposed by a committee of residents and faculty, representing all subgroups and factions. In my opinion the committee is best chaired by a woman. A way of keeping the committee from getting bogged down by the emotional reactions this issue raises is to charge it with harmonizing program policy with affiliated institutions' policies, with reviewing the program's obligations under the Family and Medical Leave Act, and with distinguishing between the program's educational obligations and those resulting from its role as employer of the residents. Other important issues that such a committee must wrestle with are whether residents may use sick leave for their time off, how much unpaid leave can be taken without requiring an extension of the resident's time in the program, whether newly adoptive mothers should be treated any differently from biological mothers, and at what point the resident is obligated to inform the training director of her pregnancy. Once the committee comes up with a policy, it should be widely circulated, reviewed, and voted upon by the residency training committee (RTC). It should then be included in every new resident's orientation packet.

The presence of this policy will reduce conflict over this issue. In our program, we require notification of the RTD at least 6 months prior to the expected delivery date. This maximizes the opportunity to negotiate any schedule changes necessary. In fact, it will usually enable the schedule for the year to be made out with the anticipated absence in mind. In addition, I have found it very helpful to counsel pregnant residents at the time they notify me of their pregnancy. This counseling includes three major elements: informing residents of what they can do to maximize the support available to them from both peers and faculty, explaining anticipated patient responses, and preparing them for how difficult it will be to return to work. Professionally oriented women, in my opinion, seem to be particularly unprepared for the emotional changes that occur within them in the presence of their first infant. For that reason, I discourage them from making any final commitment to how long they plan to be out until late in their midtrimester.

If handled well, the issue of pregnant residents can be a "problem" the entire department takes great pride and pleasure in. In our program, we post announcements of the birth throughout the department, announce it at various meetings, and send flowers.

Paternity Leave

The issue of paternity leave is similar to that of maternity leave with the additional component of it being far less accepted in our society. Thus, the reactions of both residents and faculty is much more along the lines of "Why does he need it?" and "He's getting away with something."

The solution is essentially the same as for maternity leave: Have a written policy. It is probably best to have the same committee that proposes a policy on maternity leave propose one for expectant fathers as well. This ensures a coherent proposal that, more than any other, defines the program's attitude toward gender issues. In addition, it is amazing how many of the "old boys" who resist the importance of maternity leave, no matter how much they believe in the crucial role of early attachment, will mellow in their opposition when confronted with a parallel benefit for male residents (see Appendix 21–A).

A Resident Chooses to Leave the Program

Apart from the scheduling difficulties posed by this situation, the primary problem when a resident chooses to leave, regardless of the reason, is morale among both faculty and residents. Reasons for leaving vary: decisions to change specialties, transfer to another psychiatry program, financial issues, spouse or significant other employed elsewhere, other personal reasons (e.g., to seek treatment for substance abuse), or one step ahead of dismissal. The reasons for the resident's decision may be well known to fellow residents, known only to a few, known only to the RTD and/or a few trusted faculty, or known only to the resident. A reason may be promulgated that is not the full rationale, and this may or may not be obvious to the residents and faculty. The RTD may know why the resident is leaving but not feel at liberty to convey it, which can cause tension.

Regardless of the specifics, the reaction of both the residents and faculty is most likely to be, "Is there something wrong with us?" These days, this question can include, "What's wrong with our field?" If the reason needs to be kept confidential, this stirs fantasies about what may have been going on and represents a challenge to the trust between the RTD and both residents and faculty. A further complication is that every so often a class suffers far more than its share of comings and goings. Such a class often becomes a wounded group that fails to develop class cohesion, or loses what cohesion it did have. It is hard enough on residents that they know that, as with college and medical school, they are in a situation that will entail a parting in 4 years, so that unexpected and multiple partings can become anticipatory traumas.

When a resident informs the RTD that she or he will be leaving and the reasons for it, an important part of the discussion becomes who knows, what they know, and what the resident's preferences are about what may be said about the decision. Unless it is highly predictable that the leave-taking will have a traumatic effect, it is usually best to do nothing—to leave the informing of the residents and faculty to the resident. Chief residents and assistant RTDs should be informed and consulted with about the anticipated impact of the news. The rationale behind doing nothing is the old administrative principle: *Don't just do something, stand there!* This principle embodies the notion that when one has competent, professional, well-intended people, stepping in is likely to be intrusive and destructive to their mature efforts to cope with the problem. Taking unusual action may inadvertently convey that the problem is more serious than it really is. Exceptions to this principle may be when there have been an unusual number of leave-takings in a short time, when the leaving resident holds a particularly important role in the program (e.g., a perceived "star" or class leader), or when the resident's reason for leaving involves a problem that the RTD has been attempting to address but has been frustrated about.

In small programs, the RTD will often meet regularly with all of the residents and will see most of the faculty informally. In larger programs, the RTD should meet regularly with the chiefs and with each class's elected representatives. These will be opportunities to provide information and to learn whether the news of the leave-taking is evoking a strong enough response to call for active intervention. Such intervention with the residents is usually in the form of a meeting with the entire class, and free-form discussion of the impending loss. Commonly, other issues are triggered by the news of the departing resident, issues the RTD may be unaware of or that can be worked through in an open discussion by the class and the RTD. It is common for fantasies to fly among the residents; therefore, open meetings, with information freely shared (or clear, meaningful reasons for confidentiality being expressed) are extremely useful in detoxifying these.

If the faculty is disturbed by news of a departing resident, they usually require no specific intervention as they are much less reticent about calling up, asking what's going on, expressing their worst fears, and accepting the explanations offered.

A Resident Is Dismissed

This problem is an extension of the preceding situation, complicated by the residents' feelings about one of their own being fired. Their feelings will be mixed. There is always a component of, "There but for the grace of God go I," but most residents know who the weaker members of the class are and have no wish to have incompetent psychiatrists counted among their colleagues. This side of the ambivalence is often expressed as relief or anger that the faculty waited too long to act! A common compromise formation may involve questioning the process, though not necessarily the outcome. Was the dismissed resident dealt with fairly? Given fair warning? Fair opportunity to remediate deficiencies? And were the resident's rights respected in the process?

The faculty can be at odds over a dismissal as well. Many faculty members regard themselves as experts on teaching and evaluating residents. They are often unaware of the evaluations on other services or, if aware, may have their own opinions about the prejudices or blind spots of their colleagues. Thus, they may be all over the map, from "I told you so; what took you so long?" to "This resident has been treated completely unfairly and was a good resident."

This is one of those situations in which the process must not only be fair, but be seen to be fair. A clear procedure for handling deficient residents is crucial. An element of this procedure must be the recognition that at some point, as a problem resident is dealt with, the RTD and, one by one, the faculty members shift from an education-based, "let's help out this resident" view to an employer-based, "let's put pressure on this resident to improve or else" stance. The procedure begins with a well-written, clear, due process document. In our program, we asked our forensic psychiatrist to write the first draft. This was then circulated to all faculty and residents for comment, rewritten, and then submitted to the RTC for approval. That approval was contingent on review by the university attorney, who recommended substantial revision. The RTC then re-reviewed and reapproved the procedure. Every incoming resident receives a copy of this due process document, and all faculty and residents involved in a potential administrative action are offered copies to refresh their memories (see Appendix 21–B).

A good due process is only the beginning. Every program must have a committee that implements the due process, reviews all resident evaluations, and recommends action to the RTD. The composition and procedures of the evaluation committee must be thought through carefully. Faculty members who are perceived to take evaluation seriously, hold high standards, yet are humane, discreet, and of high integrity should be appointed. Every affiliated institution should have some representation, lest a hospital or agency feel that its observations and opinions may not be taken as seriously as are those of others. The chair should probably not be on the committee because almost every due process will have the chair as the final level of appeal, and his or her impartiality needs to be protected. One can debate whether there should be resident representatives on the committee. Many faculty argue that evaluation is a pure faculty function. On the other hand, without some resident participation, the evaluation committee becomes a "black box" in the eyes of the residents and, thus, the object of projections. I have found it most effective to have the chief resident sit on and be a full participant in this committee. Input from the resident's perspective is often very useful, especially since the residents often know of a peer's deficiency even more clearly than the faculty. Further, the chief will be in a position to say, "I was there and the resident was given a fair review/ hearing."

Once the decision to dismiss a resident has been made, the RTD is in a bind. Open information would be most effective at alleviating resident anxiety and enlisting faculty support, yet ethical and legal considerations require restraint and protection of the dismissed resident's privacy. There is often the potential for legal challenges that may not be apparent for months. I was once cited by the Equal Employment Opportunity Commission for being prejudiced against older East Indians a year after a resident's dismissal! Although the residents will often pressure you for details, they are usually understanding of the need for judicious protection of this sort of information. This is one of those situations where one must simply take the heat if the dismissed resident chooses to slander you and the department. In the long run, the residents will appreciate your perspicacity, even if they get taken in by the whisperings at first. A simple "How much would you want me to say about you, were you in a similar position?" usually gets the point across.

There are times when *an RTD's job is to take the heat,* and this is one of them. The heat can be shared, however. The chair and the associate dean for house staff should collaborate in reviewing the due process and should be kept fully informed, especially if there is any hint that legal action might result from the dismissal.

Residents Who Have Chronic Illnesses or Disabilities (With Special Note of HIV Issues)

I may be naive, or it may be a product of my role as a psychiatric consultant to an AIDS clinic, but HIV seems to be much less of an issue among residents than it once was. There is no longer the terror and prejudice about HIV-positive individuals that existed 5 years ago. At that time, residents and faculty had enormous countertransference issues with patients. At this point, I rarely find faculty or residents stirred up by having to care for AIDS patients. If they are, one handles it no differently from the entire range of countertransference problems that daily arise in residency: There must be adequate didactics, appropriate supervision, and available psychotherapy.

A situation in which everyone gets distressed is when a resident or faculty member has a clinical encounter in which they may have been exposed to HIV (usually a needle stick). Panic runs wild among the residents, and the faculty often feel guilty. The RTD is aided in this situation by the fact that virtually every hospital now has standard procedures for responding to such situations. The more one approaches the event in a professional manner, emphasizing the known risks, the known preventive measures (acknowledging that no prevention is foolproof), and the well-established procedures for follow-up, testing, and counseling, the more settled everyone will become. A meeting with the residents emphasizing the "known risk" aspect of the event may be useful. I try to encourage the residents, as part of their professional growth, to take pride in those aspects of their chosen profession that are special by virtue of the risks and responsibilities undertaken in the cause of caretaking.

The final, and potentially most controversial, issue that can arise is whether to consider a candidate for the program who is HIV-positive, and how to react if it becomes known that a resident has become infected. The RTD should be aware of existing legal ramifications. Specifically, the Americans with Disabilities Act probably precludes any attempts to exclude HIV-positive residents from the program. But that is unlikely to mollify feelings. Residents are likely to be primarily supportive, yet also resentful of any special needs an infected resident may have (e.g., easy fatigability that may influence ability to take call). Faculty may also be supportive, but even more resentful than the residents. Part of the pleasure of teaching residents is the fantasy of reproducing oneself and seeing residents identify with you. Any resident who is clearly "different" challenges this gratification. The faculty may present the issue in terms of rationalizations about the resident's ability to do the work, to be a full team member, to practice enough to warrant the time and effort invested. On the other hand, some faculty may see such a resident as an asset, bringing a unique and creative perspective to the field and to the other residents.

I see the issue of the HIV-positive resident as a special case of any resident with a disability. In our program we have considered applicants who had multiple sclerosis, muscular dystrophy, chronic back problems, myocardial infarction, chronic heavy metal poisoning, sequelae of polio, psychiatric disorders, and Friedreich's ataxia. But this can only occur after the faculty has engaged in an ongoing dialogue about the program's values. *The faculty must consider who they are, their vision of the field, and the balance between humanistic values and standards of excellence* in working with residents. Only then can applicants with disabilities be considered solely on their ability to become an effective psychiatrist and to perform the functions of a resident. Once the faculty has made these decisions, they will be implicitly conveyed to the residents as part of their socialization into the program. The values of the program need not even be articulated by the RTD, for they will permeate the system. But *the RTD must see the need for and initiate the faculty dialogue.* The dialogue is often not explicit but implicit in discussions that occur in a variety of situations: the recruitment committee, evaluation committee, RTC, and in individual discussions with faculty about a whole host of issues. In these forums, as the program's values are being established, the RTD is in a strong position to influence the direction, but there must be a feeling of consensus. The Americans with Disabilities Act lends a legal dimension to this discussion, as this law cannot be broken in the application process. But the legal prescription should not preempt the departmental values dialogue.

In our program, after such a dialogue, we accepted the applicant with Friedreich's ataxia, but only after she had demonstrated how she would use her motorized cart to handle an aggressive patient. She performed well but ran into some resistance from a subgroup of her classmates who didn't want to share one particular rotation with her. The chiefs handled this with a class meeting. This psychiatrist is now chief of a unit that specializes in psychosocial rehabilitation of the severely regressed, chronically mentally ill. She has been uniformly beloved by her patients who sense her deep empathy for those afflicted with a chronic disability. My hunch is that her very presence is an inspiration for many of her patients. We have had brighter residents and others more skilled in certain areas of psychiatry, but I doubt there is any resident of whom we feel prouder. An HIV-positive resident would be no different.

Patient Suicide

There are probably some psychiatrists who, in their entire careers, have no patient commit suicide, but if there is any universal tragedy that psychiatrists must endure, this is it. Every psychiatrist must make peace with the likelihood that it probably will happen. One of my own teachers once said, "If a psychiatrist never has a suicide, he is not treating very sick patients." I quote this often to residents who have endured their first patient suicide.

In some ways, a patient's suicide must be understood as the way psychiatrist's patients are most likely to die. Deaths of patients is an issue all physicians must face. To the extent that residents can appreciate this fact, a patient's suicide is another part of the experience of practicing their profession. The willfulness of the act, in the face of the resident's efforts to help the patient find meaning in life, is what makes it difficult for residents to find peace with the event.

The resident whose patient commits suicide is likely to feel guilt beyond that associated with the failure of treatment efforts. This guilt involves whatever unresolved countertransference issues existed in the treatment relationship. A resident may feel overly guilty about the suicide of a patient at whom the resident was angry, or whom the resident especially liked. It is the level of emotional investment, positive or negative, that makes this so difficult an issue. It may be evident to everyone, faculty and fellow residents alike, that the dead patient was an extraordinarily high-risk, chronically suicidal patient, but that is often cold comfort to the resident.

The rest of the resident group will almost always be supportive and also experience a sense of relief that it wasn't their patient. The faculty, most of whom will have been there before, will be uniformly supportive, sometimes overly solicitous. Excess solicitude gives the resident the message that the event is of more magnitude than is realistic.

It is important that three things occur to help the resident and the entire group process a suicide (see Table 21–2). First, there should be a psychological autopsy, which reviews the case and treatment and pays attention to the feelings of everyone involved in the case. I encourage every site to have a standard procedure in place for dealing with suicides. An outside consultant who acts as facilitator who summarizes the case and brings closure at the end of the discussion is optimal (see Appendix 21–C). Second,

Table 21–2. What to do when a resident's patient commits suicide

1. Have a site-based, standard procedure for a psychological autopsy.
2. Be sure the resident has an available confidante.
3. Let the resident and the entire group know that you know what has occurred.

the resident needs an expert confidante. This will usually be the supervisor on the case, the resident's therapist, or some other trusted faculty member. It can be, but need not be, the RTD. The resident will also need a peer confidante, who will usually emerge from the resident's friends, family, or peers. The RTD should be alert to the vulnerability of those residents who are socially isolated. Asking the chief resident to check in on such a resident can be helpful. Finally, the entire resident group, and the resident, need to know that the RTD *knows* what has happened and is *attuned* to the issues. A note, a brief remark in the hall, or an invitation to drop by and visit about the suicide may be all that is necessary. Rarely, a formal meeting with the RTD may be appropriate.

A Resident With Legal, Ethical, or Malpractice Difficulties

It used to be very uncommon for legal complications to arise during residency. That is no longer true, partly due to the general increase in litigation in our society, partly due to the field's greater attention to ethical and forensic issues, and partly due to the increased severity and acuity of patients seen during training. It is now fairly common for residents to be named in malpractice suits arising from emergency room encounters. This is quite a shock for a young resident the first time it occurs. The RTD must balance three separate functions in these situations: the supportive/educational role, the legal role, and the administrative role.

If a resident has transgressed a doctor-patient boundary, made a serious medical error, or otherwise compromised clinical care, the RTD's first legal and administrative responsibility is to prevent harm to patients. If the severity of the error is not such that immediate administrative action is required, then the RTD can assume a more supportive, educational stance. Optimally, this is done through the site where the problem occurred; otherwise formal counseling, provision of additional supervision, getting the resident into psychotherapy, and gearing up the standard administrative procedures at their usual pace become necessary. It must be clear to the resident that this is not simply a routine matter of learning and developing clinical skills. At the same time, if the problem is regarded as remediable, adequate support should be provided. The RTD must make a complicated judgment as to the origins and remediability of the transgression. Does it reflect naivete? Personality problems? A temporary aberration? Major cognitive deficits? Serious knowledge deficiencies? This judgment will determine how much one assumes a supportive versus a potentially punitive administrative stance.

Residency training directors are constantly making decisions of this type. If a resident runs into conflict with a faculty member, which generates an angry memo, should the memo go into the resident's file or should it be held, awaiting other evidence of problems? An RTD must know the faculty as well as the residents in making this decision. Beginning a paper trail has repercussions for the resident and can be difficult to stop once started. It is important that a personality conflict with a particular attending not escalate into multiple memos that the evaluation committee must then react to. On the other hand, failure to start a paper trail can make administrative action impossible, despite widespread faculty conviction that a resident is incompetent or pathological. Thus, it is important to make an early judgment as to the significance of a serious clinical error. In some instances, a supportive, mentoring role is indicated. In others, one must request documentation in writing from faculty, place one's own memos of record in the file, and lower one's threshold for further administrative action.

Some clinical errors are so egregious that they must be acted on immediately; for example, sexual contact with a patient or wanton negligence. The due process must be written so that the RTD has the ability to immediately suspend a resident's clinical activities pending further documentation, information, and action by the evaluation committee. More difficult is the situation in which one concludes that a resident's problem is not likely to be remediated, but does not yet justify administrative action. Here, the RTD must move carefully but firmly and persistently in documenting the deficits so that the evaluation committee will be able to act without fear of lawsuit or other repercussions from the resident in question. Residents' rights must be sincerely respected by making their files available to them and allowing the insertion into the record of any material residents may wish on their own behalf. Faculty must be alerted to potential problems, but it must be done in such a way that fairness is observed and the program is not left open to charges of conspiracy or bias. Documentation must be assiduous. To accomplish this, the RTD must have worked extensively with the faculty about their feelings as evaluators. The most common problem I have observed is when faculty see a problem but are reluctant to document it, especially in the early years of residency, rationalizing to themselves that the resident is "still new," "will learn more," or will "grow out of it." No one is served well by reluctance to identify failing clinical accomplishments early. A problem that does not begin to be documented until some time in the PGY-3 is likely to place the program in the position of having a senior resident everyone is embarrassed by but fears to fire. The resident's complaint that "No one told me" seems confirmed by the written record and opens the possibility of a lawsuit.

The RTD must lead persistently in this area. Whether dealing with an egregious violation, a remediable error, or an evolving movement toward administrative action, the RTD must face the dilemma of how much to share, and with whom. I almost always share full information with the chief resident and the assistant training director, not only for their information but also for their input and advice. If I foresee any potential for legal or administrative entanglements, I *always* inform the chair of what is going on. These are people whose discretion I trust. The dilemma comes with regard to protecting the resident's rights and privacy and avoiding the appearance of a conspiracy. I never share anything with additional residents until some official action occurs, and, even then, it may be necessary to withhold information (as with a dismissal). The faculty at the site where the transgression occurred invariably are fully informed and consulted about what action to take, but I rarely inform other faculty except to ask the supervisors on the next rotation to let me know if there are any problems. I take considerable heat from some faculty for this stance, although others appreciate it. The case for full disclosure to future supervisors of a resident who has made a serious and dangerous error is compelling. At the same time, the need for fully independent observations is also important. Either choice will put the RTD in a difficult position and require taking some flak.

A more pleasant task awaits the RTD when a resident is sued but not deemed to be weak clinically by the program. Here, the RTD's entire energy can be directed toward supporting a young colleague-to-be in coping with every physician's worst nightmare. The most important thing is to have resources and support available to the resident. In addition to counseling and supervision, every hospital and medical school has an attorney, and every program must have a forensic psychiatry expert, if not immediately on faculty, then by consultation with other programs. I find that sending the resident to speak with these people is enormously reassuring to them. They immediately realize they are not in this alone, that they have expert support, and it rapidly becomes apparent that many other residents have traversed this path. I often tell residents that although it may not be pleasant, being sued while still a resident offers them the maximum support possible and is much better than encountering their first suit all alone. It can be a tremendous learning experience, one that they share with their peers, as they learn extensively about the interactions of the medical and legal systems. The hospital attorney turns out to be much better than I at convincing the residents that they are not being personally or professionally attacked by a suit. There is a lot to learn about how and why people get named in suits, as well as who gets eliminated from a suit. Some residents have even developed an unexpected interest in forensic psychiatry as a result of being sued.

Midyear Changes in Faculty or Sites

One of the most shocking discoveries I encountered as a new RTD was realizing that the most conservative group I had to deal with were the residents. I had expected the residents to be natural allies in changes, especially forward-looking, progressive changes in the program. In fact, residents almost invariably react to any proposed programmatic change negatively, even suspiciously. Faculty tend to react egocentrically, "How will it affect me and my service?" Residents also become tied to the schedule as originally published. Any alteration to it, even one that residents want, is often viewed with anxiety. My best understanding of this process is that it reflects the residents' feelings of helplessness and lack of control of their lives. No matter how understandable, sensible, constructive, and positive, a midyear change of sites or faculty stirs much distress. Further, the residents often feel they have been promised a certain program. They view changes to that program as violations of a contract, as a betrayal. Theirs is a short-term perspective, solely related to immediate training expectations. The faculty's perspective is long term, knowing the program must evolve and change.

Training directors need to be well plugged into the departmental grapevine so that they know in advance what is happening or likely to happen. This is not always easy. I recommend to new RTDs that before accepting their positions, they negotiate to be part of whatever formal or informal "kitchen cabinet" the chair uses to help run the department. Regular meetings with the appropriate service chiefs is also crucial. Attendance at staff meetings of all important affiliates is useful. This way, any service-driven structural or faculty changes will be well known to the RTD early. This gives the RTD an opportunity to inform the service of the expected impact of contemplated changes. Over time, it has the effect of encouraging affiliated sites and services to factor the educational impact and likely reaction of the residents into their decision making. I have been able to convince sites to delay changes until the beginning of the next academic year, when they can be included in the new schedule, for example. There is nothing more embarrassing than having a resident ask you about some faculty member leaving or restructuring of a service and you have no idea what is going on, or that anything was afoot.

Once you learn that a change is likely, the timing of the announcement is crucial. During the talking and planning phase, when there is much uncertainty about whether a change will occur or what form it may take, there is no point in stirring up the residents' "change anxiety" unnecessarily, especially if that period includes recruitment interviewing. Applicants will hear about the still-uncertain changes, or simply sense the residents' anxiety. However, as the decision-making process goes forward, it is wise to inform the chief residents and assistant RTDs to get as much feedback as possible about the projected impact of any changes. It is also important that the chiefs inform the RTD as soon as rumors begin flying among the residents. It is important to formally inform the residents as soon as they start hearing rumors or at the time the decision definitely to make a change is made. Typically, this will be several weeks or months before the actual change will occur, and time is afforded to process the change and respond to anxieties.

In addition, there is often a lag between the decision to make some change and the determination of what form those changes will take. Residents should be placed on the committee(s) or consulted by the decision maker (as should be the RTD) during this time period. The helplessness of the residents is part truth and part myth. Knowing of the RTD's involvement, the chief resident's involvement, and their peers' involvement helps to demythologize residents' feelings of being out of control. The announcement should be made either to the residents' entire group, or to the class involved. A series of meetings might be necessary to ensure the ongoing flow of information, especially the reasons for the midyear change, the shape of things to come, and to provide opportunities to assuage the residents' anxieties.

In the end, however, the RTD is going to have to come up with a new schedule, or endorse restructuring an old rotation, and may have to endure the residents' rage, paranoia, and accusations, even with the maximum preparation. Take the heat! It comes with the job. Further, if you see an unavoidable negative change coming up, caused by forces beyond your control, there is an old administrative saying, "It is easier to ask forgiveness that to ask permission." Do what you can to make the best of it for the residents, make your decisions on your own, tell it straight out to the residents. Then take the heat. The residents will feel more secure with an RTD who acts and owns up than with one who seems as helpless and out of control as they feel.

In the case of a faculty member leaving, especially a beloved teacher, the residents' reaction is parallel to that of the faculty when a resident transfers electively, "What's wrong with the program?" Being in the transitional stage of not yet full-fledged working people, yet hardly students anymore, residents are not yet aware of the complexities involved in career decisions. Inform them as best you can. Most will accept your explanations, but some won't. In our program we have one or two older residents in every class, often physicians retraining from other specialties. They are often more convincing about the career issues than I am. In the event that the faculty member's leave-taking does reflect a problem in the program, there is no point in hiding it except to protect the privacy of the faculty involved. Always indicate your awareness of the problem and your plans to address it.

Changes in or Absence of the Chair or Residency Training Director

At the Tarrytown Conference, sponsored by Albert Einstein College of Medicine, which most chief residents from U.S. psychiatry programs attend, a sophisticated introduction to group process, management, and leadership is begun by assigning groups a task but not designating a leader. Subsequently, the same task is assigned after a leader has been selected. The chiefs learn vividly the importance of an identified leader, and that a bad leader is invariably far more effective than no leader at all. Most of us intuitively understand this basic phenomenon of small social group behavior. Few experiences are more threatening than news of the leader's demise, no matter how intense the antipathy may have been. This is what the impending or actual absence of the chair or RTD means to both residents and faculty.

The reaction is intense and unpredictable. Among the residents there may be anxiety that borders on terror, anger that verges into rage, fear that turns into paranoia, relief that becomes euphoria, or disinterest that is probably a form of denial. The faculty will be having similar reactions, although their greater experience with institutional transitions may make them more modulated, and their focus will be more on the future role of their particular services. The residents are more likely to experience their world falling apart, whether it is or not. Rumors and fantasies run wild. I have seen residents pick up and transfer to far inferior programs because they simply could not tolerate the uncertainty of lacking or changing a leader.

Oddly enough, this may be one of the easiest "special" problems to solve. If the anxiety is born of the absence of a leader, then the clear visibility and active leadership of the RTD best assuages the feelings. In so doing, the RTD becomes a lightning rod for all feelings, but this will likely reduce acting out and keep everyone focused on their training. Then take the heat. Because residents are rightly regarded as novices at institutional life, some RTDs have a tendency to withhold or otherwise manage information they receive about the transition. To my way of thinking, this infantilizes the residents and encourages regression in such times. I prefer to educate them about the nature of institutional transitions, informing them fully of all that is going on, the good, the bad, and the ugly. This treats them like junior colleagues and invites them to behave accordingly.

A special complication comes when one is either the outgoing or incoming RTD. These are positions that every RTD will assume in his or her tenure. If one is the outgoing RTD, there can be a perceived hypocrisy in continuing to act the leader while awaiting one's successor. However, the stance of, "We go about our business as usual while awaiting my successor, at which time I will happily hand over the reins to a colleague I respect," can go a long way toward assisting the next RTD, even if one is leaving unwillingly. Helping the residents with their grief, whatever form it takes, idealizing one or vilifying one, is the primary task. If an RTD is leaving to take a position elsewhere, the RTD should call a meeting of all residents as quickly as possible to break the news. The residents most affected by this transition will be the PGY-2s. They consider themselves as belonging to the old RTD, yet will spend most of their training under the new one. Their professional identity is just enough formed yet not sufficiently secure to see them through the change. The PGY-4s already see themselves as finished and thinking about their life after residency. The PGY-3s very much belong to the old RTD, but usually feel secure enough in their identities to regulate their reactions. The PGY-1s are likely to feel betrayed, recruited under false pretenses, yet their need for a clear leader will be strong enough that they will readily look for the best in the new RTD.

Incoming RTDs in such a transition get their first lesson in taking the heat. Connections must be made with the residents; they need to know who the RTD is, that the RTD will be their leader, yet won't upset their applecart by making wholesale rapid changes. New RTDs must be visible; speak openly and positively of their predecessor; be cautious in any changes, addressing first those that the residents have wanted but that the old RTD was unable to make; and accept the residents' projections, good and bad. No matter how well incoming RTDs handle the change, there will come a time, best delayed by 6 months or so, when they do something that makes it clear to everyone that a new hand is on the tiller. Uproar will ensue. The RTD shouldn't try to make sense of it. Things will settle down, at which point a new and mutually comfortable homeostasis will take hold.

Mergings, Closings, Downsizings

All of us who work within institutions have thought about and made our peace with the fact that, when push comes to shove, the institution will invariably do what's best for it, regardless of the impact on individuals. We have accepted this insecurity, calculated our own likelihood of becoming a casualty, developed ways of functioning that we believe minimize our risk, and created whatever safety net we deem necessary. Residents have not done this. Some are aware of and deeply worried about this aspect of being part of an institution, a few to the point that we regard them as paranoid. Others (most of them) are oblivious to this fact of life and are viewed by the paranoid residents as naive. When a training program merges with another, downsizes, or closes, it almost never does so in a positive educational spirit. Invariably, the program feels forced to take drastic action due to outside influences beyond its control. Residents are brutally confronted with their ultimate unimportance to the life of an institution. The faculty, facing their worst, dreaded nightmare, generally do not feel or act a whole lot better than do the residents. Their livelihoods and careers are on the line.

The administrative problem raised by this restructuring is that the entire training program usually has to be redesigned. Once the shock of the announcement has worn off, this task, which logically falls to the RTD, can be used to help channel the reactions as constructively as possible. Most people will be either paralyzed by their feelings or fleeing for safer pastures. Others will be fighting a rear guard and almost always futile action to reverse the decision. Some will be channeling their energies into maneuvering themselves into what they perceive to be "safe" situations. By swiftly setting up a process for redesigning the program based on the new realities of available services and residents, action can be shaped constructively.

A detailed procedure for this can be found in Yager et al.'s (1998) paper on downsizing. Similarly, Tasman and Riba (1993) have written of their experience with a merger. The key elements involve the inclusion of everyone in a process for adapting to the new environment. They need to be involved in small workable groups. The support of the chair and service chiefs for the process is crucial, yet everyone must understand that, in the end, the chair has final decision-making responsibility. The RTD needs to be involved in all work groups and lead a steering committee that sifts and evaluates ideas emerging from each group. Feedback to each group about what ideas are emerging from other task forces is also important. A fair and perceived-to-be-fair process can generate a good deal of excitement as people realize they are involved in designing a whole new clinical curriculum that is liberated from the constraints of past ways of doing things. Above all, the RTD must be very visible to all, leading and facilitating the process. If the problem was that of a potentially leaderless group, this problem involves the group threatened with annihilation by decisions of the leader. Social cohesion must be rebuilt. The chair/potential destroyer is ill placed to do it. The RTD is ideally suited and must attend every meeting possible. The threat to the process is paralysis and passive aggressive behavior by both residents and faculty. One must meet, and meet, and meet some more. The RTD should be the rock around which the faculty and resident group redefine their cohesion and ideals by turning a decision that involved no concerns for education into an opportunity to improve the program. It is not a joke to suggest that the groups need to become so sick of seeing and being nagged by the RTD that they make some decisions in spite of themselves!

Finally, in the end, some very difficult decisions will have to be made. Some services will lose residents, some residents will go to institutions they never wanted to, and some institutions with which both faculty and residents have identified will lose their identities. As the dust settles, take the heat. That's what we get paid the big bucks for!

In recent years there have been outright closings of training programs. All evidence suggests there will be more in the future. These closings have tended to be abrupt, with short notice, giving no consideration to contractual or educational obligations to either residents or faculty and usually instigated by outside administrators. The residents and RTD are in the same boat. It is important, at a time when it seems that the world has become arbitrary and malignant, destroying their lives, that the RTD maintain some model of integrity and stability, even though she or he is probably also looking for a job with some degree of panic. Using the RTD network through the American Association of Directors of Psychiatry Residency Training and the American Psychiatric Association clearinghouse, the residents can all be placed in a suitable and congenial program. Their world has been destroyed, but they themselves survive, and can prosper, supported by their RTD's last official acts in that role.

Conclusions

What ties these disparate problems together is their potential or real traumatic qualities. They have the ability to tear a program apart, literally or emotionally. I go back to the introduction. If, taking into consideration the many roles of the RTD, you establish a system and set of procedures that are not only fair, but perceived to be fair, they can become opportunities for strengthening and building a program. I must confess that when I began as an RTD and one of these special problems arose, I would approach it with dread and a sense of crisis. Experience has transformed my response into a zest for grappling with difficult issues. Wrestling with these special problems can be the most exciting, meaningful, and important aspects of being a residency training director.

References

Jensen PS: The transition to residency seminar. Journal of Psychiatric Education 7(4):261–267, 1983

Lomax JW: A proposed curriculum on suicide care for psychiatry residency. Suicide Life Threat Behav 16(1):56–54, 1986

Phelan ST: Pregnancy during residency. II. Obstetric complications (review). Obstet Gynecol 72(3 Pt 1):431–436, 1988

Stewart DE, Robinson GE: Combining motherhood with psychiatric training and practice. Can J Psychiatry 30(1):28–34, 1985

Tasman A, Riba M: Strategic issues for the successful merger of residency training programs. Hosp Community Psychiatry 44(10):981–985, 1993

Wagner KD, Pollard R, Wagner RF Jr: Malpractice litigation against child and adolescent psychiatry residency programs, 1981–1991. J Am Acad Child Adolesc Psychiatry 32(2):462–465, 1993

Yager J, Burk V, Mohl PC: Downsizing psychiatric residency programs: a pilot study. Acad. Psychiatry 22(2):127–34, 1998

Young-Shumate L, Kramer T, Beresin E: Pregnancy during graduate medical training. Acad Med 68(10):792–799, 1993

Guidelines for Resident Parental Leaves

1. Four weeks of unpaid parental leave are available to each resident during the duration of the residency without educational pay back obligations.
2. Parental leave must be initiated within 6 months of the arrival of a new child.
3.. In addition to parental leave time, unused vacation time from the current academic year may be utilized as paid parental leave, and unused sick leave from the current academic year may be utilized as paid parental leave. Each resident is entitled to a total of 12 weeks of parental leave per 12-month period under the Family Medical Leave Act.
4. Any leave time not covered by sick leave, vacation, or the 4 weeks of parental leave must be made up at the end of the residency, in order to assure proper educational achievement and credentialing.
5. With the permission of the Residency Training Director, leave time may be extended to a total of 26 weeks per parental leave, with the extended portion to be made up at the end of the residency. Any time in excess of 26 weeks seriously engenders the risk of request of the resident's resignation and must be discussed individually with the Resident Training Director, who holds the authority to make all decisions regarding extended leaves. Any time to be made up will be done on a site at the discretion of the Resident Training Director and conforming to the requirements for board eligibility.
6. Although salary to cover the time made up at the end of residency cannot be absolutely guaranteed, every attempt to work out scheduling on an individual basis will be made.
7. Although this is the department policy and is compatible with Parkland's policy, other hospitals' policies may preclude payment derived from vacation or sick leave.
8. To facilitate scheduling, residents are encouraged to notify the Resident Training Director of an anticipated parental leave as early as possible. Failure to give adequate notice may compromise the availability of leave. *Six month's notice* must be given before the arrival of a new child, and any changes in length of leave must be negotiated on a case by case basis with the Resident Training Director. Changes cannot be guaranteed but are more likely to be possible with more advanced notice.
9. All final decisions regarding leaves will be made at the discretion of the Resident Training Director.

Guidelines for Resident Personal Leaves

1. No guaranteed personal leave is available during the residency.
2. All decisions regarding personal leave will be made at the discretion of the Resident Training Director.
3. Emergency leaves of less than three days duration may be facilitated through the site attending after coverage arrangements are made by the resident.

Guidelines for Resident Sick Leaves

1. Two weeks of paid sick leave are available each academic year.
2. Although this is the department policy and is compatible with Parkland policy, other hospitals' policies may preclude payment for sick leave.
3. An additional 4 weeks of unpaid sick leave are available during the duration of the residency without educational pay back obligations.
4. Any sick leave time exceeding the above 6 weeks must be made up at the end of the residency to ensure educational achievement and credentialing. A total of 12 weeks sick leave per 12-month period is available to each resident under the FMLA. Any time to be made up will be done on a site at the discretion of the Resident Training Director and conforming to the requirements for board eligibility.
5. Sick leave may be used for the care of immediate family members who become ill.
6. Documentation *may* be required at the discretion of the Resident Training Director.

Reprinted with permission of Texas Southwestern Department of Psychiatry.

Due Process Procedures for Psychiatry Residents UT Southwestern Medical Center at Dallas

Resident Assessment

1. Each resident will be assigned a faculty supervisor on each rotation or clinical experience. The level and method of this supervision will be consistent with the ACGME Special Requirements for Residency Education in Psychiatry.
2. Each resident will be given written evaluation by supervisors at the end of each rotation, or twice a year in the case of psychotherapy supervisors, or yearlong rotations.
3. The program director, and/or his/her designee, will meet with each resident at least twice yearly concerning evaluations of his/her performance and, with the resident's input, shall make recommendations for resolving deficiencies and improvement of the resident's general skills and knowledge. In the event deficiencies are identified, the program director may meet with the resident in addition to the two scheduled meetings. The program director shall document each such meeting.
4. The Progress and Evaluation Committee (the "Committee") is comprised of selected faculty of the adult, child, geriatric, and forensic psychiatry divisions, the training directors and chief residents, and is chaired by the program director. The Committee shall meet annually, or at the request of the program director, to discuss the progress of each resident. The Committee shall identify any areas in which the resident may improve his/her skills or knowledge, and any deficiencies in the resident's performance, or impediments to the resident's progress toward professional competence, and make recommendations for improvement. These recommendations shall be communicated to the resident in his/her meeting with the program director, and the resident may also meet with the Committee if disciplinary action is included in the Committee's recommendation as described more fully below.
5. The program director shall advance residents to positions of higher responsibility on the basis of the combined evaluations of the resident's readiness for advancement.
6. Each resident shall be given the opportunity to give a written evaluation of supervisors, clinical rotations, and courses at the end of each rotation.

Disciplinary Action

1. The Committee, either at its regular meeting or a specially scheduled meeting, may additionally recommend that disciplinary action be taken. Recommendations for discipline may include: formal letter of warning; suspension from clinical duties, with or without pay; probation; or, in the most extreme situations, nonrenewal or termination.

2. Notice of disciplinary action shall be prepared by the program director and provided to the resident. Such notice shall include: the reasons for the disciplinary action, the length of time the disciplinary action will be in effect, and the corrective action the resident is required to make (unless the recommendation is termination.)

3. After the program director has met with the resident regarding the recommended disciplinary action, the resident may appeal the recommendation of the Committee by giving written notice to the program director within 10 working days from the date of his/her initial meeting with the program director.

4. In cases of appeal, the program director shall convene a majority of the Committee as soon as reasonably practicable to meet with the resident requesting the appeal. Resident members of the Committee may attend and have voting privileges. The resident requesting the appeal is encouraged to bring any additional information to the Committee's attention, including other opinions that the resident believes were not sufficiently appreciated in the previous deliberations.

5. At any time during the appeal of a disciplinary action, the resident may choose to be represented by an attorney to ensure that his/her rights are appropriately protected, but must notify the program director no less than 3 working days before the date of any hearing at which an attorney shall appear on a resident's behalf.

6. After the meeting of the Committee regarding an appeal of a disciplinary action, the Committee shall provide a written response to the resident within 5 working days.

7. In all cases except for termination, the Committee's determination upon appeal shall be final. All recommendations for termination or nonrenewal, however, are subject to review by the department chair.

Suspension of Patient Care Responsibilities

1. A supervisor or director of a clinical service who believes that patient welfare may be jeopardized because of a resident's performance may request the program director to temporarily suspend the resident's clinical activities.

2. If such a suspension is determined to be warranted by the program director, the program director shall inform the resident in writing of the nature

of the observations that caused temporary suspension of clinical privileges and shall convene a meeting of the Committee as soon as is reasonably practicable. In such an event, the resident is encouraged to invite any members of the faculty, staff, or residents to provide information to the Committee for consideration.

3. The recommendation of the Committee, including the recommendation for any disciplinary action, shall be provided to the program director within 5 working days from the date of its meeting, which shall be promptly communicated with the resident. The resident may appeal this recommendation as described above.

Morbidity and Mortality Conferences

Suicides and attempted homicides by clinic patients are reviewed regularly. The purpose of the conference is resident support, continuous quality improvement and education. The focus is placed on the precipitating event, some of the ways family and environment may have encouraged suicidal crises (interaction of patient's psychopathology with family dynamics), and professional intervention. Supporting the family and documenting events is also discussed.

22

Professional Development of Residents

Carol C. Nadelson, M.D., and Carol A. Bernstein, M.D.

This chapter focuses on the characteristics and experience of psychiatry residents as they progress through their training programs. We will consider the following issues:

1. The changing scene in psychiatric residency training
2. Common difficulties including stress
3. Safety
4. Ethics
5. Learning and supervision
6. The resident as teacher
7. Psychotherapy for residents
8. Support and training groups
9. The relationship between residents and the training director
10. Administrative issues
11. Key transitions during residency

The Changing Scene in Psychiatric Residency Training

Many factors influence the environment in which residency training in psychiatry takes place. These include demographics of the residency pool, changes in the health care delivery system, economic factors including mounting student debt, increased knowledge base, and attitudes of medical students about the profession. Demographics of psychiatric residency have changed over the past decade. The numbers of women and minority residents have continued to rise, as have the numbers of international medical graduates (IMGs). In 1995, the number of U.S. seniors selecting psychiatry as a career fell sharply (down more than 40% from 1988). This was probably a consequence of multiple factors, including increased pressure for students to enter primary care. Concomitantly, the number of IMGs entering psychiatric training increased so dramatically that more than half of first-year psychiatry residents on July 1, 1996, were IMGs. Women continue to make up more than 40% of psychiatric residents.

The effect of changes in the health care delivery system on residency has been profound. Although today's house officers work fewer hours and are paid more than those who trained a decade or two ago, the pressures of training seem to have escalated. Shorter lengths of inpatient stays have resulted in greater turnover of sicker patients and increased requirements for paperwork and documentation. These contribute to expectations for house staff performance that can be overwhelming. The imminent reduction in reimbursement for graduate medical education will decrease the availability of funds for training, particularly for residents in specialties like psychiatry, and will likely increase burdens for residents and faculty. The impact of these changes has already led to reductions in program size, mergers, and even the closure of some training programs. The characteristics of residency training in psychiatry may remain unstable and unpredictable for the foreseeable future.

In the past, most medical students who entered psychiatry expected to become psychotherapists or psychoanalysts. Career goals frequently included a primary commitment to private practice with some teaching, and perhaps a bit of clinical research and administration. Expectations have changed, along with systemic changes and the vast increase in psychiatric treatments available to patients. Shrinking inpatient services, which now function as acute, short-term intensive care units with dramatically reduced lengths of stay, expanded emergency services, and sicker patients in outpatient clinics have created a situation in which traditional learning through long-term contact with patients may not be possible. Many residents do not get to know their patients or their families during these brief hospitalizations. They rely more on outpatient contacts, which have also been curtailed by the changed health care system. These developments make it more difficult to build the kind of trusting relationships with patients and their families that evolved from the long-term contact that characterized psychiatric training and practice in the past.

As reimbursement for service is increasingly controlled by third parties, tightening financial constraints are further reducing the number of psychotherapy visits that are possible for patients insured by various systems of care. As a result, residency training programs are beginning to focus more on teaching brief treatment modalities (such as interpersonal therapy, cognitive/behavioral therapy, and brief dynamic psychotherapy) to help prepare residents for future health care scenarios. Ironically, since some of these modalities, particularly the brief dynamic therapies, require a highly sophisticated understanding of psychodynamics, they present a challenge to psychiatric educators to provide this when opportunities for residents to see patients over time have decreased, and didactic requirements for new modalities limit the time available for a comprehensive psychodynamic education.

Among the other changes brought by the health care revolution is the increasing role of the primary care or family practice "gatekeeper" and its effect on the psychiatrist. It is increasingly important to develop training opportunities for psychiatric residents in primary care clinics where these residents can work alongside their primary care colleagues, providing psychiatric services in both consultation and liaison roles.

Most medical students have had little prior experience with psychiatry or psychiatrists that is comparable to their own life experiences with pediatrics or internal medicine. Often, the image of the psychiatrist has not been the same as the image of other physicians, and choosing psychiatry may place students in an uncomfortable position within their peer group and with nonpsychiatric faculty within the medical school.

Common Difficulties for the Beginning Resident

Those beginning psychiatry residencies encounter a world that is very different from the familiar world of internal medicine or surgery. Prior experience is not a preparation. Illnesses are unfamiliar, the structure of psychiatric services are not like those the resident has learned to understand on medical and surgical services, and the nature of emergencies is confusing at best. How does one decide whether to send a potentially suicidal patient home or determine how dangerous a patient might be?

Often residents attempt to concretize the process by focusing on didactic learning, a mode that is familiar and comfortable. The clinical learning process, however, is more difficult and stressful. The resident may be tempted to retreat into silence and to mimic the stereotypes that may constitute the only image of psychiatrists with which they are familiar. A supervisor's criticism may be felt as far-reaching, and the art of learning how to ask for help or accept supervision is difficult.

One of the most challenging issues for the beginning resident is the need to deal with the inherent ambiguity in the field. Unlike many other medical specialists, psychiatrists have few lab results that enable them to even pretend that there are concrete data upon which to base a diagnosis —although more are available to monitor pharmacologic treatment. The beginner has few interviewing and evaluative skills. Different perspectives and disagreements among faculty intensify the anxiety and uncertainty of the resident, who may begin to feel more doubtful about the field. The beginning resident is also confronted with a powerful sense that there is too much to be learned and too little time. These perceptions may lead the resident to feel incompetent and to further question his or her motivation. The resident may view faculty as inadequate, insensitive, or out of touch. This is a particular issue in psychiatric training where many residents have the perception that the "experts" in human behavior should be immune from human failings. Sometimes residents will seek other outlets for affirmation and retreat even further from the clinical situation.

The training director must be aware of these stressors and be patient with occasional regressive and dysfunctional reactions from residents. At the same time, the training director cannot encourage inappropriate responses from residents by failing to be clear and firm about policies and procedures. The training director should listen to resident complaints, even if many of the underlying problems that have been identified cannot and should not be changed. In the process of ensuring that the resident has the opportunity to acquire skills in a timely fashion, the training director should be aware that residents learn fast when what they learn helps bind the anxiety of beginning clinical work. This heightened motivation can be a great ally in the learning process.

Safety

Another source of distress for the beginning psychiatric resident is the actual danger of working in unsafe situations. Patients may be violent, perhaps even armed with weapons, and security in many facilities is inadequate (Gray 1989). Residents often resist complaining, fearing that their concerns will demonstrate their inadequacies. Recent increases in numbers of female residents have led to an increased focus on safety of facilities, on-call rooms, and parking garages. Women have generally been more willing to express concerns about safety than men. Training in a dangerous environment cannot benefit residents or patients. Making an environment safe is the responsibility of the clinical program and the institution in which the clinical setting exists. Actions that reduce the risks of working with dangerous and unpredictable patient populations include providing adequate security personnel; making modifications in the physical layout to provide adequate escape routes, alarms, and rescue access; and ensuring that all personnel receive appropriate training (Halleck 1989).

The training program must provide adequate violence management training to trainees as early as possible. This should help residents develop the ability to recognize potentially violent situations, to develop preventive strategies, and above all, to learn how to be self-protective. Training programs should try to avoid the practice of having the least-experienced psychiatric residents take call in the most dangerous settings. If for some reason it is necessary for inexperienced residents to work in settings that pose risks for violent behavior, it is incumbent upon the training director to ensure the safety of the environment by providing adequate, safe physical and support resources as well as appropriate supervision and training. These issues become even more evident if a resident is injured while on duty. (Please see Chapter 21 for a more extensive discussion of handling these delicate situations.)

Clinical responsibility for patients with severe and dangerous conditions is full of contradictions for practitioners. Matters of confidentiality, duty to warn, protection of civil rights, and the duty to protect society from dangerous people with mental illness are a few of the complex situations that face residents.

Ethics

Every profession evolves a code of ethics that is consistent with its definition of its boundaries and responsibilities. The code of ethics for psychiatry derives from the principles of medical ethics codified by the American Medical Association (AMA) and revised by the American Psychiatric Association (APA) in 1995 in the "Special Annotations for Psychiatry" (American Psychiatric Association 1995). The annotations address those issues unique to the characteristics of our field and are available from the APA. They should be distributed along with the Residency Review Committee (RRC) Essentials (Accreditation Council on Graduate Medical Education 1996), at the beginning of the PGY-1 year.

For the beginning resident, the complexity of ethical issues is intensified by the nature of psychiatric illness. Since many psychiatric patients have impaired judgment and lack the capacity to understand or make informed decisions, problems of paternalism are magnified. The psychiatrist must respect patients' autonomy while protecting them from doing harm to themselves or others.

The resident is faced with decisions about patient competence and informed consent early in the residency. Documentation of observations has special significance when behavioral data and verbal productions become the primary sources of information upon which crucial treatment decisions are made, including whether the patient will be deprived of the right to make decisions about his or her treatment or well-being.

Although confidentiality is a concern of all physicians, psychiatrists are often placed in the difficult position of having to decide when to breach confidentiality. Courts have mandated reporting of clinical data in special circumstances, for example, when a patient makes a direct threat against another person or when child abuse is suspected. Residents must be aware of these issues from the beginning of their training.

The training director must ensure that residents assigned to clinical services where this knowledge is likely to be important are properly informed about the ethical guidelines and legal procedures that cover clinical documentation. These should include guidelines about the following:

1. Confidentiality
2. Reporting to third parties
3. Informed consent
4. The extent and limitation of the psychiatrist's duty, responsibility, authority, and obligation in the face of suicidal, homicidal, gravely disabled, or mentally incompetent patients
5. The nature of the psychiatrist's relationship to other mental health professionals

These issues are best addressed as part of the orientation to a new setting, since institutions have different rules and procedures governing clinical work. Residents should be given written copies of the procedures and guidelines to refer to when needed. At the same time, a small-group seminar on ethical and legal issues in psychiatry should be given before, or at least concurrently, when residents are in the position of making decisions concerning civil commitment and participating in legal procedures that affect patients' lives. Finally, these issues arise naturally during the period of clinical and administrative supervision, and faculty should be aware of this educational opportunity.

Undue Familiarity and Boundary Violations

Attention has recently focused on a serious ethical concern that is often not adequately addressed—undue familiarity and boundary violations, including sexual interaction with patients. Sexual interaction between psychiatrist and patient is always unethical, yet it occurs more often than had been suspected (Gabbard and Nadelson 1995). The special nature of the transference that develops between psychiatric patients and their therapists increases the vulnerability of inexperienced clinicians. Those new to the field may have difficulty assessing the potential for undue familiarity to occur. The resident may not perceive the danger of becoming inappropriately involved and may minimize the danger, while the supervisor's insistence on maintaining therapeutic neutrality and distance may prevent inquiry and teaching in this area. These are issues that should be discussed actively in supervision and in peer groups, as well as in organized didactic sessions.

Residents may also be unaware of boundary violations that are less obvious than sexual interactions. Not all of these are categorically damaging to patients, but they should all be understood in the context of the clinical situation. These include, but are not limited to, revealing personal information such as sexual orientation, giving patients a ride, accepting gifts, or even stating that they themselves are in psychiatric treatment. Since residents may fail to reveal such information to a supervisor, it is particularly important for training directors to work closely with faculty members on these issues.

Sexual intimacy between supervisors or teachers and residents or students is a complex and controversial subject. Some condemn the behavior, and others insist that residents are adults capable of making their own life choices. It is clear, however, that residents are also vulnerable to transference reactions to those in authority, with whom they share intimate material as part of the working relationship. The APA's statement on medical ethics warns that sexual intimacy between supervisors and residents may represent an abuse of power and can result in impairment of patient care and compromise the resident's opportunity to learn. Since the faculty member is often in a position to evaluate, grade, and write letters of recommendation for a resident, the fiduciary responsibility precludes a sexual relationship.

Learning and Supervision

The residency experience can be a very infantilizing one since, especially in the early stages of training, residents are often placed in a dependent and ambiguous position with regard to their responsibilities. The beginning PGY-2 resident has usually completed a PGY-1 year with a sense of accomplishment, mastery, and independence as a physician. As the resident enters the world of psychiatry and a new professional developmental hierarchy, feelings of frustration and even anger may emerge.

Learning takes place on many levels and in many different ways, but, from the resident's perspective, supervision is usually one of the most important aspects of training. Not only does supervision provide direction about what to do, how to talk to a patient, and how to think about problems, but it affords the resident the opportunity to get to know and to be known by a senior colleague, and to learn something of that person's adaptation and accommodation to the work. Being supervised is a complex experience and evokes many conflicting emotions.

It is essential for residents to have relationships with senior colleagues who can serve a mentoring function by providing advocacy, advice, direction, and creation of opportunities. Since this process happens more naturally in larger institutional settings where more choices are available, residents who train in ambulatory or private practice settings may have more difficulty finding mentors. Mentoring often begins in supervision, and training directors should meet regularly with supervisors and other faculty to encourage them to take on this role.

Some specific approaches can be used to provide a good mentoring system. One is to assign a preceptor or adviser to each resident. This arrangement may or may not involve supervision of clinical work (Borus and Graves 1982), depending on the structure of the program and the year of the residency. When this process begins early and offers the flexibility to change one's preceptor or adviser if it does not work out or as one's interests change, it can be a very positive experience for the resident. As a variant, an ombudsman-type system can be provided by year or interest area. Since it is not possible to regulate these types of relationships and expect they will always be successful, maximal flexibility is important. Information about faculty members' research and clinical interests can also help residents find effective mentors. The training director should encourage residents to seek out faculty, and faculty should be receptive and welcoming.

The Resident as Teacher

An important aspect of the resident's professional growth is to become a teacher as well as a trainee (American Psychiatric Association Committee on Undergraduate Medical Student Education 1988; Moffic 1982). Organizing material for others is one way that mastery is achieved. Indeed, this aspect of learning is so important that all residents should be required to have some experience teaching others. This can be gained by teaching medical students or supervising or providing medical backup to trainees from other mental health disciplines.

Although many residents assume an important role in the teaching of medical students, they may not receive adequate supervision for their teaching. Despite all of the advantages of involving residents in the teaching process, the experience can be frustrating and demoralizing without appropriate instruction and guidance. The training director should try to schedule several didactic sessions each year to define and clarify the role of the resident as teacher at each institution. Training directors should also work closely with directors of medical student education in psychiatry wherever possible. This will not only reinforce the belief that education is important, but it will provide more cohesive guidance to residents about their roles and responsibilities as educators.

Psychotherapy for Residents

Many residents seek personal psychotherapy, some because their training program encourages them to do so, others because they feel it will help them with their work or personal problems, and still others because they are curious about the process. However, they may also be confronted with financial burdens that may preclude having psychotherapy despite their interest or need. Some residents resolve this crisis by moonlighting to pay for their treatment, sometimes imposing an even greater burden on themselves. There is no easy solution, but often there are resources in the psychiatric community for payment deferral or fee reduction. Some programs encourage nonteaching clinical faculty to provide psychotherapy for residents as a means of maintaining a faculty appointment.

Support and Training Groups

Many residency training programs provide support and/or training groups for residents, particularly for those in the PGY-2 year (Siegel and Donnelly 1978). These groups vary in form and leadership, but they are almost universally experienced positively by residents. They offer an opportunity for residents to get to know their peers, to develop a support system, to solve mutual problems, and to learn something about group dynamics. These groups should not be a substitute for individual psychotherapy, nor are they group therapy, although they certainly can be very supportive and helpful.

There are some important issues to consider when instituting a plan for these groups. They are most valued if residents can speak freely and be assured that confidentiality will be maintained. Therefore, it is best to have as group leader an experienced person who is not a member of the full-time faculty. It is also helpful if the leader knows something about medical education and residency training. Most groups meet weekly for at least part of the PGY-2 year, and occasionally throughout the residency. The purpose of these groups is frequently debated. We believe that they should focus on support and problem solving and should also offer the opportunity for residents to learn about group dynamics through understanding their own group process. Occasionally, it becomes apparent to the group leader or fellow residents that a resident has a psychiatric disorder. This situation should be discussed within the group when possible. It is important, however, that the group leader feel that there is access to the training director in the event that a resident's condition is potentially dangerous or serious, for example, if the individual is suicidal.

Many programs offer process groups based on the National Training Laboratories or Tavistock Clinic models of group dynamics and group organizations. These exercises, which are designed to be neither support nor psychotherapy groups, may be conducted 1 to 1.5 hours per week for anywhere from 1 to 3 years. They are usually more stressful experiences for residents and are designed to teach group process through group self-study.

Unfortunately, residents frequently come away with the idea that the often highly aloof and intellectual techniques used by the leaders in these exercises represent the best techniques for conducting group psychotherapy with patients. Likewise, training groups that are established for learning group process may be subtly and insidiously transmuted into psychotherapy groups, which they are not supposed to be—a process that many residents justifiably resent.

It should be made clear that these group dynamic study groups are not therapy groups. To involve residents in a group that purports to be therapeutic presents many difficulties, including ethical and clinical concerns. Clearly, we cannot require residents to participate in a therapy group, and boundaries between training and therapy must be respected.

Transitions

Certain transitions in the training cycle can be particularly stressful. As mentioned, the beginning of psychiatry rotations (either in the PGY-1 year or the PGY-2 year) can cause strain after residents have mastered the skills of medicine and pediatrics. In addition, residents may be more sensitive about performance issues once they have begun psychiatry rotations. A second transition that is typically difficult is the transition from inpatient to outpatient psychiatry. Although most programs make a concerted effort to provide residents with outpatient opportunities early in training (particularly as inpatient length of stays become truncated), the shift from treating patients in a team setting where other people have direct knowledge of the patient to a setting in which a resident is alone with a patient can be quite stressful. Historically, the third year has been the outpatient year, and although residents enjoy being able to set up their own schedules, having sole responsibility can be difficult. Sufficient, intensive individual supervision is critical to the successful mastery of skills in the outpatient arena.

The use of videotapes to monitor treatment in the supervisory encounter is one way in which technology can significantly supplement educational resources. In this regard, it is particularly important to educate the supervisory faculty, since resistance to videotaping is frequently communicated indirectly. Faculty should be made aware that concerns about interference with the therapeutic process have not been borne out. Effective supervision can go a long way toward alleviating resident anxiety about the outpatient experience.

Another key transition occurs as residents prepare to leave training and enter the workforce. In the fourth year, resident cohesiveness may begin to loosen as residents prepare to leave the educational setting. In programs where support groups exist throughout training, it may not be unusual for process groups to "fall apart" as the PGY-4 year progresses. Concerns about future employment and competitiveness among residents applying for fellowships and increasingly scarce academic jobs may contribute to resident group fragmentation and, for some residents, may lead to heightened feelings of anxiety and alienation. It is important for the residency training director to be aware of these additional stressors and to help prepare residents to move out of the protected training environment. Courses on careers in psychiatry and the transition to various practice settings and the workforce can facilitate communication between the training director and senior residents as well as alleviate anxiety.

Communication Between the Training Director and the Resident Group

To facilitate communication, training directors must take an active role. Residents' associations or councils are useful for organizing and focusing the residents' experience into a collaborative endeavor (Lock et al. 1993). Large training programs probably need to have formal residents' associations more than small programs. These groups, part union, part informal support group, can be effective instruments for the articulation of the resident experience and for the mobilization of resident effort on behalf of reform and constructive change.

Another important line of communication is to the resident's family or significant other. Although programs are concerned about ways of minimizing residents' stress, they often pay insufficient attention to resident spouses and partners and to the changing realities of dual-career families with conflicting demands and time schedule constraints. In the past, those involved in graduate education have assumed that partners of residents had careers that could accommodate the inflexibility of the residency. This is no longer true, and it is important that training directors remain open to hearing from residents about their specific situations (Gabbard and Menninger 1988; Myers 1994). Partners also appreciate meeting colleagues and learning something about the program. Inviting partners to informal social events and providing access to rounds, conferences, and seminars, when appropriate, are helpful. However, the most important factor is the consideration the training director gives to these significant others.

Another means of communicating with residents is through the use of written procedures and guidelines. These communications can be collected in a formal manual or a more informal survival guide that introduces the new residents to the program and to the larger social context of the training program within the institution. However, the role of the chief resident is critical. In some programs, the chief residency is a PGY-5 position where the chief resident functions as an "assistant" to the training director and a junior faculty member. In other programs, the chief resident is a member of the PGY-4 class. Larger programs often benefit from having several chief residents in different sites, areas, or modalities. It is always helpful to have clearly delineated the roles and responsibilities of the various chief residency positions and to list the advantages of each. The selection process should be clearly spelled out.

The Choice of Chief Resident

We have found it useful to select chief residents in January or February of the preceding year. When the chief residency is a PGY-4 position, it is helpful to allay group anxieties early while simultaneously providing the incoming chief or chiefs with the opportunity to "grow into the job." Early selection also provides the rest of the resident group with the opportunity to adjust and to go ahead with elective planning.

There are pros and cons regarding the involvement of the resident group in the selection process. Although it is extremely important to have resident input (particularly from outgoing chiefs), having the entire residency group involved may lead to the appearance of a "popularity contest." It has been our experience that outgoing chief residents generally have a good pulse on the feelings of the resident cohort. It may also be problematic if the resident group decision does not agree with the opinion of the faculty.

Administrative Issues/Moonlighting

Working outside of the training program in addition to working as a resident was not permitted when general training was supported by training grants from the National Institute of Mental Health. Now, however, because of the proliferating demand for psychiatric services, and the need of many residents to have a second income (commonly because of medical school debts or personal psychotherapy), work outside of the residency has become quite common. Some programs have formal rules and regulations regarding moonlighting. Problems arise when the time and energy demanded by outside work interfere with resident education. Training directors must be alert to signs of disruption of the training task. These signs include a pattern of missed educational activities, sleepiness or signs of distraction, and frequent unavailability.

It is essential that the training director protect the resident's chance to learn because, for the majority of psychiatrists, learning opportunities missed during residency cannot or will not be made up later. Probably the best arrangement for moonlighting occurs when it is aboveboard and under some administrative and educational control by the training director. The training director can approve requests to moonlight and even insist that the experience have some educational component. In fact, the RRC requires programs to have some mechanism for monitoring outside activity (Accreditation Council for Graduate Medical Education 1996). Cohen and Leeds (1989) describe a model program for integrating moonlighting into an ongoing educational experience. Their work also addresses administrative considerations, such as the program's liability for resident moonlighting activities and the issue of credentialing for independent practice.

Conclusion

Residency training, like all graduate education, is changing along many dimensions. It takes an adaptive and quick-footed soul to keep up. Regardless of the changes in health care delivery, social forces, demographics, and content areas within the field, residency is still a time of considerable personal growth and professional development. For many psychiatrists, the residency years are the time of the greatest acquisition of skills and knowledge. The training director plays a major role in the development of the residents who pass through on his or her watch. For this influence to be maximally positive and effective, the training director must constantly attend to issues of communication and collaboration. The training director must consistently foster a learning alliance with residents and facilitate the process of keeping professional growth on track in the face of the ambiguities of training and of medical practice.

References

Accreditation Council on Graduate Medical Education: The 1998–99 Directory of Graduate Medical Education Programs. Chicago, IL, American Medical Association, 1998

American Psychiatric Association: The Principles of Medical Ethics With Annotations Especially Applicable to Psychiatry. Washington, DC, American Psychiatric Association, 1995

American Psychiatric Association Committee on Undergraduate Medical Student Education: Psychiatric Residents as Teachers. Washington, DC, American Psychiatric Association, 1988

Borus JF, Graves JF: Training supervision as a separate faculty role. Am J Psychiatry 139:1339–1342, 1982

Cohen SN, Leeds MP: The moonlighting dilemma, balancing education, service, and quality care while limiting risk exposure. JAMA 262:529–531, 1989

Gabbard GO, Menninger RW: Medical marriages. Washington, DC, American Psychiatric Press, 1998

Gabbard G, Nadelson CC: Professional boundaries in the physician-patient relationship. JAMA 273(18):1445–1449, 1995

Gray GE: Assaults by patients against psychiatric residents at a public psychiatric hospital. Academic Psychiatry 13:81–86, 1989

Halleck SL: When residents are victims of violence. Academic Psychiatry 13:113–115, 1989

Lock J, Kleis B, Strouse T, et al: The role and function of residents' organizations in psychiatry education. Academic Psychiatry 17:26–31, 1993

Moffic HS: Educating psychiatric residents to become psychiatric educators. Journal of Psychiatric Education 6:107–111, 1982

Myers MF: Doctors' marriages: a look at the problems and their solutions, 2nd Edition. New York, Plenum Publishing Corporation, 1994

Siegel B, Donnelly JC: Enriching personal and professional development: the experience of a support group for interns. J Med Educ 53:908–914, 1978

23

Special Events

Carol A. Bernstein, M.D., and Carol C. Nadelson, M.D.

This chapter addresses issues, such as orientation, retreats, social events, academic meetings, and graduation, that are less strictly educational but have a bearing on the morale and general climate of the training program.

Orientation

In the initial orientation of residents to a department, the faculty communicates both factual and nonfactual information, including values, style, and preferences as well as specific departmental details. Given the state of anticipation, excitement, and anxiety, much of what is said bears repetition, and what is important should be put into writing. Orientations should be carefully planned. Participants may come away confused or uncertain if the flow of information is not carefully managed. First-day orientations should include brief presentations by the chair and training director to offer welcoming remarks, set the tone of the program, and acquaint residents with the primary people responsible for their training over the ensuing years of residency. If possible, outgoing first- and second-year residents should also be invited to speak about the nature of their experiences, particular stresses, and so on. If the formal presentation does not provide sufficient time for them to speak, inviting all residents to an orientation lunch is a good way for such information to be shared.

Most hospitals routinely provide orientation for entering house officers. In programs where residents rotate to multiple institutions, this may involve orientation at multiple sites. Since PGY-1 psychiatry residents spend much of their first year on medicine, pediatrics, and neurology rotations, it is not unusual for departments to omit specific orientation programs in psychiatry. We recommend holding a special psychiatry orientation session for entering PGY1s to supplement hospital orientations that are provided for everyone. These can consist of a 2- or 3-hour program that includes brief meetings (5–10 minutes long) with unit chiefs from PGY-1 psychiatry rotations and that should also include chief residents from medicine, neurology, and pediatrics. This orientation is best combined with a welcoming lunch to which all faculty and residents are invited. It is often possible to hold this orientation prior to July 1, since most hospital orientations must be held before the official start date. If your program is welcoming entering PGY-2s, these residents should be invited as well. It is also helpful to give residents an "Orientation Packet" that includes the following:

1. All schedules, including on-call schedules with rules about assignments, switches, and so on
2. Faculty and resident telephone and address lists
3. Chief resident beeper and home telephone numbers
4. A map of the hospital(s) and a map of the city, including subway, train, and bus maps and schedules
5. A recommended reading list
6. A copy of the Residency Review Committee (RRC) Essentials for Residency Training in Psychiatry
7. Institutional and departmental due process policies and procedures
8. The didactic curriculum
9. The residency training program goals and objectives
10. A resident database form to be completed for the training office
11. A list of the membership of all residency training committees
12. House staff benefits and an explanation of salary lines
13. APA membership application
14. The Principles of Medical Ethics With Annotations Especially Applicable to Psychiatry

Programs with little contact with PGY-1 residents may opt to have an orientation for PGY-2s instead. As an adjunct, chief residents should consider holding monthly lunch meetings with interns when they rotate to medicine, pediatrics, and neurology services. Such lunches or potluck dinners also help interns feel more connected to the department of psychiatry during a difficult year.

In programs that have a high proportion of international medical graduates, special orientation events designed to help them become familiar with the American culture are extremely useful. A special summer curriculum can also provide entering PGYs and transferring residents from other cultures with the opportunity to discuss what psychiatry is like in their home countries, to raise questions about their new environment, and to orient them to cultural differences. Residents may also be helped to find examples of their native cultures and to meet with faculty members and other residents from their own backgrounds.

Retreats

Program evaluation should always be an ongoing process. Some programs set aside time for an annual retreat for residents or residents and faculty specifically for this purpose. These provide residents with the opportunity to evaluate the program and make constructive suggestions for change in an atmosphere that is removed from the hospital or medical center. Depending on the program structure, it is preferable to offer faculty coverage for resident responsibilities for these events. In larger or more service-dependent programs, a retreat can be held on a weekend to maximize resident participation if coverage is not possible. The most useful retreat formats provide opportunities for residents to meet alone as a group, with special times set aside for additional meetings with the training director(s) and key faculty. The residency group in consultation with the training director may wish to consider whether such a retreat should serve a more social function for residents (thus involving significant others) or should be more program oriented.

The selection of retreat topics and mechanisms for feedback will vary depending on whether the retreat is for residents alone or residents and faculty together. The primary advantage of having a "residents only" retreat is that residents will probably be less inhibited about discussing anxieties and concerns because faculty and supervisors are not present. The primary disadvantage is that residents will not have an opportunity to interact with faculty in a setting that is unencumbered by other clinical and education responsibilities. The training director should communicate with residents and faculty to see what would be optimal for the program. Either way it is important to solicit suggestions for retreat content from all participants as well as the department chair and to make sure there is a mechanism to provide appropriate feedback.

In this era of shrinking resources, it is becoming increasingly difficult for programs to find extra funding for retreats. In our experience, some pharmaceutical companies are willing to donate support for these educational activities.

Social Events

Social events during the course of the year go a long way toward diminishing potential strain, boosting morale, and dispelling the occasional misperceptions people have of one another. An early summer welcoming party is nice complement to the formality of the orientation. A regular get-together of faculty and residents, with or without some academic task, can be useful in facilitating social rapport. An annual midwinter or graduation party where the residents plan some type of humorous "roasting" or mockery of faculty is also an invaluable means of communication and morale building. These events allow residents to express to the faculty complex messages about their experience.

As in any working environment, these periodic social events enable residents and faculty to interact in more relaxed settings. Some institutions use the holiday season as an opportunity to bring the department together. Residents also enjoy coming to the training director's home for potluck dinners, picnics, or brunches. Sometimes other faculty members will also be encouraged to host similar events. Potluck suppers permit residents to participate actively and spare the training director from "too much work"!

In some areas, the local APA district branch may have an active residents' committee. This is an ideal venue for residents from neighboring programs to get together and, in some cities, has led to sponsorship of events such as a "movie night" that also provide an occasion for medical students, faculty, and residents to interact. APA committees are also natural avenues for mentorship between residents and psychiatrists working in the community whether they are academically affiliated or not.

Academic Meetings

An important aspect of residency training is the opportunity for residents to participate in and attend academic meetings. The APA and allied organizations representing various psychiatric subspecialties have annual meetings, and many of them sponsor fellowships that enable residents to have their expenses paid to attend meetings. Some departments have resources to support resident attendance if presentations are being made. Training directors usually receive announcements about a myriad of conferences and symposia, and it is useful to have a routine mechanism for disseminating this information to the resident group. Weekly resident meetings are frequently the most effective way to do this. In hospitals where there are house staff unions, there may be a means for residents to be reimbursed for conference fees through union benefits; it is a good idea to find out if these programs exist at your institution. Obviously it is important to develop a policy outlining how much release time for conferences will be permitted and who will provide coverage. In some places, institutional benefits determine how much conference time is permitted. Other programs have no official policy. The training director should consider whether one should be developed. In general, residents who win honorary fellowships and who present research or papers at academic meetings should be accommodated whenever possible. Such opportunities can then be viewed as rewards for the presenters as well as incentives to others.

Accreditation

For a physician to sit for specialty board examinations, he or she must have graduated from an accredited residency program. Accreditation is the assurance that a residency program meets certain standards with respect to faculty, facilities, trainees, and curriculum that have been established by the Accreditation Council for Graduate Medical Education (ACGME). The Council is sponsored by the American Board of Medical Specialties, the American Hospital Association, the American Medical Association, the Association of American Medical Colleges, and the Council of Medical Specialty Societies.

There are representatives to the Council from each of the sponsoring organizations, and from the federal government, as well as from the public.

The ACGME carries out its work by means of Residency Review Committees (RRCs). In psychiatry, the RRC is composed of representatives appointed by the American Medical Association Council on Medical Evaluation, the American Board of Psychiatry and Neurology, and the APA. The APA also appoints a psychiatric resident representative.

The standards for accreditation are known as the "Essentials." These standards are revised as frequently as is deemed necessary by the RRC and are published annually in a large paperback called the *Directory of Graduate Medical Education Programs*, known popularly as the *Green Book* (Accreditation Council on Graduate Medical Education 1996). One of the requirements is that a copy of the Essentials in Psychiatry be distributed to each resident upon entering the program.

The ACGME ensures that its standards are being met by performing periodic site visits to each residency program, as well as institutional site visits to hospitals and institutions that offer more than one type of training program. The standards also require that hospitals conduct periodic in-house reviews of each training program. Thus, there are three types of training program site visits: the institutional review by ACGME, the internal review conducted by the hospital, and the ACGME reaccreditation review. (Please see Chapter 19 for further information on the site visit itself.)

Fellowships

A wide variety of fellowships exist for residents. These include APA-sponsored programs such as the Glaxo/Wellcome Fellowship, the APA/Minority Fellowships, the APA Minority "Mini-Fellows" Program, the APA Bristol-Myers Squibb Fellowship and others. In addition, many allied organizations also provide fellowship opportunities such as the Laughlin and Psychiatric Resident In-Training Examination (PRITE) Fellowships of the American College of Psychiatrists, the Charter Leadership Fellowship of the American Academy of Child and Adolescent Psychiatry, the American Psychoanalytic Association Fellowship, and the Ginsburg Fellowship of the Group for the Advancement of Psychiatry (GAP). Other subspecialty organizations also have fellowship programs. Having a resident win such a fellowship not only provides the resident with an excellent opportunity to participate in national academic activities but also is a source of pride for the entire residency program. Training directors or chairs must write letters of nomination, which should be in the "Dean's Letter" format and contain extensive information about the nominee. The author should be clear that he or she is familiar with the work, interests, and talents of the resident. Although this takes some time and effort, it is the best way to help your resident "come alive" to members of any selection committee.

Some of these fellowships are more competitive than others. One issue to consider is how to disseminate information and make choices about fellowship opportunities. Although it is more "democratic" to notify the entire resident group and see who might be interested in a particular fellowship, you also want to select residents who have a chance of winning. Whereas some programs turn the process of decision making over to residents, others have a faculty committee and may or may not request volunteers or nominations. Every process has advantages and disadvantages, and there is no absolute rule about what works best. For example, peers may know the most about an individual resident's clinical skills, but they may not be familiar with the resident's background and may choose a nominee based on popularity. On the other hand, faculty may not know enough about the full dimensions of a resident's work. It is always best to maintain a system that allows for input from both sides and to set up a mechanism that is both fair and pragmatic. All fellowships and awards are special honors and opportunities and they are meant for residents with interests and talents specific for the award. Appendix 23-A provides a partial list of fellowships available for residents.

Awards and Means of Providing Special Recognition

Chief Residency

Being a chief resident is a means of consolidating generic psychiatric skills while simultaneously functioning more independently and gaining experience in leadership and clinical administration. It is important that the chief resident have real responsibilities and accountability, and also receive support. For instance, a chief resident may require assistance from a supervisor in negotiating conflict with a senior faculty member. On the other hand, the chief resident should be able to negotiate conflict with other professionals (i.e., medicine residents) and between or among other residents in the program. The chief resident experience can be a very powerful learning opportunity and can go a long way toward identifying future leaders.

Special Awards

Rewarding residents through public recognition is another way for departments to communicate values and recognize superior achievement and effort. Awards named for retired or deceased faculty are also a way of memorializing and honoring a faculty member and the values that he or she represented. Such local awards may acknowledge research productivity and accomplishment, general clinical ability, or any other skill or achievement the department wishes to recognize. It is important that the process of selecting recipients for these awards be straightforward and clear to minimize fears of favoritism and bias that so often accompany efforts to single out superior achievement.

Graduation

Graduation is an important event for all residents. There are many ways in which graduation can be celebrated, but it is important for a program to develop some kind of special event to mark the occasion. Dinners for graduating residents and faculty are common. Sometimes these include dancing, skits, and even boat rides. If it all possible, it is helpful if graduates can attend these events for free. Again, the pharmaceutical industry may be able to offer support. It is particularly important to encourage a good turnout from faculty.

In many institutions, the adult residency program is not the only training program in the department. Some programs have developed formal graduation ceremonies for all trainees (fellowships, child and adolescent residencies, other mental health professionals, etc.). Such events enable trainees to share the excitement of graduation with family and friends. These ceremonies need not be elaborate and can take the form of a simple ceremony in an auditorium where each program director and the chair introduces each graduate and presents the graduate with a diploma. A wine and cheese reception afterward is a nice touch.

Conclusion

Residency training provides many opportunities to bolster resident morale and enhance the educational environment through a series of special events. These events also provide unique opportunities for residents and faculty to interact together in more informal settings and to develop mentorship through social as well as educational arenas.

References

Accreditation Council on Graduate Medical Education: The 1998–99 Directory of Graduate Medical Education Programs. Chicago, IL, American Medical Association, 1998

Fellowships Available
for Psychiatric Residents
(Partial List)

American Association for Directors of Psychiatric Residency Training/Ginsberg Fellowship

Criteria for nomination: Residents with academic leadership potential and
   interest in education.
Contact: AADPRT, Executive Office
UConn Health Center, Dept. of Psychiatry
10 Talcott Notch Rd. East Wing
Farmington, CT 06030–6410
Tel: 860–679–6766
Fax: 860–679–6675
Email: AADPRT@Psychiatry.UCHC.Edu.
Deadline: Early November

American College of Psychiatrists/Laughlin Fellowship Program

Criteria for nomination: PGY-3 or PGY-4 or child psychiatry fellow likely to
   make a significant future contribution to psychiatry.
Contact: Laughlin Fellowship Program
Laughlin Fellowship Committee
The American College of Psychiatrists
732 Addison St., Suite B
Berkeley, CA 94710
Tel: 510–704–8020
Fax: 510–704–0113
Email: AliceACP@AOL.COM
Deadline: Mid-September

Association for Academic Psychiatry/Bristol-Myers Squibb Fellowship

Criteria for nomination: PGY-3, PGY-4, or PGY-5 resident/fellow with a
   demonstrated interest in an academic career and ability as a teacher
   prior to and during residency. (Note: Only AAP institutional members
   may nominate fellows.)
Contact: AAP Executive Office
Department of Psychiatry

Mount Auburn Hospital, Wy 2
330 Mount Auburn Street
Cambridge, MA 02238
Tel: 617–499–5660
Fax: 617–499–5498
Deadline: Mid-February

American Psychiatric Association Minority Fellowships Program

Criteria for nomination: PGY-2 or PGY-3 minority residents who are U.S.
    citizens or permanent residents with a commitment to serve
    underrepresented populations, demonstrated leadership abilities, and
    interest in the interrelationships between mental health/illness and
    transcultural factors.
Contact: Program Coordinator
APA Minority Fellowships
OMNA/APA
1400 K Street NW
Washington, DC 20005
Tel: 202–682–6096
Fax: 202–682–6837
E-Mail: mking@psych.org
Deadline: End of January

American Psychiatric Association/Glaxo Wellcome Fellowship Program

Criteria for nomination: PGY-2 or PGY-3 residents with demonstrated
    leadership abilities and potential for contributing to the APA and for
    becoming future leaders in psychiatry.
Contact: APA Office of Minority/National Affairs
1400 K Street, NW
Washington, DC 20005
Tel: 202–682–6097
Fax: 202–682–6837
E-Mail: jtaylor@psych.org
Deadline: March 31

American Psychiatric Association/Bristol-Myers Squibb Fellowship

Criteria for nomination: PGY-3 or PGY-4 residents (during the fellowship
    year) with substantial interest and significant potential for leadership in
    any area of public sector psychiatry.
Contact: APA/Bristol-Myers Squibb Selection Committee

APA Office of Psychiatric Services
1400 K Street, NW
Washington, DC 20005
Tel: 202–682–6326
Deadline: April 1

Group for the Advancement of Psychiatry/Ginsburg Fellowship

Criteria for nomination: PGY-2 or PGY-3 residents or first-year child
psychiatry fellows with demonstrated leadership abilities, commitment to
social issues, willingness to participate in a collective process, and likely
to make a significant future contribution to psychiatry.
Frances Roton, Executive Director
Contact: GAP Central Office
P.O. Box 28218
Dallas, TX 75228
Tel: 972–613–3044
Fax: 972–613–5532
Deadline: September 1

American Academy of Psychiatry
and the Law/Rappeport Fellowship

Criteria for nomination: outstanding PGY-3 residents with demonstrated
interest in psychiatry and the law.
Chair: Rappeport Fellowship Committee
American Academy of Psychiatry and the Law
One Regency Drive
P.O. Box 30
Bloomfield, CT 06002–0030
Tel: 604–733–5722
Deadline: April 1

American Psychoanalytic Association Fellowship

Criteria for nomination: Full-time general or child psychiatry residents or
fellows or psychiatrists who have become board eligible within the past
three years who will hold full-time academic appointments in an
educational institution during the fellowship year and who have
demonstrated special aptitude or interest in psychodynamic psychiatry
and psychoanalysis.
Contact: American Psychoanalytic Association
309 E. 49th St.
New York, NY 10017
Tel: 212–752–0450, Ext. 12
Fax: 212–593–0571
Deadline: Feb 1

American College of Psychiatrists PRITE Fellowship

Criteria for nomination: Current PGY-2 residents in general psychiatry who
   are interested in psychiatric education and have a strong fund of
   knowledge in the field.

Chair: PRITE Fellowship Selection Committee

ACP Central Office

732 Addison St., Ste. B

Berkeley, CA 94710

Tel: 510–704–8020

Fax: 510–704–0113

Deadline: Mid-January

Program for Minority Research Training in Psychiatry/ACNP
Travel Fellowship

Criteria for nomination: Minority medical students, general and child
   psychiatric residents, who are U.S. citizens or permanent residents.

Contact: Program for Minority Research Training in Psychiatry (PMRPT)

ACNP "Mini-Fellow" Nominations

American Psychiatric Association

1400 K Street, NW

Washington, DC 20005

Tel: 202–682–6225

Deadline: July 30

APA PMRPT Minifellowship

Criteria for nomination: Minority medical students, psychiatric residents, and
   psychiatrists who have completed formal psychiatric training in the
   previous 4 or 5 years who are U.S. citizens or permanent residents to
   attend the annual APA meeting.

Contact: Program for Minority Research Training in Psychiatry (PMRPT)

"Mini-Fellow" Nominations

Office of Research

American Psychiatric Association

1400 K Street, NW

Washington, DC 20005

Tel: 202–682–6225

Deadline: March 1

AAGP Geriatric Psychiatry Fellowship Program

Criteria for Nomination: PGY-2 residents with an interest in geriatric
   psychiatry.

Contact: American Association for Geriatric Psychiatry Fellowship Selection
   Committee

7910 Woodmont Avenue, Suite 1350
Bethesda, MD 20814–3004
Tel: 301–654–7850
Fax: 301–654–4137
Email: AAGPGPA@AOL.COM
Deadline: March 15

APA Member-in-Training Trustee Elect (MITTE)

Criteria for nomination: PGY-2 or PGY-3 resident in the summer prior to
    election to serve for 2 years on the APA Board of Trustees.
Contact: Chairperson, APA Nominating Committee
1400 K Street, NW
Washington, DC 20005
Attn: Carol Lewis
Tel: 202–682–6063
Fax: 202–682–6282
E-mail: clewis@psych.org
Deadline: Mid-August

APA Committee of Residents & Fellows (CORF)

Criteria for nomination: Residents and fellows (one from each of the APA's
    seven geographical areas) who must be in training throughout their
    tenure on the committee—must be a member of the APA.
Contact: Ms. Sherrie Batey
APA Office of Education
1400 K Street, NW, Suite 510
Washington, DC 20005
Tel: 202–682–6130
Fax: 202–682–6102
Deadline: Early January of year in which vacancy will occur.

AACAP/Charter Leadership Award

Criteria for nomination: PGY2 resident interested in child and adolescent
    psychiatry with demonstrated leadership qualities.
Contact: President
American Academy of Child and Adolescent Psychiatry
3615 Wisconsin Avenue, NW
Washington, DC 20016-3007
Tel: 202–966–7300
Fax: 202–966–2891
Email: ACADRSRCH@AOL.COM
Deadline: June 1

AADPRT IMG/Mentorship Program
Criteria for nomination: Outstanding PGY 2, 3, or 4 IMG resident who will
    still be in training during the mentorship year.
Contact: AADPRT Executive Office
UConn Health Center, Department of Psychiatry
10 Talcott Notch Road, East Wing
Farmington, CT 06030–6410
Attn: IMG Mentorship Program
Tel: 860–679–6766
Fax: 860–679–6675
Deadline: October 1

24

Subspecialization and Training After General Residency in Psychiatry

Stephen C. Scheiber, M.D.

The American Board of Psychiatry and Neurology (ABPN) is one of the 24 member boards of the American Board of Medical Specialties (ABMS) (1998; Table 24–1). The primary function of the ABPN is to certify individual general psychiatrists, adult neurologists, and child neurologists in their respective specialties and for the different subspecialties (American Board of Psychiatry and Neurology 1998). The psychiatry Residency Review Committee (RRC) is responsible for accrediting programs in general psychiatry and in recognized subspecialties (see Chapter 19) (Accreditation Council for Graduate Medical Education [ACGME] 1998).

What Training Directors Need to Know

Certification is a voluntary process. The majority of graduates of psychiatric residencies participate in this three-step process. The training director in particular and the psychiatric faculty in general have major responsibilities in assisting the residents to achieve certification upon graduation from residency programs.

The three basic responsibilities are as follows:

Table 24–1. ABMS member specialty boards

The American Board of

Allergy and Immunology
Anesthesiology
Colon and Rectal Surgery
Dermatology
Emergency Medicine
Family Practice
Internal Medicine
Medical Genetics
Neurological Surgery
Nuclear Medicine
Obstetrics and Gynecology
Ophthalmology
Orthopaedic Surgery
Otolaryngology
Pathology
Pediatrics
Physical Medicine and Rehabilitation
Plastic Surgery
Preventive Medicine
Psychiatry and Neurology
Radiology
Surgery
Thoracic Surgery
Urology

Associate Members

American Hospital Association
American Medical Association
Association of American Medical Colleges
Council of Medical Specialty Societies
Federation of State Medical Boards of the United States, Inc.
National Board of Medical Examiners

■ To provide the educational experience that is required and document satisfactory completion of training as designated in the program requirements for residency training by the psychiatry RRC (see Chapter 19). (Accreditation Council of Graduate Medical Education [ACGME] 1995)

■ To provide the necessary didactic experiences so that the resident graduate of programs will be exposed to the knowledge base in basic psychiatry, basic neurology, and clinical neurology that will be tested on the Part I written examination.

■ To provide the necessary clinical experiences so that resident graduates can demonstrate their psychiatric skills, knowledge, and professional attitude, which will be tested in the Part II oral examination.

The Certification Process

All training directors are required to be board certified by the ABPN or its equivalent and, therefore, should have as a minimum personal experience with the certification process as a former candidate. Many training directors and psychiatric faculty members have also served as examiners for the Part II oral examinations and hence have experiences that can be helpful for the residents in their programs.

The training director is key in providing information about ABPN policies and procedures. The Board office communicates directly with the training directors in writing. It is then the responsibility of the training director to post this information for residents, and it is the responsibility of residents to familiarize themselves with the material.

For instance, residents need to learn that the application deadline for the Part I examination is February 1 of the PGY-4 year for a resident who is due to complete that year of training by June 30. The resident must submit a completed application and a check for the application and Part I examination fees. The training director must submit documentation of the resident's satisfactory completion of training to the Board office between July 1 and July 15 for those residents graduating by June 30. All this information is available to training directors and residents by writing the Board office (American Board of Psychiatry and Neurology 1998). When requesting an application, residents and training directors will also receive a copy of the *Information for Applicants* booklet. This booklet is updated annually. Many training directors will actually order applications in bulk for their PGY-4 residents. Training directors do well to advise their residents to read the *Information for Applicants* booklet carefully and follow Board policies and procedures.

The ABPN relies on residency training directors to keep residents informed about ABPN policies and procedures. However, the ultimate responsibility for obtaining information lies with the individual resident and subsequently the individual applicant to the Board. In addition to sending written materials directly to training directors, each year representatives of the ABPN attend the annual meeting of the American Association of Directors of Psychiatric Residency Training (AADPRT) and participate in workshops and plenary sessions. One of the most valuable workshops, mutually conducted by the ABPN and the AADPRT on the first afternoon of the annual meeting, is the one designated for new training directors. At this workshop, the ABPN reviews details of its policies and procedures and outlines the important relationship of the training director to the ABPN. In addition, the executive vice president of the ABPN prepares a report that is distributed to the attendees of the annual meeting. The report updates the membership of the AADPRT on policies and procedures of the ABPN.

To be certified in general psychiatry, an individual must possess an unlimited license to practice medicine in a state, commonwealth, territory, or possession of the United States or a province of Canada and must have completed an ACGME-approved program in psychiatry.

Applicants need to know that the applications are reviewed in the order that they are received, and all information, with the exception of documentation of satisfactory completion of residency training for those who are completing their PGY-4 year, must be submitted to the Board office by the application deadline. Residents who have divided a training year between two programs (a split year) must submit letters from the respective training directors of the two institutions where the resident has served detailing the rotations completed at each of the training programs. Residency training directors are encouraged to submit proposals to the ABPN for split years before a resident transfers. Approval of the split training can then be obtained and a letter of approval placed in the resident's file, which can later be submitted with an application to the Board office. Between July 1 and July 15, training directors must send a letter confirming the resident's satisfactory completion of training to both the Board office and the resident who graduated. Child and adolescent psychiatry residents who apply for their Part I examination in their first year of child and adolescent psychiatry residency must have completed all their general psychiatry requirements by June 30 of the PGY-4 year.

Written Examination

The fall written examination is administered in either October or November. This is given in more than 70 locations throughout the continental United

States; Hawaii; Alaska; Ottawa, Canada; Puerto Rico; and Germany. The Board attempts to give applicants a choice of locations as to where they will sit for their examination.

A written examination consists of about 400 multiple-choice questions. About 250 items cover the basic sciences of psychiatry and about 150 items cover the basic sciences of neurology and clinical neurology. Candidates must pass both portions to pass the examination. Candidates who fail may take the Part I written examination annually until they do pass. Two failures necessitate reapplication (request for new application, copy of unlimited license, and the application and Part I examination fees).

The residency program requirements for psychiatry require that residents be administered a cognitive examination at least twice during the course of the residency. Most residencies provide for this minimal requirement by administering the Psychiatric Resident In-Training Examination (PRITE) that is a product of the American College of Psychiatrists. The results of the in-training examination correlate fairly well with the subsequent results on the Part I written examination (Webb et al. 1996). Since training directors are privy to the results of the examination, it behooves the training director and the psychiatric faculty to provide any remedial measures should residents demonstrate limited knowledge in any of the subsets of the examination. The PRITE can also serve to identify areas of common strengths and common weaknesses in the teaching in a particular program. Again, it behooves the training director to enhance the learning in areas where there may be identified deficits.

Training directors and faculty should advise residents to do their best on this in-service training examination, since the motivations may not be as strong for this educational exercise as for the certification examination.

The Part I Written Examination Committee of the Board updates its content outline approximately every five years. As part of this process, the committee asks the training directors to review the content outline and make suggested changes and revisions. These changes are brought to the Psychiatry Council of the ABPN and ultimately passed by the directors of the Board. The revised copy then becomes the outline that is used for formulating test questions. Hence, the training directors know in advance what topics the Board will cover in their written examinations. The hope is that the didactic exercises in residency training programs will address the material that the Board will cover on the written examination, and hence residents will be prepared for this examination.

Oral Examination

Those passing the written examination are then assigned to an oral examination site within 15 months. The oral examination is administered three or four times yearly in different geographical locations around the country. Each candidate takes two 1-hour examination sections. One section is for the interview of a general psychiatry patient for one-half hour followed by presentation of a summary of findings including history and mental status findings, formulation of the patient's problems, a differential diagnosis and a review of treatment, management, and prognosis. Each candidate is typically assigned to two primary examiners and a senior examiner who supervises two or three examinations. The head of the examination team is there primarily for administrative purposes. During the second hour of the examination, candidates view a half-hour videotape of a psychiatrist interviewing a psychiatric patient. The second half-hour is again spent in summarizing history and mental status examination findings, formulation of the case, differential diagnosis, treatment, management, and prognosis. Candidates must pass both the audiovisual and live patient sections at the same examination.

Beginning in the fall of 1994, all candidates who pass the oral examination are issued 10-year, time-limited certificates (American Board of Psychiatry and Neurology, 1998). Those who fail may repeat the examination two additional times within 6 years. After three failed attempts or a lapse of 6 years, they must repeat and pass the Part I examination before again being admitted to the oral examination.

The program requirements of the psychiatry RRC require that at least twice during the course of residency training the residency training program provide an exercise for evaluating clinical skills. This requirement is often met by the setting up of what are often called "mock boards." In addition to being an educational exercise whereby residents can get feedback on their clinical skills, residents can also be advised about what they may do differently in preparation for taking their oral board examinations. All training directors have their own idiosyncratic views of what should be done to help residents prepare for boards. As a former training director, I believe that an individual who dedicates himself or herself to learning in the course of the residency program and who attends didactic exercises and takes on complete clinical responsibilities in a rich learning environment will have the best preparation for passing the Board examinations.

Beyond this generalization, everything else should be geared to the individual and how that individuals learns best. Options include textbooks, journals, CD-ROMS, audiovisual tapes, group exercises, programmed learning, and so on

Perhaps the best advice for residents is to take the examination as soon after graduation as is feasible. Practical advice at the time of the examination includes getting a good night's sleep, not taking toxic substances in advance of the examination, and treating patients with humanity. The ABPN does not endorse any board review activities

Subspecialty Training in Psychiatry: Rationale for Training and Certification

Formal Criteria

In 1986 the only subspecialty recognized by the ABPN was: child psychiatry (American Board of Psychiatry and Neurology 1999). That year representatives from six subspecialties were invited by the ABPN to discuss formal subspecialty recognition. This in turn led to the ABPN formulating criteria for subspecialty certification should subspecialties wish to have official recognition by the ABPN. The criteria in turn were derived from the ABMS criteria for official subspecialty recognition. The ABPN criteria for formal subspecialty recognition are included in Appendix 24–A.

Although there are formal criteria for recognized subspecialties, there are many more subspecialty interests that individual psychiatrists can have and that departments sponsor. These do not meet formal criteria for a variety of reasons, and in other cases subspecialties may not seek ABMS recognition or request accreditation through the psychiatry RRC. Many of these subspecialty programs are small in number. They may be suitable for accommodating local situations but fail to meet national criteria. One must distinguish between a special subspecialty interest versus formal subspecialty recognition. Rural psychiatry, for instance, would be more suitable for locations like northern New England (Vermont, New Hampshire, Maine), rural Arizona, upstate New York, West Virginia, South Carolina, and South Dakota, to name a few. Local circumstances such as the presence of a major oncology center, like Memorial Hospital in New York City, M. D. Anderson Hospital in Houston, Texas, or Roswell Park Hospital in Buffalo, New York, would lend themselves to fellowships in psycho-oncology. Centers of excellence in human genetics could lend support for psychiatry subspecialty interests in psychiatric aspects of human genetics.

In the past, at the height of the community mental health center movement of the 1960s, community psychiatry fellowships were attractive. Perhaps in the future, imaginative psychiatry programs will concoct ways to make managed care subspecialty tracks look attractive.

In any single institution the rationale for offering residency training after the required 4 years in general psychiatry would rest with what is uniquely available in that institution that would attract individual graduates of general residency programs to spend additional years in training. If there are no formal criteria, this could result in an individual spending 3 months, 6 months, 12 months, 24 months, 36 months, and so on in a single institution in a program designated as a fellowship. The area of study could be very narrowly focused. For instance, it is possible to conceive of a fellowship in the PET scan studies of obsessive-compulsive disorders in latency aged children. The setting most likely today for such an experience would be the National Institute of Mental Health (NIMH). An individual, on completion of such studies, could receive a certificate from the host institution, and a graduate of such a program could certainly begin an academic research career in a child and adolescent psychiatry division at a major university program. Approved subspecialty training requires that there be standardized criteria that meet ACGME approval and in turn can result in an ABPN certificate for those who graduate from such programs. Freestanding subspecialties do not necessarily have to meet any fixed criteria (American Psychiatric Association 1995).

The rationale for setting up a post–general residency program is multidetermined. It is possible that a department chairman would restrict subspecialty training to those approved by the ACGME. This would restrict postgraduate programs in psychiatry to child and adolescent psychiatry, geriatric psychiatry, addiction psychiatry, and forensic psychiatry (see Table 24–2). This would also mean that the department chair has made a major academic commitment including the necessary resources to develop these

Table 24–2. ABMS approved areas of subspecialization for psychiatrists

Addiction Psychiatry
Child and Adolescent Psychiatry
Clinical Neurophysiology
Forensic Psychiatry
Geriatric Psychiatry

subspecialty training programs. In turn, the parent institution must also have made a commitment to these subspecialties. At a minimum, this means the department chair would support the program director and his or her work as well as a supporting faculty as outlined in the ACGME requirements. These requirements would include faculty members having active research interests in the subspecialty area and exhibiting scholarly productivity with articles accepted in refereed journals. In other words, the chair of psychiatry must be prepared to make a major commitment to any new subspecialty training programs.

For the training program director in psychiatry, any new subspecialty program must by definition enhance the general residency program. A new subspecialty psychiatry program cannot drain resources from the general psychiatry program. There must be sufficient clinical material available to general residents, otherwise the program cannot be approved. It is anticipated that faculty from this subspecialty will be available for teaching general residents as well as the subspecialty residents and doing consultations as well as patient care. This enhanced expertise in the department in turn should improve patient care as well as the teaching of general residents, medical students, and other health professionals.

General residency training directors can be extremely valuable to training directors in subspecialties recognized by the ACGME. Namely, those training directors in these recognized subspecialties can seek the advice and help of general training directors in submitting an initial application for ACGME approval as well as to help the subspecialty training director prepare for site visits.

Subspecialty Career Advice for Residents

Residents in a general program will frequently turn to the residency training director and faculty members in the department of psychiatry to obtain guidance regarding their future, whether it be in academic settings, in clinical practice, or in other pursuits. The advice given residents has changed over time and certainly no one faculty member has the precise answer for each and every resident.

These changes can be characterized as follows: In the 1960s, faculty members were likely to tell graduates that everybody had an opportunity to develop interests and pursue multiple opportunities in what was then the shortage specialty of psychiatry. However, further training in community psychiatry, psychoanalysis, consultation/liaison psychiatry, and child psychiatry could enhance professional growth and development. Graduating from a general residency program was viewed as a "ticket" to a variety of practice options: solo office practice; public mental health centers; inpatient government settings such as the military, the Veterans Adminstration (VA), and state hospitals; community mental heath centers, and academic medical centers, to name a few.

In the 1970s, graduates were likely to be advised that it was useful to cultivate a subspecialty interest during electives in the fourth or final year of general residency training. These include electives or selectives in rural psychiatry, community mental health center psychiatry, forensic psychiatry, geriatric psychiatry, addiction psychiatry, intensive dynamic outpatient psychotherapy, administrative psychiatry, research, and others. Those interested in an academic career would be told they could benefit from additional training beyond the PGY-4 year, perhaps a research fellowship. Particularly attractive was spending time at the NIMH or at a major research academic center.

By the 1980s, mechanisms were being put in place for formal subspecialty recognition, culminating in the 1986 meeting sponsored by the ABPN to review six subspecialty requests. This meant that those interested in focusing a percentage of their future professional time in a subspecialty would need to complete formal training beyond the general residency program, similar to what was required in child and adolescent psychiatry. The trends toward subspecialization followed the lead of internal medicine and pediatrics, which started the move toward subspecialization in the 1940s.

What about the 1990s? In 1992 President Clinton was elected. One result of his health care reform proposals was a shift from supporting subspecialty medicine to supporting primary care medicine. A similar shift then occurred in the support of graduate medical education. Primary care was narrowly defined as family practice, general internal medicine, general pediatrics, and general obstetrics and gynecology. The emphasis turned to the primary care doctors diagnosing and treating patients for all illnesses regardless of the initial clinical presentation. This dramatic shift has led to administration proposals whereby 50% of future graduates would be encouraged to enter primary care specialties including family practice, internal medicine, and general pediatrics. An additional 7% of obstetricians-gynecologists were designated as primary care physicians as well. This change in direction came about in spite of the defeat of the president's health care reform initiatives.

The renewed emphasis on primary care led to reexamination of new subspecialties. Indeed, the greater tendency in the last half of this last decade of the twentieth century is toward considering combined training programs in psychiatry with one of the primary care specialties rather than encouraging new subspecialty development. This leaves the final recognition of any new subspecialty in psychiatry in doubt, and residents need to be advised about this change.

Resources for Programs

For ACGME-approved programs, there must be fiscal commitment. In recent times the main source of funding has increasingly been patient care revenues. The model for this has been Medicare and other third-party reimbursements and, if not most positions, in subspecialty training programs have relied on this source. Similarly, the VA has been a huge source of support for graduate medical education in the United States, with the major exception of pediatrics. Third-party payers other than Medicare have followed the lead of Medicare and have supported graduate medical education through reimbursement. Managed care companies have typically not followed suit. Government support of graduate medical education is under review by the executive branch. Multiple threats to the continuation of this major support are upon us. Medical reimbursement has already been reduced for subspecialty training, with the exception of geriatric psychiatry, after the PG-4 year in psychiatry. Combined training programs are experiencing reductions in support particularly after completion of the number of years required for one of the primary certificates. For instance, a 5-year program for medicine and psychiatry that in the past was funded for 5 years at full-time equivalent payment has now been reduced to 4 years of full-time equivalent payment and then the last year would be at 50% full-time equivalent. The VA is also exploring reductions in its support of graduate medical education. This will undoubtedly result in the reduction of the number of trainees funded through the VA.

The fiscal support for subspecialty training may have to come from sources other than third-party payors. One possible source in the future will be faculty earnings in a subspecialty. In the current economic climate it would be easier to finance subspecialty training in forensic psychiatry than, for instance, in addiction psychiatry. This is because forensic psychiatry earnings typically are not through third-party payors but from other sources such as the judicial system.

The role of chairs of departments of psychiatry is critical in deciding the allocation of resources for subspecialty training in their departments. Compromises will have to be made. Not all subspecialty requests by interested faculty members will be supported. Hopefully, in the spirit of academic traditions, open discussions, particularly with faculty members, will be held, and department chairs will listen and respond to the collective wisdom of their faculty members.

Faculty Resources for Subspecialty Recognition

In addition to fiscal resources for subspecialties recognized by the ACGME, a program must have subspecialists who are certified by the ABPN (or its equivalent). Program directors must devote a designated percentage of their professional time to being a program training director in the subspecialty. A designated number of full-time equivalent faculty members in the subspecialty as well as allied specialists and subspecialists must be a part of the faculty to train the subspecialty resident. Academic subspecialists in the program must have active research projects leading to scholarly productivity (Tucker et al. 1991).

Manpower and Practice Issues

The manpower needs designated for the delivery of psychiatric services are in a state of flux. Needs are difficult to define and vary widely according to the source. Clearly the focus of the mid-1990s is on a managed care model with primary care health providers (one cannot assume that these are necessarily physicians) performing a gatekeeper function. This system typically eliminates the freedom of choice of patients in selecting subspecialists for initial diagnosis and/or treatment. The role of the subspecialist is then principally as a consultant to the primary care provider. In instances where gatekeepers ask psychiatrists to provide care, it is typically for the administration of psychopharmacological agents, not for treating the whole patient. If such a system became universal, the need for general psychiatrists would be dramatically reduced, and the need for subspecialists in psychiatry would also be reduced. An exception may be forensic psychiatry, where reimbursement schedules are typically not driven by third-party payers such as Medicare. Instead, they are determined by the marketplace and most particularly by the monetary value the legal system has placed on a psy-

Table 24–3. Total number of certificates issued by ABPN as of July 1998

Psychiatry	35,541
Neurology	8,853
Child Neurology	1,121
Neuropsychiatry*	1,159
Child and Adolescent Psychiatry	4,449
Addiction Psychiatry	1,776
Clinical Neurophysiology	974
Forensic Psychiatry	824
Geriatric Psychiatry	2,425

*Last certificate awarded in 1969.

chiatrist's expertise. To date the legal system has not borrowed the gate-keeper function from the medical system model.

Conclusion

Residency training directors and psychiatric faculty have a major responsibility in educating residents to meet the challenges of the future. One of the individual challenges for residents is passing the Part I and Part II sections of the ABPN examinations so that they can become board certified. Subsequently, it is the graduates' responsibility to maintain their professional expertise so that they will be able to be recertified in their specialties and subspecialties (Shore and Scheiber 1994).

Further, the training director and faculty members have a responsibility for keeping residents informed about the availability of postresidency graduate medical education experiences, some of which also will lead to subspecialty recognition by the ABPN (Table 24–3). Ideally, the training directors and the Board work closely together to help reach these goals.

References

Accreditation Council for Graduate Medical Education: 1998 Annual Report. Chicago, IL, Accreditation Council for Graduate Medical Education, 1998

American Board of Medical Specialties: Annual Report and Reference Handbook. Evanston, IL, American Board of Medical Specialties, 1998

American Board of Psychiatry and Neurology: Information for Applicants. Deerfield, IL, American Board of Psychiatry and Neurology, 1999a

American Board of Psychiatry and Neurology: Information for Applicants for Child and Adolescent Psychiatry. Deerfield, IL, American Board of Psychiatry and Neurology, 1999b

American Board of Psychiatry and Neurology: Information for Applicants for Added Qualifications. Deerfield, IL, American Board of Psychiatry and Neurology, 1999c

American Psychiatric Association: Directory of Psychiatry Residency Training Programs, 6th Edition. Washington, DC, American Psychiatric Association, 1995

Graduate Medical Education Directory 1998–1999. Chicago, IL, American Medical Association, 1996

Shore JH, Scheiber SC (eds): Certification, Recertification and Lifetime Learning in Psychiatry. Washington, DC, American Psychiatric Press, 1994

Tucker GJ, Martin MJ, Scheiber SC: Subspecialization in psychiatry. Am J Psychiatry 148(11):1463–1465, 1991

Webb LC, Juul D, Reynolds CF, et al: How well does the psychiatry residency in-training examination predict performance on the American Board of Psychiatry and Neurology Part I Examination? Am J Psychiatry 153(6):831–832, 1996

ABPN Criteria for Subspecialty Recognition

1. ABPN will review applications from recognized organizations widely representing psychiatry or neurology or subspecialty organizations comprised primarily of members certified by ABPN.
2. In addition, strong evidence must be given that this will not dilute the general fields of neurology or psychiatry and that the function cannot equally be met by other means.
3. Must be a minimum number of physicians for critical mass. This should be no less than 100 for neurology and generally no less than 500 for psychiatry.
4. Current programs are distributed in all general geographic regions.
5. The number of people and programs must be continually increasing over a 10-year period.
6. There must be at least one national society for the subspecialty.
7. Academic degrees required must be identified.
8. Training sequence and program essentials must be specified. Minimum length of training must be 1 year.
9. Subspecialty must be practiced by physicians.
10. Absolute minimum number of programs can be no fewer than 15 in neurology and 25 in psychiatry. Fewer than 25 will not be considered without special justification in neurology.
11. Absolute minimum number of training positions can be no fewer than 15 in neurology and 25 in psychiatry. Fewer than 25 will not be considered without special justification in neurology.
12. Absolute minimum number of trainees completing training each year can be no fewer than 10 in neurology and 20 in psychiatry. Fewer than 20 requires special justification in neurology.
13. Documentation of the need must be based on objective data, not subjective impressions.
14. There must be objective evidence from institutions documenting intent to develop additional educational programs.
15. Faculty engaged in training must participate in research as well as clinical activities.

CHAPTER

25

Training in Child
and Adolescent Psychiatry

William M. Klykylo, M.D.

The History of Child Psychiatry Training

Child and adolescent psychiatry serves as a prototype for psychiatry sub-specialty training since it was the first subspecialty to be accredited by the American Board of Psychiatry and Neurology (ABPN), and since it predates board certification in psychiatry itself (Krug et al. 1964). Training in child and adolescent psychiatry began and for many years was undertaken in the context of child guidance homes or clinics, facilities with little medical identity or affiliation. The first of these is reckoned to be the Chicago Juvenile Psychopathic Institute (now known as the Institute for Juvenile Research) which was founded in 1909. By the 1920s, a number of similar facilities were established around the country. Psychiatrists began to serve in an unofficial apprenticeship basis in these facilities, with no set standards or coordination. Psychiatrists who had gone through such experiences frequently went on to other cities to establish additional clinics. By 1940, more than 600 such facilities had been established, and many of them offered training experiences for various professionals, including psychologists and social workers. In this context was evolved the classical team of child and adolescent psychiatrists, psychologists, and social workers. By the 1940s, the term *child psychiatrist* was frequently used although there was not yet any official definition for such a professional subspecialty.

Training in child and adolescent psychiatry in the late 1930s and early

1940s was supported by 1-year training fellowships from the Commonwealth Fund (Cohen and Dulcan 1987). After the World War II, Public Health Service fellowships were available, commonly for 2 years. This is the origin of today's 2-year child and adolescent psychiatry residency. At the same time, psychiatric training was offered briefly to pediatricians with the intent of developing "pediatric psychiatrists," but this effort was eventually abandoned. The federal government began offering more extensive support for child psychiatry residency training through the National Institute of Mental Health, funding some 72 trainees per year in 1962. In all, by the early 1960s, nearly 200 child psychiatry trainees were noted nationally. In 1959 the American Board of Psychiatry and Neurology began examining candidates for certification in the subspecialty of child psychiatry. The growth of the field in the last 35 years has been fitful, at times modest and at times dramatic. At this writing, more than 100 residencies in child and adolescent psychiatry were accredited and graduating in excess of 200 residents per year.

Program Administration

Child and adolescent psychiatry is a discipline that grew, evolved, and developed many of its standards outside the context of medical facilities. However, in the last 2 decades, divisions of child and adolescent psychiatry have become attached and integrated into larger departments of psychiatry, often in major medical centers. Frequently these divisions received support for their clinical and scholarly activities from sources other than those supporting general departments of psychiatry, often from direct clinical service in affiliated institutions. These sources of funding have frequently been challenged or obliterated in recent years. This combination of circumstances, divergent origins, and extramural funding have frequently created a tension between divisions of child and adolescent psychiatry and the departments to which they belong. Because of the unique nature of child and adolescent psychiatry, both as the first psychiatric subspecialty and because of its special responsibility to children, many academic child and adolescent psychiatrists approach their work with a belief that theirs is the most important of all specialties. At the same time, their general psychiatric colleagues may feel their own work is equally valuable. These tensions have consequences for child and adolescent psychiatry residencies and their relationships to general psychiatry departments and training programs, especially as they relate to competition for funding.

The administration of these programs varies among institutions. Not infrequently the training director may also be the division director of child and adolescent psychiatry. In such settings it is essential that an assistant training director be appointed and empowered, both to share the workload and to relieve the division director of inevitable tensions that arise between training and other administrative issues. In all cases, Residency Review Committee (RRC) requirements mandate that the identified training director have at least half-time (typically 20 hours per week) to devote to the residency. Ideally, the division director should answer directly to the chair of the department, in a position equal to that of heads of other major divisions. Similarly, the training director, if a separate person, should answer directly to the division director. The training director should not be equally beholden to the general psychiatric residency training director, except in regard to the training of general psychiatry residents. If any of these conditions do not obtain, there is a strong tendency for the position of child and adolescent psychiatry residency training and for child and adolescent psychiatry division itself to be devalued.

In some programs, perhaps as a result of the strong commitment of child and adolescent psychiatry to education, one individual may serve as training director for both general and child and adolescent psychiatry residency programs. Such an arrangement provides both obvious challenges and tremendous opportunities for the integration and coordination of training. More often, programs are separately administered. The disadvantage of separate training hierarchies for general and child and adolescent psychiatry residencies is that such programs can become separated, often into jealously guarded fiefdoms. In such a situation, duplication of efforts can ensue, and the cross-fertilization that should occur among colleagues of different disciplines may be hampered.

Program Collaboration

Perhaps one positive effect of today's scarcity of educational resources may be the encouragement of training and curricular collaboration between general and child psychiatry. In a well-functioning program, qualified faculty from both areas are involved in the training of each others' residents. This may be seen in particular in the PGY-4/PGY-1 year. Many general residency programs have "special topic" seminars during this period with subject matter chosen by residents. More-advanced presentations in such topics as statistics, research design, biological psychiatry including molecular biology, history of psychiatry, psychiatry in literature, health care policies and systems, and transition to practice may be offered. All of these topics are very appropriate for both general and child psychiatrists; in many cases they could be taught by faculty from both sides. Usually, general residencies contain didactic and practical instruction on human development, child and adolescent psychiatric assessment, and psychopathology. These are all topics that ideally should be taught by child and adolescent psychiatrists. In some cases, child residents, particularly advanced ones, may be able to serve as instructors or "teaching fellows" in these activities, thus serving a set of mutual needs. Some teaching activities such as rounds and seminars within a child and adolescent residency may also be appropriate as electives for PGY-4 residents.

There are many opportunities for administrative collaboration as well. Most residency programs have an administrative coordinator or assistant or executive secretary. These persons are invaluable to the operation of any residency program, for both their daily efforts and the great amount of knowledge and institutional lore that they collect. It is nearly impossible for training directors themselves to maintain all of the documentation, coordinate didactic activities, distribute paper, and serve as "mother hen" to residents. Administrative coordinators possess equanimity and diplomacy, and these qualities are far more important than specific training. Since the administration of child and general residencies is so similar in regard to documentation for accreditation and resident advancement, the expertise of these persons and at times their efforts can be usefully shared.

Some particular tensions inevitably ensue between general and child and adolescent psychiatry residencies. The most common of these center around workforce issues. From the standpoint of child psychiatry, the ideal situation is one in which the fourth year of the affiliated general psychiatry residency is entirely elective. In this case the program is not so dependent on the service and fiscal production of the residents that the entry into child and adolescent psychiatry is perceived as a stress to the general program. Many institutions are not so fortunate. In some settings the expression of an interest in child psychiatry on the part of a general resident may even be discouraged, lest it occasion a burden to the department as a whole. When such stresses are unavoidable, policies should be elaborated well in advance of recruitment of residents, jointly by the general and child and adolescent residency training directors. Where sufficient collegiality or support does not exist for this to happen between the training directors themselves, these issues should be mediated, again in advance, at the highest level of an institution or department, typically by the chair. If such tensions are left unresolved, they will affect morale not only among the faculty but among the residents themselves, who may feel as though they are recipients of a "bait and switch" in regard to training experiences. It is in the interest not only of child and adolescent psychiatry programs but entire departments to avoid such situations. The situation of happy equitable collaboration between divisions enhances both morale and residency recruitment, as does the presence of a vital program in child and adolescent psychiatry.

The Residency Review Committee Special Requirements

Graduate medical education in the United States is overseen by the Accreditation Council for Graduate Medical Education (ACGME), which is sponsored by the American Board of Medical Specialties (ABMS), the American Hospital Association (AHA), the American Medical Association (AMA), the American Association of Medical Colleges (AAMC), and The Council of Medical Specialties Societies. Training in psychiatry, as in all medical specialties, is supervised by an RRC sponsored by the American Board of Psychiatry and Neurology, the American Psychiatric Association, and the AMA Council on Medical Education. This committee establishes and regularly updates program requirements for residency education in psychiatry, including child and adolescent psychiatry. These requirements are available in the annual ACGME *Essentials* (Accreditation Council for Graduate Medical Education 1996) directory and should be familiar to all persons involved in the direction or administration of residency education. The RRC requirements in many respects are quite specific, yet open to interpretation and elaboration according to the needs and resources of a particular site (Schowalter 1996).

The RRC Site Visit

Training sites are accredited after site visits by ACGME personnel or, in some cases, specialist site visitors. In preparation for a site visit an exhaustive program description is completed according to a format specified by the RRC. When a new program applies for accreditation or when the accreditation of an existing program requires renewal, a site visitor, who is typically a specialist in graduate medical education but usually not a psychiatrist, reviews the application, visits the training site for 1 or more days, and then prepares a report for the entire RRC. In certain cases a specialist site visitor, in this case a child and adolescent psychiatrist selected by the RRC, may be sent to conduct the site visit. Indications for a specialist site visit include a new program applying for full accreditation after an initial period of provisional accreditation, a program that has been on probation after deficiencies discovered in an earlier site visit, or a program that has undergone significant administrative or facilities changes. Preparation for a site visit or other RRC proceedings is frequently an arduous and stressful activity. The scope of such efforts are beyond this article but have been described elsewhere. In a positive sense, a site visit encourages training directors both to rededicate themselves to particular goals and objectives and to reorganize the many details of a training program. In my experience, attention to detail with clear and lucid documentation can remove much if not all of the anxiety of a site visit.

Program Components

The RRC requirements include statements of *program length and prerequisites, institutional organization,* and *faculty qualifications and responsibilities.* These are straightforward and generally unvarying. Child and adolescent psychiatry residencies are 2 years long. Today's demands for alternate career paths have led to provisions that residencies may be completed in as many as 4 years at half-time, or in two blocks no more than 5 years apart. Other RRC requirements such as affiliation agreements, the requirements of participating institutions, and the appointment of residents are similar to those in general psychiatry. A somewhat controversial requirement is the "critical mass" rule, that a program must have at least two residents in each of the 2 years of training. This rule has been elaborated to ensure peer interaction and group discussion in seminars and conferences. Some academic child psychiatrists today have noted that no program requirements for any nonpsychiatric residency contain such a rule, and that it may be impractical for many programs; but it is uncertain as to whether this rule will be modified. Finally, the RRC requirements address faculty qualifications and responsibilities, stating there must be a single program director devoting at least half-time to the training program and a faculty that includes at least three full-time equivalent child and adolescent psychiatrists as well as other mental health professionals.

The requirements for *facilities and resources* and for the educational program are much more variable, in recognition of the variations among institutions in our pluralistic nation. Incidental but important requirements include office space, space for physical and neurological examinations, facilities for seminars and lectures, teaching aids such as one-way mirrors and audiovisual equipment, and extensive library and data processing resources. Residents and faculty alike spend less time in the physical environment of a library and more time than ever on-line; thus, "computer literacy" for residents is essential, as well as access to appropriate facilities and databases.

Inpatient/Acute Care

The RRC requires "24 hour responsibility in working with acutely and severely disturbed" patients. This has typically occurred in the context of an inpatient setting, but in today's world, settings such as residential treatment centers, partial hospitalization units, or day treatment programs are also acceptable and appropriate (Klykylo et al. 1996). The requirements demand that residents spend no less than 4 months and no more than 10 months full-time equivalent in such a setting. This is to ensure that residents derive adequate training in this area but not become servants of institutional "cash cows." Some program directors in the past have been tempted to disguise these types of experiences as outpatient or other training experiences, but such attempts have generally not been successful and have frequently backfired. Work in such settings should be undertaken by residents only in the context of serving with an attending physician, who has both clinical responsibility and authority within the service site and status as a faculty member within the division and department. When this is not the case, both the educational experience of the residents and the liability of all parties involved may be compromised.

The specific didactic and educational activities on an inpatient unit will vary with the setting and patient population. At a minimum, regular rounds should take place. These include both "card rounds," wherein attending physicians, residents, and unit staff review the course of each patient on a regular and timely basis; and patient rounds wherein attending and resident physicians can actually observe each other interacting with individual patients. Each resident should also receive individual supervision, both around interactions with individual patients and their families and addressing resident participation in groups and other unit activities. Whenever possible, residents should lead or co-lead therapy groups and participate in other therapies and activities on the unit. Finally, the inpatient unit affords an opportunity for didactic teaching in conference or seminar format. We have found useful a program of weekly to semi-weekly conferences of which approximately half of the topics are pre-arranged with the other being determined by current clinical presentations, needs, or resident interests. Figure 25–1 depicts a typical schedule.

Therapeutic Modalities

The RRC requirements address a need for training in many therapeutic modalities that are typically administered on an outpatient basis. Such training can occur in a variety of settings. Traditionally, residents spent at least a portion of their time through much or all of their residency in an outpatient office, conducting individual, family, and group psychotherapies. The requirements continue to mandate experience in short- and long-term individual psychotherapy, psychodynamic psychotherapy, family therapy, crisis intervention, and pharmacological therapies. They also require work with at least some outpatients for at least a year's duration. Today such work is undertaken in a variety of settings. In addition to the traditional academic outpatient dispensary, these settings may include community mental health centers, day treatment and outpatient affiliates of residential

	Monday	Tuesday	Wednesday	Thursday	Friday	Saturday or Sunday
A.M.						
8–8:45 Card rounds	- ->|					On-unit time
9–9:30 Unit meeting	- ->|					On-unit time
10–11:00 Attending rounds	- ->|					On-unit time
11–12:00	Residents' didactics	Off-unit didactics	Unit in-service	Family therapy conference	Residents' didactics	
P.M.						
1–2:00		Off-unit didactics				
2–3:00	Intake conference	Off-unit didactics	Family therapy	Professor rounds		
3–4:00		Off-unit didactics	Family therapy			

Figure 25–1. Resident schedule adolescent inpatient unit.

treatment centers and other multimodal systems, schools, clinics run by other mental health professionals, and even shelters. In most settings, the provision of a variety of treatments including combined psychological and somatic treatments is not as problematic as the maintenance of long-term treatment in today's managed care environment. Often this is accomplished by the resident providing continuity; that is, the resident may transfer a patient as the resident rotates from one setting to another. This requires oversight from the training director as to the case load and appropriateness for long-term therapy for each resident's cases. It is very useful in documentation of these matters for each resident to prepare a log, including demographic information, diagnoses, treatment modalities, and course of treatment, for each patient seen throughout the residency.

More and more outpatient psychiatric work both in academic and private settings is conducted through specialty clinics. These may address such entities as attention deficit hyperactivity disorder, affective disorders, trauma and abuse, or developmental disorders. These clinics tend to follow a more traditionally medical than psychodynamic model, with patients and families being served by multiple professionals outside the context of the 50-minute hour. These settings afford a special opportunity for faculty and resident physicians to observe one another's clinical work. They also provide an opportunity to derive revenue from residents' clinical activities, which is otherwise becoming more difficult given the reluctance of many of today's public and private payers to support therapy such as psychodynamic psychotherapy when conducted exclusively by trainees alone.

Pediatric Consultation

In addition to standard inpatient and outpatient experiences, the RRC imposes several special training requirements unique to child and adolescent psychiatry. Of crucial importance is the consultation experience, since it is paradigmatic for much of child psychiatry practice. Consultants "do not primarily engage in treatment but use their specialized knowledge and skills to assist others to function better in their roles." Consultation experiences are required in pediatric outpatient or inpatient medical facilities, and in schools. Training and experience in legal issues relevant to child and adolescent psychiatry is also required. Many of these requirements can be fulfilled through a rotation in a pediatric hospital, where ongoing programs involving the education and legal protection of children take place. In many residencies, residents spend anywhere from 3 to 12 months or more in a full- or part-time rotation in pediatric services. This is best undertaken in a hospital setting where a child and adolescent psychiatrist is on staff and, preferably, on the faculty of the department of pediatrics as well. In such a setting, residents can work under supervision in inpatient and outpatient clinical facilities, developmental disability clinics, and pediatric neurology services. They also have the opportunity to participate in emergency evaluations, either by being on call to an emergency department or to participate in an existing psychiatric emergency service.

The relationship of child and adolescent psychiatry and pediatrics is complicated beyond the scope of this article. Many (though by no means all) of the historical turf battles have lately burned themselves out, and in most settings child and adolescent psychiatrists who are collaboratively and collegially minded (and who are secure in their own identities as competent physicians) can function effectively with the appreciation of their pediatric colleagues. What is much more problematic is funding for such activities in already stressed pediatric institutions. Such pressures often make psychiatric rotations in these facilities shorter than might be desired. Nonetheless, even short rotations can be useful if they are conducted under the supervision of a child and adolescent psychiatrist who is dedicated and involved on-site.

School Consultation

School consultation is one of the oldest activities of child and adolescent psychiatry but can be problematic in today's environment. While ever more lip service is being given to increased involvement by child and adolescent psychiatrists on-site in schools, more and more school districts, struggling under today's financial constraints, find it difficult to maintain what they regard as supportive services for pupils. In the context of relatively affluent and progressive school districts, existing on-site consultation activities may be available in which residents can participate. More often, however, such activities need to take place in the context of a program sponsored or administered by a medical or mental health facility. For example, some community mental health centers may have contracts with severe behavioral handicap (SBH) or severely emotionally disturbed (SED) programs in a given local or district school system. Mental health facilities may offer case-centered consultations, which are conducted through diagnostic evaluations. Many pediatric hospitals have on-site classrooms or schools where residents can be involved. The multidisciplinary diagnostic center, included in university-affiliated facilities (UAFs), can be a particularly productive venue for teaching educational consultation, since such facilities frequently employ diagnostic special educators as part of the multidisciplinary team.

Forensic Consultation

The degree of training in forensic child and adolescent psychiatry is extremely variable among programs. In many cases, such work is conducted through court-affiliated clinics, a proud tradition going back to Chicago and the Institute for Juvenile Research. In other areas such work may be conducted by individual practitioners who qualify themselves by interest, training, or experience. The degree of interest or support for such activities by the legal system varies among jurisdictions. In some settings the same practitioners or facilities may provide consultation in both civil and criminal proceedings, whereas in other settings these activities may be entirely separate. In my experience the development of a service in either a juvenile or domestic relations court depends entirely on the attitude and inclinations of the judges. Those practitioners desiring to develop such a service are best advised to cultivate their relationship with judges and magistrates in the first place. In the absence of an existing "court clinic," such training for residents may best be pursued through "tagalong" apprenticeship-like experiences with practitioners experienced in this work. The RRC requirements include experience in court testimony, but this is simply impossible in many jurisdictions where the testimony of trainees is not admissible as evidence; and it is most likely undertaken where possible in the context of a court clinic. The elements of a training program in this area and possible venues for it are discussed in detail by Nurcombe (1993) and others.

Two examples of resident rotations are presented in Figures 25–2 and 25–3, one from a community-based program (Wright State University) and one from a program based in an academic medical center (University of Illinois—Chicago). These are offered as stimuli rather than recommendations; many other arrangements are feasible.

Program Staffing

There is extreme variation in faculty and staffing of child and adolescent psychiatry residencies, as noted earlier. The RRC Essentials requirements mandate a faculty that includes a total of at least three full-time equivalent, fully trained child and adolescent psychiatrists who devote "substantial time" to the residency program. These faculty may have ABPN certification

Year I

4 H/10%	Residents' Clinic	Rosary Hall	Outpatient
36 H/90%	*Childrens' Medical Center*	*WPAFB Medical Center or Mental Health Center SJCTC*	*Franciscan Medical Center*
	Primary: Pediatric Consultation	Primary: Outpatient Dx & Rx in multidisciplinary team	-Adolescent -Partial
	Secondary: Developmental and Behavioral Peds. Clinic	Secondary: Infant visits	
	4 Months	4 Months	4 Months

Year II

8 H/20%	Residents' Clinic—Rosary Hall, Including 2 hours/Week in Diagnostic/ Consultative Clinic			
32 H/80%	*Children's Medical Center*	*Franciscan Medical Center*	*Community Psychiatry*	*Elective*
	Primary: Senior Pediatric Consultation Secondary: Developmental and Behavioral Peds. Clinic Outpatient Neurology Clinic	Senior and Administrative Residency, Adolescent Day & Inpatient Unit	SJCTC 6 hours Learning Center 8 hours Dayton Mental Health Center Forensic Unit 8 hours Substance Abuse 10 hours	
	3 Months	3 Months	3 Months	3 Months

Figure 25–2. WSU-SOM child and adolescent psychiatry clinical rotations: block diagram.
Source: William M. Klykylo, M.D.

or equivalent qualifications and demonstrate a strong interest in resident education. Furthermore, a member of the teaching staff at each participating institution must be designated to assume responsibility for educational activities at that site. The participation of professionals from other disciplines, including neurology, pediatrics, psychology, social work, special education, and speech and language pathology, is also essential to produce comprehensively trained child and adolescent psychiatrists. Often such fac-

Year I	3 Months	3 Months	3 Months	3 Months
	Metro C. & A Inpatient Unit and UIC Consult-Liaison 40% each × 6 mos.-80% total		Forest Child Inpatient Unit 80% × 3 mo.	Allendale Residential Treatment Unit 80% × 3 mo.

UIC/IJR Outpatient Clinic 20% × 12 mo. (Includes Family Systems Program live group consultation × 12 weeks in summer.

Year II Community Mental Health Clinic (at DuPage County or UIC) 20% × 12 mos.

UIC/IJR Outpatient Clinic 30% × 12 mos. (Includes giving 1-hour lecture to third-year medical students every 8 weeks, and supervising a psychiatry resident.)

Group Research Practicum: 10% time × 9 mo.

Electives:
20% × 2 mo./
35% × 1 mo.   10% × 3 mo.   20% × 3 mo.   40% × 3 mo.

Cook County Juvenile Court Consults 15% × 2 mo.	Special Ed District of Lake County School Consultation	Pediatric Neurology	Custody Evaluations
Outpatient Group Leader			
15% × 3 mo.	30% × 3 mo.	20% × 2 mo.	20% × 1 mo.
3 mo.	3 mo.	3 mo.	3 mo.

Figure 25–3. UIC/IJR child and adolescent psychiatry clinical rotations: block diagram.
Source: Courtesy of Geraldine Fox, M.D.

ulty must serve on a voluntary basis, so the greatest challenge of the program director is to stimulate and maintain the morale and enthusiasm of these individuals. Fortunately, many individuals still consider it an honor to educate medical residents. Regular public recognition of these efforts, including adjunct faculty appointments, can be very helpful. Many faculty in a general psychiatry residency may already be conducting didactic and other activities suitable for child and adolescent psychiatry. A close integration of conferences and seminars, particularly among first-year child residents and fourth-year general residents, is usually productive.

Didactic Resources

The stresses on faculty time in today's environment are thankfully somewhat mitigated by the increasing availability of didactic resources. For example, it is possible for virtually any program in any setting to have access to the same library and reference materials as those of any other program through interlibrary loans, on-line databases, and searches. Medline and other literature search facilities are available at essentially all medical libraries. Through such programs as Grateful Med, individual physicians can conduct their own electronic literature searches. Even more up-to-date information can be acquired from Internet news groups, wherein clinicians and academics from around the world can communicate. In years past, child psychiatrists had to content themselves with only one or a few textbooks. Now there is a wide choice of textbooks coming from both North America and Europe, and today at least one new comprehensive textbook seems to be released every year. The quantity and quality of our journals has increased dramatically. In 15 years, the *Journal of the American Academy of Child and Adolescent Psychiatry* has gone from a quarterly to a monthly publication. Other publications such as the *Child Psychiatric Clinics of North America* and the *Journal of Child and Adolescent Psychopharmacology* have also appeared. Other journals such as the *Journal of Autism and Developmental Disorders* and *Child Psychiatry and Psychology* continue to prosper. Outside of child and adolescent psychiatry, many other relevant publications are available representing disciplines including child psychology, developmental and behavioral pediatrics, and speech and language pathology.

The curriculum modules for child and adolescent psychiatry residencies developed by Martin Drell and others, headquartered at the American Association of Directors of Psychiatric Residency Training (AADPRT), deserve special note (Dulcan 1994). These allow faculty to develop teaching competence in areas outside their particular subspecialties and allow programs that in the past might have been regarded as small or physically isolated to provide an adequate curriculum in broad areas of the specialty. The situation of a very few centers that have experts in virtually every subspecialty area is to be envied but is no longer necessary to produce well-trained child and adolescent psychiatrists. What is of greater importance is the intelligence, dedication, and enthusiasm of faculty and residents who are willing to learn together. Moreover, such a model inculcates in residents the habit of continuing self-education and lifelong learning.

Perhaps the foremost pedagogical requirement for a child and adolescent psychiatry program in these times is creativity. There is much to be taught, but there are many ways to learn. Programs that are short of more traditional resources can more than compensate by the clever and enthusiastic use of alternatives. Finally, the utility and productivity of such resources can regularly be assessed through trainee assessment devices such as the Psychiatric Residents In-Training Examination (PRITE), Child-PRITE, and PKSAP. These instruments are best used as assessments not so much of individual residents as of the performance of entire programs.

Workforce Issues

Estimates of future workforce needs, both nationally and in a given locality, should be of prime importance in planning and developing residency training programs (Enzer 1989; Yager 1989). Unfortunately, in today's changing climate of health care delivery, such estimates are varied and uncertain (Verhulst and Tucker 1995). At this writing there are roughly 5,000 clinicians in this country who are identified as child and adolescent psychiatrists. The GMENAC Report of 1980 (Graduate Medical Education National Advisory Committee 1980) suggested that by 1990 we should have had 9,000 practitioners, a tripling of the 1980 workforce. Few practitioners today report insufficient demand or clinical need for their services; however, sources of financial support are much more uncertain and changeable. At this writing it would appear that most child and adolescent psychiatrists entering practice are seeking either institutional employment or membership in multispecialty or multidisciplinary group practices. Outside of the public sector, the bulk of patients seen by most child psychiatrists today are enrolled in HMOs or other integrated health care delivery systems. If anything, child and adolescent psychiatry has been at the forefront of medicine in confronting and adapting to systematic changes. However, our experience has not given us any particular advantage in predicting future trends. Some observers have speculated that, in a model of medication management and consultative practice only, approximately 2,500 child and adolescent psychiatrists would be employed nationally. However, whatever pattern emerges within the private sector, it would appear that there will be a burgeoning need for practitioners within the public system in schools, residential treatment centers, juvenile detention facilities, and related outpatient programs. As of this writing, there has been no report of a competent child psychiatrist anywhere in the United States unable to find full employment through some combination of various public and private endeavors. Although many are advocating a downsizing of the number of training sites, and it is possible that funding for postgraduate medical education could be reduced, there seems to be no clinical need for this type of downsizing in the foreseeable future. It is in the nature of institutions to perpetuate themselves, and few, if any, programs will voluntarily spontaneously dissolve themselves. For this reason, program directors must develop strategies for the enhancement of existing residencies.

Recruitment

Recruitment of personnel, both residents and faculty, is the sine qua non of program development and maintenance. Both these topics are discussed in detail elsewhere in this text, and those principles relevant to general psychiatry also apply here. However, recruitment of residents to child and adolescent psychiatry is often complicated by the demand for an extra 1 to 2 years of training. Residents today are often burdened by debt incurred in their medical education. In addition, many residents are unwilling or unable to defer the demands of domestic life, including childrearing. These issues will not disappear, nor are residents likely to be dissuaded as to their importance. Therefore, program directors must mitigate the problems that emerge from these issues. Residents must pay off their debts and would usually be able to do this only through moonlighting. It is unrealistic in today's environment to oppose or even ignore moonlighting, as has been frequently the case in the past. It is rather more sensible to help establish "approved" or "supervised" moonlighting activities in connection with the sponsoring departments and institutions. Such activities may be an extension of the resident's regular work or related work in adjoining facilities. Such an arrangement offers an a number of advantages. First, it may mitigate the potential liability that programs incur when residents moonlight, since presumably they would be working in established clinical settings of known quality. Second, such activities can be more closely supervised and coordinated with residents' rotations so as to be more educationally productive. In addition, program malpractice insurance may cover residents' activities in some settings, making it unnecessary for residents to work extra hours to pay for outside insurance. Such work, in the same settings as residency training, may be incorporated into the residents' daily or weekly schedule with less disruption of other activities. Finally, such activities, especially when conducted by advanced residents, can provide the community with useful clinical services at a reasonable rate, enhancing both the clinical care of patients and the reputation of the program.

Recruitment activities among general residents, like voting in certain large cities, should be done early and often. Program directors should lobby for training experiences, both didactic and clinical, as early as possible in general residency programs, and they should participate and support these activities with enthusiasm. Such experiences offer not only exposure to children and child psychiatry, but also an opportunity for mentorship, which many believe to the single most important factor in recruitment of residents.

Recent work at Wright State University (Klykylo and Dunseith 1995) has addressed the "attrition" of general psychiatry residents: Whereas 30% of entering general psychiatry residents express an interest in child and adolescent psychiatry, typically only about half of them actually enter child and adolescent psychiatry residency. This study suggests a number of reasons for this, not the least of which is simply the emergence of other interests. However, it appears likely that a significant minority of these "dropouts" may be discouraged by the typical challenges of today's population of seriously ill children in multiproblem, socially distressed families. The most effective antidote to this is the opportunity for residents to observe settings such as residential treatment centers, where children are followed for an extended period of time and where they do, in fact, improve. It is also some consolation that today's entering child and adolescent psychiatry residents seem very realistic about the nature of contemporary clinical work and appear much more willing to "get their hands dirty" than others might have been (Varley et al. 1996).

Transition From General Psychiatry

Another issue specific to child and adolescent psychiatry recruitment is the identity of the entering resident as a general psychiatrist. Some studies (see, e.g., McConville and Klykylo 1989) have suggested that residents may be fearful about losing their identity and skills as general psychiatrists, including practical fears about their performance on general psychiatry boards. These fears may be accompanied by fears that they may lose contact, social and professional, with their general psychiatric colleagues from residency. Finally, residents entering child and adolescent psychiatry often experience a sort of *anomie* as their role changes from experienced residents to, once again, beginners. They may envy their general psychiatric colleagues who are chief residents, practicing largely on their own. All of these issues can be addressed by ongoing collaboration between general and child and adolescent residency programs. In particular, the participation of first-year child and adolescent psychiatry residents in PGY-4 general activities such as seminars, case conferences, and meetings can be very important and useful. This underscores the previously stated need for collaboration between programs within the department of psychiatry.

Consolidation of Workforces

Another important strategy that child and adolescent psychiatry residencies should consider is that of consolidation with other programs. This does not necessarily mean a merger, although in some cases this may be the most productive measure, but rather a collaboration in didactic and clinical teaching activities. Two programs in the same city or general area may be able to offer joint conferences or clinical rotations. Individual supervision may be offered by faculty members with particular areas of competence in one or another program. Although institutional resistances have made such efforts difficult in the past, today's dire straits may accelerate them, especially if department chairs can recognize how such efforts amplify the results of existing expenditures. Where geographical distances are too great for residents or faculty to commute, today's opportunities for teleconferencing, videotaping of presentations, and on-line communication present attractive alternatives. In a number of areas, programs are presently collaborating in offering "mock boards" (clinical examinations for residents), and this is a promising development.

The Future

Today's stresses on program development and residency training in child and adolescent psychiatry are undoubtedly severe and at times disheartening. However, they also offer an opportunity to train practitioners better suited for the realities of twenty-first-century medicine than would have been produced in the past. Child psychiatrists of the future will retain a strong commitment to the needs of children and families but will recognize that these needs must be met concurrently through a variety of methods and services. They will be broadly trained and conversant not only with multiple modalities of assessment and treatment, but with their integration. The child psychiatrist will be much less of a "lone ranger" and more much the member of a team. While leadership of the team is no longer the innate prerogative of a physician, properly trained child and adolescent psychiatrists may often be able to assume leadership because of merit, if they are comfortable with change in both strategies and roles. If anything, this comfort should be our heritage as clinicians dedicated to children who are constantly changing and growing. The stresses on our training programs today for flexibility, fluidity, and creativity within the traditional context of devotion to children and their needs offer an example to the clinicians of the future.

References

Accreditation Council for Graduate Medical Education: Essentials and Information Items 1996–1997. Chicago, IL, American Medical Association, 1996

Cohen RL, Dulcan MK (eds): Basic Handbook of Training in Child and Adolescent Psychiatry. Springfield, IL, Charles C Thomas, 1987

Dulcan MK: Frequently asked questions about education in child and adolescent psychiatry. Academic Psychiatry 18(1):46–49, 1994

Enzer NB: Recent trends in the recruitment of child and adolescent psychiatrists: an overview of general and faculty needs. Academic Psychiatry 13:176–188, 1989

Graduate Medical Education National Advisory Committee: Summary Report to the Secretary, Vol 1 (Publ No HRA-651). Washington, DC, U.S. Department of Health and Human Services, 1980

Klykylo WM, Dunseith N: Career choices regarding and adolescent psychiatry among residents. Paper presented at the 42nd meeting of the American Academy of Child and Adolescent Psychiatry, New Orleans, October 1995

Klykylo WM, Baren J, McConville BJ: The crisis stabilization unit and its community relationships. Paper presented at the 43rd meeting of the American Academy of Child and Adolescent Psychiatry, Philadelphia, PA, October 1996

Krug O, Gardiner G, Hirschberg J, Third Author, et al (eds): Career Training in Child Psychiatry. Washington, DC, American Psychiatric Association, 1964

McConville BJ, Klykylo WM: Transition from general resident to child resident. Paper presented at the meeting of the American Academy of Child and Adolescent Psychiatry, New York, 1989

Nurcombe B: Forensic consultation, in Child and Adolescent Mental Health Consultation in Hospitals, Schools, and Courts. Edited by Fritz GK, Mattison RE, Nurcombe B, et al. Washington, DC, American Psychiatric Press, 1993, pp 187–289

Schowalter JE: Recruitment, training, and certification in child and adolescent psychiatry in the United States, in Child and Adolescent Psychiatry, A Comprehensive Textbook, 2nd Edition. Edited by Lewis M. Baltimore, MD, Williams & Wilkins, 1996, pp 1205–1208

Varley CK, Calderon R, Vincent JG, et al: A survey of child and adolescent psychiatry residents. Academic Psychiatry 20(1):15–25, 1996

Verhulst J, Tucker G: How many psychiatrists do we need? Academic Psychiatry 19(1):219–223, 1995

Yager J: Issues in general residency training pertinent to the recruitment of child psychiatrists. Academic Psychiatry 13(4):202–207, 1989

26

Recruitment of Residents

Sidney H. Weissman, M.D., and Nyapati Rao, M.D.

Recruitment of trainees into psychiatry initially consists of developing strategies to interest diverse populations of physicians and medical students.

Recruitment usually focuses on a given year's class of senior U.S. medical students (USMGs). It also includes other groups of physicians. The total number of trainees from the non-U.S. seniors interested in psychiatry has varied markedly over 2 decades. This pool includes:

1. International medical graduates (IMGs). This group is further subdivided into U.S. citizens who have obtained their medical education outside of the United States and citizens of other countries.
2. Transfers to psychiatric residencies. This group consists of physicians who transfer into psychiatric residencies while still in residency training in other medical fields. This group includes both USMGs and IMGs.
3. Practicing physicians. These are physicians in practice who change medical careers.
4. Graduates of osteopathic medical schools.

Each group of potential trainees has special needs and interests. The recruitment of each group into a given residency calls for unique strategies for each category of potential trainees. Not all residencies attempt to attract members of each group. However, as the number of USMGs entering psychiatry residency in the July after they graduate from medical school has declined, the reliance on other groups of potential trainees has increased. By 1996, the majority of residency programs have some trainees from the non-U.S. senior student group. Each residency training director will need to know which group of potential trainees are most likely to be interested in training in their program. Following this, the training director must then develop recruitment strategies that relate to the identified groups. It is possible and probably essential for effective recruitment of the non-U.S. senior group for programs to develop, in addition to recruitment strategies to reach each group, tracks, or elements in the program that relate specifically to unique training needs of each group. The issue in developing recruitment strategies is not simply developing a marketing or communication program, but the critical development of elements in the actual training program that focus on the needs of each group, and to then communicate effectively with trainees. An initial successful marketing of a program without the capacity to deliver to trainees what was promised will, in the long term, not be helpful to the program's survival.

As this volume is being prepared, the United States is undergoing a major reassessment in determining the essential size of the nation's physician workforce. An additional national study addresses the mix of physicians between specialists and generalists. Numerous reports have been written, including one by the Institute of Medicine that calls for a reduction in the number of physicians in graduate medical education (residencies). The studies, although they vary in mechanism, endorse a position of the Association of American Medical Colleges that would call for limiting the number of graduate medical positions (residency slots) to approximate the number of graduates of U.S. allopathic and osteopathic medical schools. Training positions would not be available in the most rigid of these proposals for IMGs or to physicians in practice who wish to change their specialty.

Although the most rigid of these models is not likely to be implemented, we can anticipate in upcoming years a major push to decrease funding by the federal government of graduate medical education. Various scenarios have been proposed to implement this policy. One uses 1996 as a modal year. In this scenario Medicare would only fund a number of first-year resident positions equal to new U.S. graduates entering psychiatry. With this model, the number of new psychiatric residents supported by Medicare would fall to the range of 500 to 550. This is far below the projected 800 needed to retain current workforce numbers. A 25% reduction in the total number of all first-year residents would reduce the number of psychiatry residents to approximately 900 but would continue to require major numbers of non-U.S. seniors to fill all available positions in psychiatry. The proposed 25% reduction in total first-year residency positions reduces the number to 18,750 from the current (1996) 25,000. This is a reduction supported by the Association of American Medical Colleges. If reduction of residency positions is implemented in the U.S. graduate education system, the reduction will have a significant impact on psychiatric residents' training. It will necessitate that departments of psychiatry reduce their number of trainees and develop new methods of delivering service. It should be noted that it is unlikely that there will be a final one-step resolution of the number of graduate medical education positions, but an ongoing and evolving policy shift that will deal with the changing political and economic realities of medical practice. In this light, the training director in the next decade must be prepared to respond to these shifts when they occur in terms of the resources of their programs and the unique needs of the community in which they are located. There will not be a recruitment strategy of one size fits all. We would, however, suggest that the number of psychiatric residency trainees at the beginning of the next century may be similar to the numbers of the early 1980s. That is 15% to 25% fewer than we have today.

Recruitment Strategies

We will first discuss issues in recruitment that are the same for whichever group of potential trainees you are seeking.

1. *Structure:* Be clear on the strengths and weaknesses of your program. Review in depth the structure of your program with your faculty, and clarify and distinguish between educational and service requirements. Make sure that there is an appropriate balance. We will assume you have met the Residency Review Committee (RRC) requirements; but since the RRC has broad guidelines, you must be clear that what may be acceptable to the RRC will not necessarily attract trainees. For example, how often are residents on call in your program as compared with other programs in your region? What is the mix of public sector rotations and academic medical center or private hospital rotations? All will meet RRC requirements, but the mix will determine how you are perceived or how you wish to be perceived. There is not a right mix,

but be clear how your residency is constructed and how this construction relates to the potential trainees you wish to recruit.

2. *Morale:* Morale is determined by both the faculty and staff and the residents. It is essential for the training director to keep a close watch on the program's morale. Alteration in morale in either group demands immediate attention. Obviously, as many programs struggle with the complex issues created by managed care and faculty members find their time intruded upon as they must alter their practices and research activities to enable their department to survive, this influences their performance and morale. It is not simply putting the best face on a bad situation. The department must not experience itself in a constant crisis. It must organize itself such that the faculty feels that as the department responds to pressure that, although they may not like all of the changes occurring, they are able to maintain their core identities as academic psychiatrists. Loss of the connection to the faculty's core identity will lead to alienation and a deterioration of morale among staff and faculty and the creation of a destructive environment for recruiting. Although it is impossible to have a positive resident morale in the absence of a positive faculty morale, the converse is not true. Departments can be constructed to support faculty activities at the expense of resident educational experience. One could attempt to base the economic survival of a department on resident service. Some say that this is especially true in hospitals that predominantly train IMGs. If this is done and this is quickly learned by applicants—and it will be—with a declining pool of potential trainees, these programs will not be able to fill their positions; or if they do, it will be with trainees not accepted elsewhere. Finally, if resident morale is poor, it will immediately be communicated to applicants when they interview at the program.

3. *Marketing:* It is with some reluctance we address this issue. If one has a fine program, why must one market? Perhaps the problem is a confusion between advertising, which is one form of marketing, and the general concept of marketing. Marketing of a residency means you are making sure that the potential groups of trainees you wish to attract know about the existence of your program and its strengths. Each training director needs to examine for approximately a 10-year period the source from where their trainees have been recruited. They then need to assess whether they wish to alter the source of trainees or maintain their current position. Either way, depending on their location

and resources, they must develop or maintain a strategy to ensure that potential trainees know what the program is about. Sometimes, this may mean reaching out to students from medical schools in other cities. Sometimes medical school–based programs must develop programs to reach their own students. It does not follow that the students in a given medical school are aware of the strengths and values of the residency in their own school or its affiliate hospitals. Some programs have developed relationships with premier medical schools in foreign countries.

Special marketing issues exist for a residency that is not the residency of a medical school department of psychiatry. Even if the residency's hospital is affiliated with a medical school, it does not follow that the medical school's students will be encouraged to enter a residency at an affiliate. The affiliated hospital will need to establish its own relationship with the medical school's students. It will also be necessary for the freestanding program or affiliate hospital program to establish effective communication with other medical schools. Frequently, medical school core faculty, when asked by students about residencies, will suggest medical school programs but not others.

Market Uniqueness

As commented upon in "selling" your program identity, your program's unique capabilities are what makes your program special. All programs meet RRC requirements, but you must identify and communicate to potential residents and medical school faculty at other schools the special elements of your program that distinguish it from competitors.

The Brochure

Frequently the first direct connection by a potential applicant to your program, other than talking to a residency staff member, is the written material describing your program. Programs vary from the kind of material they send. Some use Xeroxed sheets while others use glossy paper brochures with photographs. Some give detailed accounts of learning objectives, clinical rotations, and seminars while others include friendly photos and general information. There is, of course, no correct answer regarding what you should include, but you must consider what you want to communicate. A brochure will not ensure recruitment, but a poor presentation in what the applicant receives will likely cause a potential applicant to apply and go elsewhere.

The Applicant Interview or the Program Preview

The applicant interview by the residency faculty offers the faculty the opportunity to assess the applicant's abilities. Interviews also offer the applicant an opportunity to preview the residency. It is the latter function we will explore. The qualified applicant wants to learn about the residency. This includes curriculum issues, the faculty, the program's residents and its location, as well as the possibility for doing research. The applicant's day visiting your program must give the individual an opportunity to learn about each dimension of the program. Personal style and your preference will determine how you will structure the interview day. An important aspect frequently ignored is the time spent with residents in the program. Just as not all faculty members are effective applicant interviewers, not all residents can effectively interact with applicants. Selection of residents to meet with applicants is best done by the training director, who knows the strengths and weaknesses of each resident, not the chief resident or a secretary. If you have a resident who has graduated from the applicant's medical school, it is useful to have that resident also meet with the applicant.

Dual-Career Couples

Dual-career couples include couples where both partners are graduating from medical school and seeking residencies or any couple where each member of the couple has specific career needs. Many of these couples will seek programs located in major metropolitan areas because of broader career opportunities for the nonpsychiatrist member. Programs in large cities need make few special arrangements, but programs in smaller cities need to be available to offer potential assistance to land these individuals. The intensity of the assistance will, of course, vary in each situation.

The Match

The National Residency Matching Program (NRMP) serves as the route to connect nearly all U.S. senior students and varying numbers of all other applicants with their residencies. Individual residencies do not sign contracts with the NRMP. Rather, hospitals sign contracts to offer their first-year residency positions through a notification and selection system administered by the NRMP. When a hospital joins the "Match," so do all of its residencies.

Senior U.S. students usually join the Match. When they join the Match, they may only withdraw under special circumstances. All the applicants to residencies may also utilize the Match. International medical graduates, for example, may enroll in the Match. Unlike the situation for U.S. seniors, however, IMGs may withdraw at will from the Match. This is so because, unlike with U.S. seniors where the Match can enforce their remaining in the Match with their medical school for other applicants, the Match has no such enforcement authority with regard to IMGs. Therefore, a program can offer an IMG a position outside of the Match and, if they accept, reduce the number of positions requested in the Match. Each program will need to assess its situation in deciding how to proceed. At this time the NRMP is considering changes in its system for IMGs. The proposed change would not allow MG applicants to accept positions outside of the "Match" or programs to change the number of positions offered to accommodate these IMGs.

The Match List

After completing interviews, it becomes necessary to rank order your applicants for your Match list. You may tell applicants you will rank them in your assured acceptance group, but you cannot require them to commit to your program prior to the Match. Generally speaking, since most students, with the possible exception of applicants to the most prestigious programs, obtain their number one choice, students interested in a program usually maintain contact with the program director of their desired program.

It is usually among non-U.S. seniors where the training director does not fully know their preference or standing in other programs that the Match list becomes more important. Indeed, it is useful to maintain contact with all the IMGs you may be interested in recruiting to make sure that they have not accepted positions outside of the Match and have, therefore, withdrawn from the NRMP.

The Faculty Interview

The faculty interview of residency applicants requires a degree of diplomacy on the part of the training director. Not all faculty members are effective interviewers or evaluators of candidates. Further, some feel they have special abilities as interviewers and feel they should use the interview to stress the applicant to "learn" more about them. Others feel that any aspect of the applicant's life is open for their review. While the nature of our field means that knowledge of the potential resident's psychological functioning is important, the training director must work with the faculty to be sure that interviews obtain only appropriate data in a supportive fashion. Although stress-inducing interviews were once in vogue, they have no place in the assessment of applicants. Besides being inappropriate, such interviews will cause applicants to go elsewhere.

The Psychiatry Transfer Resident

Although we have been discussing the recruitment of trainees directly into psychiatry from medical school or from nonpsychiatric residencies or practice, the same general principles apply when addressing residents transferring programs. Reasons for residents transferring programs are diverse. The one essential element to be addressed when a resident transfers programs is communicating directly with the training director of the sending program. Although this is an RRC requirement, applicants may give reasons they do not want you to communicate with their training director. Although the situation may be difficult, this information is essential in evaluating the transferee. Of course, you must obtain the information in a tactful way that does not subject the potential transferee to undue pressure.

Special Recruitment Issues

U.S. Senior Medical Students: Although generally the largest single group of potential trainees, U.S. senior medical students are the most difficult to recruit because they have the most options. All residencies will offer qualified U.S. seniors positions. Following the general principles outlined will be essential for recruiting this pool of applicants.

If your program is a medical school–based residency, your parent medical school graduates should be your first potential applicant pool. If you are not a medical school program, establish links by way of residents or faculty members and cultivate other schools. Finally, remember, of all applicant groups, U.S. seniors are the most concerned about other residents in the program. They see these residents as their lifelong peers and friends. Keep this in mind as you talk about what career paths graduates of your program follow.

U.S. Medical Graduates Who Are Not Currently Seniors: Responding to this pool, whether they are currently in other residencies or are in practice, requires that the residency has flexibility in how they can be scheduled into the program. For example, if an internist wishes to enter a program, how easily can the residency schedule a 2-month neurology rotation? The department secretary needs to be able to tell these potential applicants that the program is flexible.

Recruitment and Selection of IMGs

What Training Directors Need to Know About Obtaining and Interpreting Academic Records, Reference Letters, and Other Data for International Medical Graduates (IMGs)

In this section, we describe the strategies that we use to effectively evaluate IMGs.

This is by far the most difficult group to evaluate; therefore, we explore the IMG recruitment process in greater depth. International medical graduates are a diverse group culturally and linguistically. They come from very diverse medical education systems and at widely differing stages of their lives. U.S. training directors are frequently unfamiliar with ways of obtaining information about the applicant's medical school and their performance. There are certain basic data that the training director will find useful in assessing IMG applicants.

Since IMGs' reference letters may be bland and uninformative, and the medical schools and their transcripts unfamiliar to you, you may be tempted to rely heavily on qualifying exam scores in screening applicants to interview (Rao et al. 1991). However, other methods will yield important additional information (Rao et al. 1994):

1. Ask IMG applicants to submit a focused autobiographical statement about themselves and their interest in psychiatry. Such statements can give a three-dimensional picture of the applicant. The statement will also provide a very quick assessment of the applicant's writing skills. The training director may talk to the applicant during the interview about the personal statement, which will fulfill a number of functions. It can verify the statement as the applicant's own writing, it will provide openings for a deeper discussion of the applicant's life issues and path to psychiatry, and will serve as a dynamic example of the applicant's communication skills.

2. Further information about language skill may be obtained by asking the applicant to discuss a favorite piece of English literature, and to show any examples of creative writing (poems, essays, etc.).

3. The applicant may be asked to view a videotaped psychiatric interview and discuss it with the interviewer(s). This can provide a rich source

of information about the applicant's language and communication skills within the clinical and simulated supervisory setting, as well as offering a sample of the applicant's interpersonal observation skills.

4. In addition to the specific focus produced by the preceding techniques, the entire interview, including lunch with a current resident, provides material for assessing the applicant's interpersonal and communication skills.

5. Educating oneself about foreign medical education systems and specific schools requires input from many sources as there is no single reliable, comprehensive source. Look up the medical school in the WHO "World Directory of Medical Schools." Ask colleagues and residents from the country in question about that school and the medical education system. Training directors may find some useful chapters in Khan (1995).

6. For the many IMG applicants who have worked in health-related fields in the United States before applying to residency positions, question their supervisors about their performance. We do not favor only those IMGs with American hospital experience. However, we have found that having an American hospital experience will make the IMG's orientation to the residency experience less problematic.

7. Become familiar with the issues and procedures involved in J-1 and H-1 visas. Please see the section toward the end of this chapter for a more detailed discussion of the visa issues.

8. Create a selection committee composed of members who have all demonstrated good interviewing skills and sensitivity to IMGs' cultural issues and the phase-specific issues of immigration. Such a committee can be very helpful in educating its members to the cultural contrasts IMG applicants encounter in the United States with respect to formality/informality, confrontation/politeness, and individual-competitive versus group-cooperative norms.

9. Try to have each candidate seen by at least one interviewer who is familiar with the candidate's culture. This is very important in enabling the selection committee to interpret the interview data.

10. The average IMG residency applicant in psychiatry has been out of medical school longer than his or her USMG counterpart. Assess the applicant's experience during these extra years with respect to gaining practical knowledge of medicine, biomedical research, and life in the United State. Inquire about migrations on the way from the home country to the United States.

11. Assess the applicant's motivation for entering psychiatry, including the individual's knowledge of what the field is like here in the United States and motivation for undertaking a second residency, if this is the case.

12. Ask about any experiences with psychiatry or psychiatric patients. Many IMGs do not have a well-rounded exposure to psychiatry in their undergraduate years as do USMGs. This is due to a lack of emphasis on psychiatry in foreign medical schools' curricula as a result of workforce and educational priorities determined by their societal needs. Thus an IMG may be applying for postgraduate training in multiple specialties. The training director will be challenged to choose the potentially good psychiatric resident from this group and avoid those who are just seeking an entry into the U.S. graduate medical education system.

13. Assess the applicant's humanistic interests, the degree of acculturation, and the status of any possible value conflicts relevant to the practice of psychiatry in the United States. For example, the U.S. subcultures are characterized by a strong emphasis on individuality, whereas in many traditional societies loyalty to the group takes precedence over one's own individualistic needs and aspirations. Similarly, value judgments regarding religion, spirituality, sexuality, gender roles, and cross-generational ties in a family may cause conflicts for the IMG and must be explored in the interview.

14. Questioning candidates about immigration-related experiences, and their feelings about the process they had gone through, can be a very productive approach to obtaining a fleshed-out picture of the IMG applicant.

In the preceding, we have described certain strategies that will help training directors choose the most-qualified IMG for their program. One must note that the Equal Employment Opportunity Commission (EEOC) requires that no job applicant be asked questions about their national origin or their marital status. Any questions or procedures used to assess an IMG must be used to assess a USMG as well. Our recommendations follow the EEOC guidelines (see the website http://www.eeoc.gov).[1]

---

[1] Because of the requirements of the Equal Employment Opportunities Commission (EEOC), to ensure fairness for all residency applicants, we asked a number of attorneys familiar with EEOC requirements to review our initial recommendations. Questions or procedures they felt might be perceived as violating EEOC guidelines were deleted from our final proposal. All

Sometimes we are asked the question whether there is a weighting or ranking of characteristics that will predict future performance. We have no research to suggest any differential weighting of these data, but we can offer an order based on our experience: A well-written autobiographical essay that fully describes the individual, passing the qualifying exam creditably in as few attempts as possible, previous training in psychiatry, medical school honors, American hospital or research experience, and freedom from significant psychopathology usually are associated with successful performance as a resident.

Visa and Immigration Issues

The Accreditation Council for Graduate Medical Education (ACGME) permits foreign-born IMGs with provisional Educational Commission for Foreign Medical Graduates (ECFMG) certification to enter U.S. residency programs if they are naturalized citizens, hold a permanent resident (immigrant) visa or either one of the temporary visas J-1 or H-1B (exchange visitor), or a federal work permit. Those possessing J-1 exchange visitor visas can only enter residency programs in medical school hospitals or hospitals affiliated with medical schools. The J-1 permits the candidate to reside in the United States to acquire medical training for a maximum of 7 years or until completion, whichever is shorter.

In addition, J-1 visa holders must obtain permission from their governments to undertake training in a specialty that is in short supply in their native country. They are also required to commit themselves to return to their native country after completion of training in the United States to practice their specialty for at least 2 years. There are exemptions possible for this return rule, but the procedures are extremely lengthy, costly, and uncertain in outcome.

The H-1B visa was originally intended only for research activities, but it has recently been broadened to include clinical training. The H-1B visa

---

EEOC fairness requirements apply to all applicants, USMG or IMG. No one can be asked questions about national origin or marital status. Any questions asked of an IMG must be asked of a USMG. One area of disagreement existed with our consulting attorneys. One felt that policies could be established for psychiatry residency applicants even if the in-depth review of performance was not followed in other departments for their residency applicants. Another attorney felt the same general procedures must be standard throughout the institution. We urge that, prior to establishing your own protocol, you have it reviewed by your own EEOC counselor.

permits candidates to undergo medical training without placing any restrictions on their length of stay in the United States. However, candidates musthave passed the Federation Licensing Examination (FLEX) or United States Medical Licensing Examination (USMLE)-Part 3 and hire their own attorney to process the paperwork and follow through with a labor certification process with the U.S. Naturalization and Immigration Service. The training institution hiring a candidate must participate in the certification process. The H-1B visa can eventually be converted to permanent resident status without the need to exit the United States for a period of time as the J-1 requires (Perlitsh 1997).

Qualifying Examinations

To undertake graduate medical education in the United States, an IMG must be certified by the Educational Commission for Foreign Medical Graduates (ECFMG). ECFMG certification requires passing the qualifying examinations and documenting completion of educational requirements to practice medicine in the country where they attended medical school. Also, most states in the United States require ECFMG certification for licensure.

The ECFMG exam includes a medical science exam and an English language proficiency test. Past medical science exams included the Visa Qualifying Exam (VQE), which was last administered in September 1983; the Foreign Medical Graduate Examination in the Medical Sciences (FMGEMS), last administered in July 1993; the National Board of Medical Examiners examination (NBME), last administered in April 1992; and the Federation Licensing Examination (FLEX), last administered in 1993. Currently, the United States Medical Licensing Examination (USMLE) is given to both USMGs and IMGs. Effective July 1998, to obtain a new ECFMG certificate all IMG's must successfully complete an additional examination. This is a Clinical Skills Assessment that uses standardized patients, given by the ECFMG currently only in Philadelphia.

Applicants may present with complicated permutations of these exams. For example, an applicant can be eligible for ECFMG certification by having passed a part of the Foreign Medical Graduate Examination in Medical Sciences (FMGEMS) and a part of the National Board of Medical Examiners (NBME) examination or a part of the USMLE. As of 1993, the USMLE replaces all other qualifying exams, but those IMGs who have passed the previous examinations and have acquired the provisional ECFMG certificate will still be eligible to enter residency training.

The ECFMG encourages training directors to verify an applicant's performance with the Commission. The training director must also be aware that the ECFMG process of collecting documentation from the IMG's medical school will begin only after the IMG has passed the qualifying examination. This process can be subject to considerable delays from the applicant's medical school. If time is at a premium, it may be a useful practice to interview only those candidates who have acquired the provisional ECFMG certificate and have a valid visa.

The future number of IMGs in training in the United States, as noted earlier, will depend on the political resolution in the United States of the question as to how many physicians the United States needs. As this volume is being prepared, we have no answer to the country's resolution to the workforce issues. We believe it is likely that there will be changes in the number of psychiatric trainees as well as the content and process of psychiatric education. For these reasons, it will become increasingly important for all of psychiatry to present our field as an exciting career opportunity to all U.S. medical students.

References

Khan F (ed): International Medical Graduates in U.S. Hospitals: A Guide for Program Directors and Applicants. Philadelphia, PA, American College of Physicians, 1995

Perlitsh SM: Negotiating the immigration maze: updates on current immigration issues. January 15, 1997

Rao NR, Meinzer AE, Primavera LH, et al: Psychiatric residency selection criteria for American and foreign medical graduates: a comparative study. Academic Psychiatry 15:69–79, 1991

Rao NR, Meinzer AE, Berman SS: Perspectives on screening and interviewing international medical graduates for psychiatric residency training programs. Academic Psychiatry 18:178–188, 1994

27

Continuing Medical Education in Psychiatry

John B. Herman, M.D., and Nancy L. Bennett, Ph.D.

"Lifelong learning" is the paradigm for medical education encouraged from the first days of medical school. This message serves early notice that practitioners in the art of medicine must commit themselves to remaining abreast as scientific advances ever more rapidly translate from research into the "community standard" of clinical practice. In this chapter, we review the many benefits of Continuing Medical Education (CME), CME program planning, and the "nuts and bolts" of producing a CME event in psychiatry.

The Purposes of CME

Institutional Rationale for Sponsorship of a CME Program

Sponsorship of a CME program is a public demonstration of an institution's commitment to the process of learning and its role as a promoter of education. Every flyer, poster, published advertisement, or public announcement of CME activity attracts positive public attention to its sponsoring institution.

Such endeavors enhance the academic identity of the sponsoring institution, and at the same time affirms a department's commitment to state-of-the-art clinical practice.

Regional professional colleagues can be particularly appreciative of CME opportunities. By learning about and attending such activities, appreciation for your department and the sponsoring institution is enhanced in the eyes of professional groups such as other academic institutions and state and local medical and psychiatric societies.

Faculty Rationale for CME Contribution

The opportunity to teach colleagues is greeted as a compliment and can boost individual and departmental morale. Although much effort may be required to prepare an effective presentation, it is unusual for individuals to decline the offer. Indeed, such a request is rightly viewed as an endorsement of a clinician's abilities. The effort that faculty members take to prepare a presentation contributes to their mastery of a topic and their professional growth and, consequently, enhances the overall quality of a department. Individuals who might not otherwise consider themselves capable of a "teaching standard" may find such efforts extremely satisfying, often serving to stimulate ongoing professional growth as teacher-clinicians and even as clinician-researchers.

The Benefit of CME to Communities

CME activities enhance relationships with a host of outside individuals and agencies. Community agencies, schools, and special interest groups (such as the Alliance for the Mentally Ill, etc.) learn of a department's interest in education through its CME activities and may solicit help for their own projects, oftentimes inviting a program's featured speakers to their local meetings. Additionally, engaging in CME projects may lay the groundwork for mutual collaboration in educational, research, and even treatment projects.

The Benefit of CME to Individuals

Institutions, organizations, and state and local agencies require and increasingly audit compliance with CME requirements.

Most hospitals now require their staff to demonstrate CME activity in order to retain hospital privileges. Hospitals are themselves accredited by the Joint Commission on Accreditation of Healthcare Organizations (JCAHO), whose oversight in recent years has increasingly focused on employee quality assurance and quality improvement procedures. Thus, hospitals are called on to demonstrate the competency of their professional staff. Participation in CME programs is a standard yardstick used to measure professional quality.

Most managed care companies require that physicians document participation in CME. These companies promote their physician panel by guaranteeing minimum standards of professional quality demonstrated not only by board certification and state licensing but CME activity as well.

In the United States, physicians are licensed by state-controlled licensing authorities. Currently 23 states require demonstration of CME credits to obtain periodic recertification. This trend is growing. Currently 2 states (Florida and Massachusetts) have special requirements for demonstration of CME in "Risk Management," designed to reduce professional liability in areas such as domestic violence, HIV, and patient confidentiality. Other states are currently considering adding these requirements as well.

Lifelong Learning and the Acquisition of Knowledge

Far beyond the pressures generated by hospitals, managed care companies, and state and federal agencies, the quest for ongoing education for physicians is personally driven and highly honorable. The pursuit of postgraduate learning long preceded the imposition of such activities by outside authorities. Clinicians' concern for their own competence and the wish to deliver the best care to patients remains the overriding driving force for CME.

CME seminars and conferences offer clinicians the opportunity to step back from the pressures of everyday practice and slip into the "mind-set" of learning. Participants enjoy these experiences of learning and reflection as contributing to their own personal practice standard and enhancing their professional identity. Continuing education conferences allow participants an opportunity to compare themselves to the "experts." For most clinicians, every conference is a "win-win" opportunity: If the material presented is fresh and practical, clinicians leave the conference reinvigorated with new tools to employ in their practice. If the materials presented seem familiar and reflect the clinician's own individual practice, the participant experiences a comforting affirmation that his or her clinical work remains contemporary and in "the community standard."

Thus, CME activities represent an opportunity for clinicians to recalibrate their practice against the high standard that they themselves (more than even their patients or outside agencies) require for comfortable, competent practice.

In our oftentimes highly stressful and sometimes isolating vocation, the opportunity for clinicians to socialize and to establish or reestablish relationships with colleagues is one of the best reasons for attending a CME activity.

CME Program Planning

The following section outlines the traditional model of CME program planning that most policymaking and certifying CME accrediting bodies use.

CME Accreditation

Most professional groups requiring continuing education assign responsibility to an accrediting board to oversee quality standards in CME. Generally there are fees associated with applying for or obtaining granting status certification.

For physicians, a national organization, the Accreditation Council for Continuing Medical Education (ACCME), establishes program guidelines (such as conflict of interest standards and curriculum specifications) and approves institutions such as medical schools, state medical societies, and other organizations to administer the approval process for every program seeking to give American Medical Association Physician Recognition Award "category 1" CME credit. Likewise, for psychologists, the American Psychologic Association allows local delegation of the accreditation process in a similar fashion.

Generally these local organizations are experienced and can be very helpful in helping mount a program that adheres to defined standards. The ACCME and the American Psychologic Association maintain lists of local accrediting agencies. For nurses and social workers' accreditation, independent state and local organizations usually must be contacted directly, and rules vary widely.

Commercial Support and Faculty Disclosure

Industrial sponsors often offer financial or "in-kind" educational grant support for CME programs. Such funding has attracted increasing concern because of the potential for undue commercial influence on educational content. Although commercial sources are allowed to provide educational grants for programs, all planning activities must be controlled by the CME sponsor. To ensure this policy, the ACCME has developed standards of compliance requiring a written agreement between sponsor and funding source whenever funds or in-kind services are accepted. Additionally, faculty members must disclose any financial interest or relationship with a manufacturer of any commercial products discussed in their presentation.

Professional Licensure

The necessity of securing professional recertification has inspired the proliferation of CME course offerings throughout the country. Becoming familiar with the recertification rules and regulations in your own state or local area is important as you plan a CME course. For physicians, accreditation requirements for CME in risk management (including HIV, substance abuse, domestic violence, etc.) is increasing and should be considered for inclusion in courses.

Although newer educational models have garnered much attention recently, this section outlines the currently accepted sequence required by the ACCME for program accreditation. State medical societies and the American Academy of Family Physicians may vary slightly in their requirements for accreditation of CME programs. Continuing quality improvement techniques, individualized study, and distance learning have also provided variety in ways to approach appropriate CME activities that are meaningful to individuals.

Needs Assessment

For the individual charged with the opportunity and responsibility for developing CME programs, needs assessment is the first step. Although this element of program planning is often intuitive or obvious ("I notice most clinicians out there seem to be way behind in their clinical practice of X"), a thoughtful, deliberative process will improve the chances that your efforts in developing a CME program will be rewarded with appreciation from the sponsor and by a course enrollment large enough to justify the efforts made.

CME program planning is motivated by the perception of a gap between a professional community's current practice and the state of the art in field or discipline. To confidently seek the endorsement of a sponsoring institution for a CME activity, program planners must try to determine the nature of this "gap."

If necessary, local or national experts in a given discipline can be consulted to help establish the need for training or advanced course work. Such discussions should refine the focus of program content (basic research vs. clinical trial results vs. practical and clinically applicable information) and suggestions for course faculty. A questionnaire canvassing your own faculty and the target audience provide supportive data demonstrating the need for a program. The use of national statistics can also support a program proposal. Gleaning information through a literature search serves to support the argument in favor of "closing the knowledge gap" locally. Surveying CME programs offered by other groups locally or in other geographic areas may underscore the need for a CME program.

Developing Program Objectives

Having established the need for a CME program, explicit course objectives must be established. Such objectives ensure concordance between the course curriculum and the audience's expectations. It is essential that the course planners make clear to the course faculty the results of the needs assessment surveys. For example, a faculty member should not extend efforts in preparing a lecture focusing largely on new findings in neuroscience research when the learners are drawn to a course promising a curriculum in practical applications of new pharmacologic agents. Likewise, prospective learners must receive a clear statement of what they should expect to learn from a course. Course objectives assist the course planners in negotiating with the faculty (who may have other areas or prepared lectures they prefer to present) and consequently protect both the faculty and planners from a dissatisfied audience.

Developing a CME Format

An educational offering may take place in a variety of settings and through a number of methods: standard lecture hall, small seminar rooms, on-site clinical demonstrations/observation, mail or e-mail correspondence, audiotape or videotape and, more recently, closed-circuit video teleconferencing and the Internet. Each of these can be effective means of conveying information and closing the gap of knowledge that motivates the drive for CME. It is essential that the format selected allows the faculty and learners to meet the program objectives. For example, planning a weekly evening seminar can be prohibitively impractical for a course whose target and audience is a widely dispersed group of suburban and rural practitioners. In this case, a daylong, weekend conference would more likely achieve the objective.

On the other hand, if an educational objective involves enhancement of collaborative clinical problem solving among a hospital's subspecialists, a weekly grand-rounds-type conference within that hospital would be appropriate.

Faculty Selection

The ability to convey knowledge in a clear and entertaining fashion is the key to the success of a good teacher, and a collection of good teachers is the key to the success of a CME program. Just as the program format must match the program's objective, so too must the faculty match the format into which you place them. For example, a highly regarded and gifted supervisor might appear wooden, dull, tongue-tied, or anxious when appearing in a lecture hall at a podium behind an amplified microphone. Likewise, a gifted speaker able to enthrall a large audience may have difficulty handling the spontaneous, give-and-take, open-ended style of an ongoing seminar. The course planners must "cast" the right faculty member for the role they expect the individual to play. Ideally, faculty members should come from within the sponsoring department. This is good for a faculty and good for a department. Such selections should not, however, be made at the expense of the course objectives and the learner's experience. Experts from near or far often improve a course, add luster, and boost enrollment. They can offer added benefit by allowing the local faculty to become learners themselves, inviting the guest to a specially arranged lunch or dinner seminar for faculty members only.

Program Evaluation

Once up and running, course participants must be repeatedly encouraged to collaborate with the course planners and faculty as constructive critics. Audience members on the receiving end of the course are in the best position to report on the success of the effort. Collectively, the objective reports of each learner can define how well the course has achieved its objectives. A written questionnaire (see Figure 27–1) should be distributed to each course participant at the beginning of a course. Course participants must be encouraged earnestly and often to help by suggesting to the course planners how to improve the next CME presentation. Course faculty can improve teaching from evaluations about their own individual presentation (see Figure 27–2). Evaluations are useful to improve specific lectures and become an invaluable resource for future program planning. It is not at all unusual

Name _____

Address _____

_____

_____

Program Title

1. Overall Course Evaluation	Unacceptable		Average		Outstanding
Curriculum/Topics	1	2	3	4	5
Discussion/Panels	1	2	3	4	5
Faculty	1	2	3	4	5
Question Time	1	2	3	4	5
Organization	1	2	3	4	5
Syllabus	1	2	3	4	5
2. Facility Evaluation					
Meeting Rooms	1	2	3	4	5
Sleeping Rooms	1	2	3	4	5
Hotel Location	1	2	3	4	5
Meals	1	2	3	4	5
Food at Breaks	1	2	3	4	5
Audio-visual Materials	1	2	3	4	5

3. How will this program enhance your professional practice?

4. Have you learned or refined a skill as a result of participating in this program?

Figure 27–1. Attendance documentation and program evaluation.

Please circle one answer for each of the following questions.

P = Poor   F = Fair   G = Good   E = Excellent

		Comments
1. Lecture on Pharmacological Treatment of Depression Dr. Jones		_____ _____ _____
Quality of Presentation	P F G E	_____
Relevance to Practice	P F G E	_____
		Comments
2. Lecture on Alternative Treatments of Depression Dr. Smith		_____ _____ _____
Quality of Presentation	P F G E	_____
Relevance to Practice	P F G E	_____

Figure 27–2. Individual faculty lecture evaluation.

for a course teacher to note improved ratings as a consequence of incorporating the suggestions and criticisms of course participants. Such feedback can have a major role in the professional growth of individual faculty members and consequently the quality of the course and, eventually, the reputation of a department.

Analysis of course evaluations can serve a number of purposes. In addition to evaluating each individual teacher, other questions may be included in the evaluations as to preferences for changes in the course format (time of year, time of day, duration of course, etc.). Space should be provided for open-ended comments from course participants can provide a range of ideas from learners (see Figure 27–3). Evaluations may be helpful to the department chair or hospital administrators as they determine the need for further CME offerings. Many departments utilize CME directorship and faculty participation as criteria for promotion and academic advancement.

The course director or course planning committee should review the course evaluation forms. Individual faculty members should be warned that the solicitation of anonymously submitted critiques can sometimes result in either exaggerated praise or undeserved criticism. It is not unusual for the same speaker to receive comments such as, "exceedingly useful and applicable to my practice! A wonderful presentation by an obviously sea-

1. Clarity of course objectives	not clear	somewhat	very clear
2. Accessibility of faculty	not accessible	somewhat	very accessible
3. Time for questions	not enough time	somewhat	enough time
4. Helpfulness of handouts	not helpful	somewhat	very helpful
5. Overall quality of teaching	poor	average	excellent
6. Overall quality of program	poor	average	excellent
7. What are the strengths of this program?			

8. What changes would improve the program?

9. What pieces of information from this program will you use in your practice?

Figure 27–3. (Program title)—evaluation.

soned clinician" and, from another member of the same audience, "The speaker's awkward presentation of irrelevant minutia was thinly veiled defense of his insecurity about the subject. You really should ask someone else more senior to present this lecture." Course planners should include in their evaluation not only the opportunity for such comments but also an objective "scoring" system that allows for quantitative averaging of a single lecture and between other lectures (Figure 27–3).

The evaluation that solicits responses regarding the course organization and facility (hotel, lecture hall, food and beverage, registration, the syllabus, etc.) will provide information and future planning. The course faculty, your most important resource, should themselves be solicited for their comments for improvement.

Course Administration

The great effort required to coordinate the administrative tasks in planning, preparing, executing and evaluating a course must not be underestimated. If course faculty are "cast" to be the right players "onstage," so too must any course planner pay careful attention to "backstage" operations. Failure to attend to the details can bedevil a course and make the difference between success and failure.

Budgeting

Planning checklists for categories to be considered in a typical CME program are included in Figure 27–4. Many new and smaller programs will not have expenses in each of these areas.

The budget of a course generally corresponds directly with the course duration and the number of learners expected to attend. For example, a weekly or monthly 1-hour lecture series intended for clinicians within your own department, taught by your own faculty and in space provided by your own hospital, would have little cost beyond photocopying and secretarial support. Courses intended for a national audience numbering in the hundreds may require months of planning and the full-time administrative support of one or two staff members.Numerous consultants also may be needed to advise planners about advertising and marketing as well as coordination of accreditation, faculty scheduling, quality control across faculty member presentations, compilation of an integrated course syllabus, coordination of conference facility, catering, audiovisual equipment, and parking and hotel accommodations for course faculty and participants. Such

Program Title _____

Date _____

Site:

Representative _____

Phone/fax/e-mail _____

_____

Confirmed _____

A. SPACE

Anticipated number of participants ____

Meeting Room Set-up:

____ Classroom Style   ____ Lectern

____ Theater style   ____ Microphone

____ Screen   ____ Projector

____ Registration table   ____ Other

____ Other   ____ Other

Emergency phone number _____

B. Food Service

• Registration

　Time _____ Number _____

　Menu/cost _____

• Breaks

　Time _____ Number _____

　Menu/Cost _____

• Meals

　Time _____ Number _____

　Menu/Cost _____

C. Exhibits

　Group Name _____

　Table size _____

　Other _____

　Fee _____

　Confirmation _____

Special Arrangements

D. LODGING

Participants: Hotel _____

Rooms Reserved _____

Date _____

Other _____

Speakers: Hotel _____

Date _____

Transportation _____

Other _____

Other _____

E. Equipment

　Audiovisual equipment

　　____ Slide projector/clicker

　　____ Carousels (# _____)

　　____ Overhead projector

　　____ Pointer

　　____ Video player

　　____ Tape recorder

　　____ X-ray viewer

　　____ Other

_____

_____

_____

_____

_____

_____

_____

_____

(continued)

Figure 27–4. Facilities and equipment checklist.

PROGRAM TITLE _____ DATE _____ BUDGET		Estimate		Actual
	Low	Middle	High	
Attendance				

Income
  Participant Fees   @
  Other				

Total Receipt				
Refunds @				
Total Income				

Expenses
  Instructional Staff
  Travel				

Subtotal				

Promotion
  Development
  Printing
  Mailing lists
  Mailing
  Other advertising				

Subtotal				
Instructional Supplies				
Subtotal				
Facilities				
Subtotal				
Food Service				
Subtotal				

Administrative Costs
  Records
  Overhead
  Credit application
  Travel/Food Service
  Correspondence
  Other				

Subtotal				
Total Expenses				

Grand total
  Income
  Expenses				

Difference				

Figure 27–4. Continued

enterprises may require a significant commitment of resources and may put the sponsor at risk for financial loss if paid attendance revenues or outside sponsorship do not meet course costs.

Revenue support for CME programs may be underwritten by your department or hospital, by nonprofit community organizations or from corporate sponsors (managed care organizations, or pharmaceutical companies, etc.). The choice of whether and how much to charge a participant may be determined by the institutional and departmental goals for presenting a course. For example, to enhance community or collegial relations, courses may be offered at no charge or nominal charge. These courses can be seen as a community service that enhances the reputation of your department and the relationship with outside agencies and professional colleagues.

Budgeting for courses that are designed to gain financial rewards for your department require considerable attention to cost projections and careful marketing. When costing-out a CME program for the first time, it is essential to attempt "what if" estimates of the number of participants and the price individuals might be willing to pay for a course. Although estimates are guesswork at best, this allows a financial calculation of your break-even point and can establish your threshold for loss. Courses presented on evenings or weekends may be more attractive to a clinician who is unwilling or unable to leave a busy practice. Comparing course fees against local and national standards is essential.

CME Program Marketing

To whom and *how* to publicize your program represent crucial decisions in the successful marketing of a CME program. This strategy must be guided by the findings of the needs assessment activities. If your target audience is small (e.g., on-site mental health clinicians), the word can be spread through departmental notices, posters in the hospital, e-mail, and announcements at meetings. As the scope of a CME program increases, marketing choices increase in cost and can often evoke some anxiety about misspending scarce resources.

For most CME programs, the two primary avenues of marketing are professional periodicals and direct mail. Periodicals in which to advertise must be chosen carefully to maximize exposure to a target audience. Most periodicals will share demographics and other details of their readership. The content and form of your advertisement is a big decision, and its importance as a marketing device should not be underestimated. Care must be taken not to spend significant sums procuring advertising space only to place a dull or visually unappealing announcement. Advertisements serve as a symbol and presage the quality of the course. Desktop computer design by graphic professionals is a fast and economical means of producing an attractive product and should be considered a minimum standard. The design of an advertisement in a periodical is limited to including the course title, location, date, and a brief course description. A tear-off coupon included allows readers to request your course flyer (with registration information).

Direct mail is perhaps the most effective means of marketing a CME presentation. As in the design of the advertisement, use a professional to create your course brochure or flyer. Most hospitals or medical schools have an on-site graphic artist available for this task. In addition to the cost of producing and mailing the flyer, the mailing list becomes one of the most critical facets necessary for a successful marketing campaign. If you have presented CME programs in the past, the list of past participants is your most valuable resource. Mailing lists are generally available from professional organizations, periodicals, and so on for a fee. "Mail houses" are a widely utilized direct marketing tool. These for-profit businesses maintain relationships with a vast array of organizations. After carefully selecting the groups to whom you would like to send a flyer, the mailing houses can arrange for the procurement of mailing labels (for a onetime use fee) and may also be able to stuff the flyers into envelopes, affix the labels, and handle bulk mailing. Mailing labels are often not sold directly to individuals or organizations. Additionally, most mail houses provide the service to "merge and purge" mailing label lists, to avoid duplicate mailings to individuals who may appear on more than one list.

Partial lists, limited to specific states or geographic regions, professional degree, and even the recipient's expressed "area of professional interest," are generally available. If the scope of your course is more limited, you can contact publications and professional organizations directly to inquire regarding their mailing list policies.

In large-sample experience, the rate of enrollment following a large mailing can be as low as 0.5%. Thus a typical, well-placed mailing of 10,000 flyers might yield only 50 participants for a highly priced course. On the other hand, a course offered for free with mailings to a carefully targeted audience might yield a 10% or greater course enrollment.

When considering the cost of promotional material, note that your sponsoring institution, department and faculty all benefit from the distribution of news of a course offering, independent of its success in attracting course enrollment. Offering special fee "group enrollment" or tuition-free registration to selected participants (residents, department members, selected community representatives) can also promote goodwill of significant benefit.

Designing a CME Program Brochure: The Basics

Like the invitation to any important event, the brochure sets the tone for your program. It must stimulate immediate interest if your intended guest is to accept your offer. Thus, a graphic designer can be a critical feature of effective brochure design. Assume you have only seconds to visually attract the attention of your clinician-target after the envelope is opened. Some brochures choose to describe program contents broadly, mentioning general course features without many specific details. Given the investment in time and money that the competitive CME market requires of its discriminating audience, little opportunity should be left for the chance criticism of a cautious brochure recipient. Some brochures feature extracurricular recreational activities and regional points of interest accessible to participants and their families. Highlighting such activities may attract one group of learners while it may discourage those with a more hearty academic appetite.

Essential elements of a course brochure include:

1. *Identification of sponsoring institution and your department*—prominently featured and highlighted.
2. *Course title*—develop a course title. The title must be a well-written, straightforward "headline," capturing the essential educational element of the conference at a glance. A title may be "catchy," but take care not to descend from the edges of clever to the nether region of "cute."
3. *Date of the conference*—include the day(s), date, and year.
4. *Name of the course directors*—consider including your departmental chief and/or institutional sponsor.
5. *Course location*— list by city and meeting facility name (brief).
6. *Description of course*—ACCME regulations require that the course description must include a clear statement of course objectives (e.g., "the objective of this course is to review exciting and new developments in the diagnosis, course, and treatment of psychiatric syndromes associ-

ated with reproductive function in women"). Additionally, a concise and easily readable course description will excite interest in your prospective audience member. It is helpful to design the brochure and course description with the understanding that the average physician may focus only seconds of attention on your mailing among the scores she or he receives every year.

7. *Course schedule*— detail a schedule for the course including the time and duration of each lecture, its title, and the name of the presenter.

8. *Faculty description*—list the name, professional degree, and academic and clinical appointments of each faculty member.

9. *CME accreditation*—elaborate accreditation for physician, psychologist, social work, and/or nurses organizations must be included in the brochure. Many participants are interested in CME credits and look to the brochure for confirmation of course accreditation.

10. *Registration information*—put in information relative to registration including course fees, method of payment, address to send registration, and necessary telephone numbers (with hours of availability).

11. *Refund policy*—clearly state the policy to avoid confusion.

12. *Course location*—describe the location of the course site including telephone number and/or reservation number if held at a hotel. Map "graphic" if appropriate.

13. *Accommodations*—specify accommodations available in the area when courses intend to attract an out-of-town audience (chamber of commerce/bed and breakfast, telephone numbers, etc.).

14. *Travel*—describe methods of travel to the course location.

15. *Tear-off registration form*—require the full name, daytime phone and fax number, mailing address, degree, and a statement regarding the requirements for a full payment to accompany application (if payment is required).

Facilities Management/Contracting

Whether conducting a large or small program in CME, another element required for the success of any program includes careful attention to "hospitality." It is prudent to determine course needs and to secure a reservation for an adequate facility prior to advertising your course. Whether within your own hospital, in a hotel, or in a conference center, it is essential to personally visit on-site to assess seating capacity, acoustics, audiovisual capability, break-out facilities (small seminar rooms and coffee break areas), accessibility to transportation and parking, handicap access, and so on (Table 27–1). Question the manager of the prospective facility regarding available services, technical staff, and catering capacity. Obtain past references regarding experiences with conferences, audiovisual equipment, and so on. If you plan to conduct your program in a conference facility or hotel, inquire about the schedule of other, concurrent events scheduled for the same time. Attempting to conduct a medical lecture is difficult when noise from the preparation of the Junior Prom competes for the attention of the course participants.

Planning at this level cannot be too detailed. After "walking through" your event with the facility manager, include each detail should be included in a written contract. In some metropolitan areas, hotel and convention contracts must sometimes be reserved 5 to 10 years in advance. Soliciting the assistance of your department's or hospital's business manager or counsel may be very useful, especially for those unfamiliar with the complexities of contracts and contracting. If contracting with a hotel and expecting out of town course attendees, it is wise to secure a block reservation for rooms, often available at a reduced fee, which can be an incentive to prospective course participants.

The cost of catering services can be a significant course budget item. Seriously consider including meals with courses. Depending on its location, course participants often prefer to "get away" during the lunch and/or evening breaks. Serving a continental breakfast and including a coffee break midmorning and liquid refreshment break midafternoon are standard and must be budgeted in the course costs. Careful food selection can reduce these costs. In the course lecture hall, providing water at all times is very much appreciated by course participants.

Running a CME Program

You know, we should really give a course on that!!! —Anonymous

Genius is 1% inspiration and 99% perspiration.—Thomas A. Edison

Delivering the right educational "product" to a "physician/consumer" eager for the opportunity to learn requires attention to the elements described in the last section. Determining whether to give a local and smaller course

Table 27–1. Facility site visit checklist

1. **Accessibility**
   - To public transportation
   - Parking
   - Handicap access
2. **Amenities**
   - Catering costs
     — coffee by the cup, by the pot, or by the audience size
     — catering "menu" with costs
     — availability of adequate catering staff during scheduled breaks
   - Availability of "break-out rooms" for small seminars
   - Availability of "conference suite" for course directors and staff
3. **Seating**
   - Capacity
   - Quality of chairs: padded vs. hard
   - Aisle placement for easy crowd egress and collection of questions
   - Layout and sight lines relative to speaker
   - "School room" (with tables) vs. theater style
4. **Podium**
   - Location
     — elevated in easy sight of audience
     — clear sight line for speaker to view to projection screen
   - Microphone (flexible gooseneck mount preferred)
   - Remote controller for slides
   - Laser or other light pointer
   - Timer clock in easy view for speaker
   - Reading lamp for speaker notes
   - Fresh, cool water available for speaker
5. **Acoustics**
   - Sound system
     — speaker placement
     — easy access to controls
     — technician on-site at all times
   - Adjoining spaces (hallways, service corridors, function rooms, street noise)
6. **Audio/Visual Capacity**
   - In-house staff and equipment vs. need to hire outside specialists
7. **Lighting**
   - Room lighting that can be dimmed for slide/video viewing
   - Controls convenient for AV technician
   - Spotlight that remains on speaker even with room lights dimmed

versus a national (and larger) course, to give an expensive versus an inexpensive course, to recruit outside faculty or use internal resources—all affect program planning significantly. Past experience in planning and executing CME programs should be a significant determining factor. "Trying out" an inexpensive, local course can help to gain valuable experience in course administration while helping test the waters for interest in a course topic. Such a trial run also allows a faculty to gain experience in public speaking, and for a faculty "audition" in a real-life environment.

The Course Syllabus

After you have determined the need for a course, completed the design of a course, invited a faculty member to present, and determined the location and marketing strategy for a course, the "nuts-and-bolts" decisions for the actual lecture or seminar presentation must be considered.

It is usually helpful to require faculty members should be required to prepare a handout or syllabus material to accompany each lecture, whether for a lecture seminar series or for a large multilecture course. The faculty must be strongly encouraged to prepare an outline that closely follows the sequence of their own lecture notes. This allows course participants to easily follow along with the lecture and to take notes. These outlines should be reviewed by the course director for quality standardization. If the lecturer plans to show 35-mm or overhead transparencies, course participants enjoy having copies of the slides to follow along with the lecturer. The inclusion in the syllabus handout of one, or at most two, relevant chapters or papers is often very much appreciated. Careful attention must be given to obtaining copyright release permission for these reproductions, for which the textbook or periodical company may charge between $25 and $400.

Visual Aids

It has often been said that the worst extemporaneous lecture is preferable to the best read lecture. It is difficult to engage learners by reading a lecture. By far the most common standard teaching tool in CME is the 35-mm transparency. Such transparencies, preferably produced by a desktop computer software (Microsoft Powerpoint©, Aldus Persuasion©, Harvard Graphic©, etc.), significantly enhance an audience's ability to follow along with the lecturer, and they allow the lecturer to speak in a lively and spontaneous fashion, promoting audience interaction. Simple slides containing as few words as possible, using "bullets" (outline formatted text) are easiest to read.

A standard rule of thumb suggests that a slide should be easily readable when held at arm's length.

Considerable progress has been made in the technology integrating graphic presentation elements into CME. Hardware and software tools are advancing our capacity for eye-catching motion and "live video" teleconference presentations. Such advanced tools offer promise, especially as they become less costly and more user-friendly. Faculty need sufficient "real-time" experience and hands-on practice with these new media well before a professional presentation.

For larger audiences in big spaces, a greater sense of "being with" a speaker can be achieved through the use of a large (4 to 8 feet) closed-circuit rear-projected video projection screen. As mentioned earlier, constant on-site technical support personnel attending all such equipment is important.

Faculty Interaction

Course participants enjoy interacting one-on-one with faculty members and often desire the opportunity to ask specific clinical questions. When inviting faculty members to speak at a course, it is reasonable to ask if they might plan to stay for 15 or 30 minutes after their lecture to answer questions as they arise.

Questions From the Audience

Course participants often are eager to ask questions as they arise in the lecture. Generally speaking, speakers should reserve the last 10 or 15 minutes of a 60-minute lecture to entertain questions. In a small seminar format with 50 to 75 attendees, questions might be asked spontaneously from the audience. In larger courses, some course directors prefer to place a microphone in the aisles and ask participants to line up at the microphone. This method can sometimes discourage less-inclined audience members from participating. Other course directors prefer collecting and screening questions on 3 × 5 cards. This allows the course director greater control of the content and quality of the presentation, screening out the esoteric while advancing the repeatedly asked questions.

Adhering to the Schedule

Faculty members, especially those less experienced with public speaking, frequently underestimate the amount of time their lecture requires. Therefore, encourage faculty members to practice their lecture several times before their presentation. A course director takes full responsibility for maintaining a prompt schedule, especially in multispeaker half-day or daylong CME programs. Course participants regularly express gratitude for keeping to the schedule and view promptness as a courtesy to both the audience and to faculty members who might otherwise be forced to start late and rush their own talk.

Course Coordinators

For larger, especially daylong or longer, courses, the continual presence of a knowledgeable, mature, and responsible coordinator with full knowledge of the course program, the meeting facilities, course faculty, and so on is a "must." Many courses receive low ratings based on the poor administration of unforeseen but inevitable glitches, such as the late or "no-show" lecturer, the errant fire alarm, the emergency call from a course participant's office, equipment failure, or an audience health problem. The larger the audience, the longer the course, and the greater the size of your faculty, the greater the likelihood of these unforeseen events. The steady, unflappable administrator is invaluable in these moments; when they are well handled, such events can win commendations and a loyal audience eager to return next time.

One seemingly minor but essential task for the course coordinator is the "reminder call" to each course faculty member in the days immediately prior to the course. Through the careful attention to this single detail many courses can be saved from the embarrassment of a no-show speaker.

If your course is being held in a larger convention facility or hotel, request the same communication device/walkie-talkie carried by the facility managers. This allows immediate contact with facility managers in the event of a problem. Post messages for course participants on a bulletin board.

Additional Learning Materials

For many educational programs, course participants appreciate the opportunity to view or purchase additional educational materials, such as books, videotapes, and so on. Procuring the services of a local book merchant who offers carefully selected relevant texts is viewed as an important addition to many course offerings.

Conclusion

For the practicing clinician, teacher, and researcher, CME is more than a requirement, it is a fact of life. Most professionals need very little encouragement and wish only for the opportunity to participate as learners. The ability to recognize the knowledge gap and to efficiently and effectively provide the educational service to the appropriate audience in a comfortable, well-organized setting can be a gratifying endeavor and a valuable service, benefiting your institution, your department, your faculty members, and, ultimately, the patients we all serve.

For Further Reading

Bennett NL, LeGrand BF: Developing Continuing Professional Education Programs. Urbana-Champaign, IL, University of Illinois Guide Series, 1990

Caffarella R: Experiential Learning: A New Approach (New Directions for Adult and Continuing Education, No 62). San Francisco, CA, Jossey-Bass, 1994

Caffarella R: Planning Programs for Adult Learners: A Practical Guide for Educators, Trainers, and Staff Developers. San Francisco, CA, Jossey-Bass, 1994

Davis BG: Tools for Teaching. San Francisco, CA, Jossey-Bass, 1993

Davis D, Fox R: The Physician as Learner: Linking Research to Practice. Chicago, IL, American Medical Association, 1994

Davis DA, Thomason MA, Oxman AD, et al: Changing physician performance. A systematic review of the effect of continuing medical education strategies. JAMA 274:700–705, 1995

Fox R, Mazmanian PR, Putnam W: Changing and Learning in the Lives of Physicians. New York, Praeger, 1989

Merriam S: Updating our knowledge of adult learning. Journal of Continuing Education in the Health Professions 16:136–143, 1996

Rosof AB, Campbell Felch W: Continuing Medical Education: A Primer, 2nd Edition. New York, Praeger, 1992

Stross J: The educationally influential physician. Journal of Continuing Education in the Health Professions 16:167–172, 1996

Psychiatric Administration

28

Development as a Psychiatric Administrator

Larry R. Faulkner, M.D.

Psychiatric administration has been the subject of regular discussion in the literature for at least the last 4 decades (Barton 1962). Although a thorough review of this work is beyond the scope of this chapter, three consistent themes do emerge that form the foundation for my discussion. First, there is widespread acknowledgment of the need for psychiatric administrative expertise and leadership in the management of mental health service delivery systems that are growing more and more complex (Barton 1973; Cozza and Hales 1992; Freedman 1972; Greenblatt 1972; Levinson and Klerman 1967; Reese 1972; Talbott 1987). Second, there are inadequate numbers of competent psychiatric administrators who are ready, willing, and able to meet this need (Barton 1973; Freedman 1972; Greenblatt 1972; Levinson and Klerman 1967; Reese 1972; Talbott 1987). Third, there are insufficient opportunities for promising young psychiatrists to obtain well-designed training experiences in administration (Barton 1973; Freedman 1972; Greenblatt 1972; Levinson and Klerman 1967; Reese 1972).

If these three themes are indeed accurate, then it seems logical to conclude that adequate numbers of competent psychiatric administrators to fulfill the growing need for them will only be achieved by careful attention to the process by which these individuals are produced. Since this is a handbook on psychiatric education and faculty development, I will approach the process of becoming an effective psychiatric administrator from

549

an educational perspective. I begin by outlining a framework for this educational approach and then describe the specific components of that framework in some detail. I conclude by using this educational framework and my own experience to outline several common mistakes that make a successful administrative career less likely.

My comments will be most relevant for young psychiatrists who are perhaps considering whether an administrative role is an appropriate career option for them. I believe the educational approach I describe can provide a model for understanding what a psychiatric administrator actually is and what one must be willing and able to do to become effective in that role. It is important to emphasize that this chapter is not a summary of an empirical study, but rather an expression of my own opinions. I will draw heavily on the work of others who have directly and indirectly influenced my career. I thank them for their help and guidance, and I apologize for any insights I now claim as my own that they might well have expressed years ago.

An Educational Framework for Becoming an Effective Psychiatric Administrator

Taking an educational approach to the process of becoming an effective psychiatric administrator requires the articulation of a framework with three separate components: a specific goal, a willing and capable trainee, and a sound curriculum. The goal is obviously to become an effective psychiatric administrator; the trainee is a psychiatrist with potential who decides to pursue the goal; and the curriculum is the means whereby the goal can be accomplished. Having a clear framework in which to approach the task of becoming an effective psychiatric administrator is not only helpful in identifying specific components that must be addressed, but, as I discuss later, it is also useful in understanding where problems might arise along the way.

For clarity of presentation, the three components of the educational framework I have described might be rephrased into specific questions. To set a goal of becoming an effective psychiatric administrator, one should be able to answer: What is a psychiatric administrator? To assess whether one has the potential to become an effective psychiatric administrator, the individual should be able to answer: What are the characteristics of effective administrators? To know whether one is pursuing a sound educational curriculum, the individual should be able to answer: How does a capable person become an effective administrator? In the next three sections of this chapter, I will consider each framework component and question in turn.

Setting a Specific Goal: What Is a Psychiatric Administrator?

A number of authors have attempted to clarify the definition of a psychiatric administrator. In the process, some have chosen to describe different levels of administration. For example, Levinson and Klerman (1967) make a distinction between "executive positions" and "administrative positions." They note: "Executive positions are ordinarily defined as those at the highest level of organizational authority, with responsibility for making and changing policy. Administrative positions are a step lower; the administrator has major responsibilities but his task is primarily to implement rather than to make policy. *The distinction is not an absolute one, however, and the terms are often used interchangeab*ly" (Levinson and Klerman, p. 54; emphasis added).

Dressler (1978) states: "Management positions can be clustered into three separate levels, defined by differences in authority and responsibility. These consist of top management (executive), middle management (supervisor), and lower management (clinician)" (p. 357). The executive "determines institutional policies and priorities and ultimately is responsible for all activities conducted by the organization" (pp. 357–358). The supervisor "develops procedures for implementing institutional policies and is responsible for the operation of a particular service element or elements" (p. 358). The clinician "delivers clinical services to patients and is responsible for rendering treatment" (p. 358). Dressler also points out that there is a *"tendency in mental health organizations to minimize the hierarchical distinction among management positions"* (p. 357; emphasis added).

Talbott (1987) discusses the differences between "management," "administration," and "leadership," stating: "The word *manager* implies involvement with some small area (say the production of widgets) and the term *administrator* implies involvement with a larger, complex organization . . ." (p. 61). He goes on to note that "management" is a "hands-on function," "administration" is an "executive function," and "leadership" is a "visionary role" (p. 65). Talbott acknowledges the overlapping components of the administrative role when he describes the process of running a mental health program: "I would argue that, at the very minimum, *we are managing.* If we are competent, we *are administrating*. But if we and our organizations are to survive and grow, *we must be leading*" (p. 65; emphasis added).

Cozza and Hales (1992) also make a distinction between "managers," "administrators," and "leaders." They draw upon the work of McConkey (1989) who writes: A "manager . . . is primarily concerned with efficiency, whether things are being done right," an "administrator . . . carries out policies formulated by someone else . . . ," and a "leader" is mainly concerned with "effectiveness and whether the right things are being done, the proper vision and directions have been established, and the right atmosphere has been established to encourage people to live up to their full potential" (p. 16). Cozza and Hales (1992) note that some functions of these roles "*may overlap*" (p. 34; emphasis added).

The opinions of the preceding authors, as well as others I have not cited, clearly establish the complexity inherent in the definition of a psychiatric administrator. The administrative role appears to have at least three overlapping aspects. I would suggest that an administrator must be able to perform *each* separate component as well as integrate them into a coherent whole that is greater than the sum of the parts.

Turning to the dictionary definition of an administrator provides additional support for this position. According to *Webster's* dictionary, an "administrator" is "one who administers"; "to administer" means "to manage"; "to manage" means "to direct"; "to direct" means "to guide"; and "to guide" means "to lead" (Neufeldt 1990). Reese (1972) captures the essence of this opinion well when he writes: An administrator "is usually servant to some, master to others, and peer to many . . . An administrator may be a charismatic leader, a stimulating catalyst, a slave driver, a popularity seeker, a latent paranoiac, or a plodding caretaker. *He may need a slight touch of each . . .*" (p. 1252; emphasis added).

In summary, to clarify the goal of our educational approach and to answer the question posed by that goal, I would suggest that a psychiatric administrator is a psychiatrist who manages, administers, *and* leads a mental health organization. It naturally follows that I believe that young psychiatrists who aspire to become effective administrators must be willing to endorse this goal and all that it entails. They must be willing to assume the roles of manager, administrator, *and* leader and to integrate those roles into a coherent administrative style. I also believe this is true no matter how simple or complex the mental health system that one aspires to lead. To be maximally effective, both individual clinical services as well as entire complex organizations require an administrator who is willing to manage, administer, *and* lead. Although it may be true that the scope of each of these activities is less in simpler units and systems, I believe the tasks are still present nonetheless.

Assessing Administrative Potential: What Are the Characteristics of Effective Administrators?

Once a young psychiatrist decides to become an administrator, how does the individual know whether he or she has the potential to become effective in that role? What are the requisite characteristics of success? This question has preoccupied many authors over the years. Suffice it to say that there is considerable opinion about this subject, but very little empirical evidence. Much of the debate has centered on the question of whether leaders are "born" or can be "made" (Cozza and Hales 1992). As is usually the case in any discussion with such divergent perspectives, the truth is probably somewhere in the middle.

Greenblatt (1972) states: The "character requirements of a good administrator" include "high energy and drive, physical endurance, high maturity, robust health, great intellectual ability, high capacity for concentration, the ability to appraise people without sentiment, the capacity to encourage and tolerate change, great resiliency, flexibility, creativity, steadfastness, determination, tough-mindedness, etc." (p. 379). Barton (1973) reports a similar list of some of the "personality traits . . . frequently attributed to executives": "physical endurance sufficient to meet the stresses of the job; abundant energy and drive to work problems through to a solution; ability to pick up cues quickly and deduce relationships from unrelated events; flexibility and the capacity to encourage and tolerate change; determination and tough-minded perseverance to fight to achieve an objective, unswerving from the goal as others advance distractions in substitute ideas or compromise goals; high capacity for concentration and low tolerance for ambiguity; ability to appraise people without sentiment" (p. 11).

While noting the validity of many of these characteristics of good administrators and executives, both Greenblatt and Barton also caution against making too much of them. For example, Greenblatt (1972) notes: "The characteristics are probably an idealized projection of what the writers would like to see in themselves," and "no totally virtuous executive exists: all have some limitations and drawbacks" (p. 380). Barton (1973) also writes:

"There is no convincing evidence that a stereotype of traits characterizes the successful administrator. Executives have no more traits in common than do other groups in society" (p. 11).

One logical approach to help clarify the characteristics of effective administrators would be to return for guidance to our definition of a psychiatric administrator. In doing so, we realize that effective administrators should have the personality and characteristics to enable them to "manage," "administer," *and* "lead." This requires an impressive array of innate abilities and learned skills, and it partly explains the difficulty in identifying adequate numbers of qualified administrators to meet the need for them. At the risk of making the same "idealized projections" that Greenblatt cautions against, I would suggest that an effective psychiatric administrator needs to possess many of the innate and/or learned characteristics listed in Table 28–1.

It should be obvious that most of these characteristics are inherently subjective. No two psychiatric administrators will possess all of them to an equivalent degree, and it may even be possible for an administrator to succeed while appearing to be somewhat lacking in one or more of them. It is my opinion, however, that serious deficiencies in these characteristics will ultimately result in major administrative problems. This is true because it is just these characteristics that enable psychiatric administrators to fulfill effectively their management, administrative, and leadership tasks. For example, Cozza and Hales (1992) mention many of these characteristics as being closely related to the skills they consider to be "essential to competent leadership," including "reaching for goals, establishing a trusting environ-

Table 28–1. Characteristics of an effective psychiatric administrator

Above-average intelligence	Good judgment
Energy	Integrity
Drive	Generosity
Endurance	Flexibility
Good health	Creativity
Organization	Resiliency
Determination	Empathy
Decisiveness	Humility
Self-confidence	Friendliness
Responsibility	Sense of humor

ment, using effective communication, making decisions constructively, developing subordinates through delegation, being aware of and managing group process, utilizing and resolving conflict, and using power productively" (p. 45).

It is probably easier to assess whether individuals have skills like those described by Cozza and Hales than it is to determine whether they possess those types of characteristics I list in Table 28–1. In essence, identifying the specific skills helps to operationalize the required characteristics of effective administrators. To that end, I would suggest that any young psychiatrist who contemplates becoming an administrator should be willing and able to develop the skills listed in Table 28–2. These skills are not offered as a unique or exhaustive documentation of each and every aspect of an administrative role. As noted previously, other authors have developed similar lists. There is obvious overlap among many of these skills. I am sure that an intense debate could occur concerning whether specific skills I have

Table 28–2. Skills required of an effective psychiatric administrator

Develop a strategic vision and plan
Manage within a budget
Approach tasks in an organized manner
Follow tasks through to completion
Pursue multiple tasks simultaneously
Use authority and power productively
Delegate authority and responsibility appropriately
Make timely decisions
Give others credit for organizational success
Consider the opinions of others
Manage conflict constructively
Recruit competent subordinates
Be generative in relationships with subordinates
Inform and support supervisors
Assess personal strengths and weaknesses realistically
Accept and give consultation, supervision, and continuing education
Accept constructive criticism
Communicate effectively in writing and speaking
Use varied administrative styles as necessary
Be a constructive role model
Participate in organizational social and ceremonial activities
Be sensitive to political processes

listed are indeed crucial to administrative effectiveness and also whether other skills I have not listed might be even more essential. It is also important to note that most of the skills I have simply listed here are complex issues that have been the subject of extensive study in their own right (e.g., strategic planning, the use of administrative power, administrative styles, etc.). Unfortunately, a thorough discussion of these skills is beyond the scope of this chapter. These apologies aside, I do believe that to be an effective administrator, young psychiatrists should have the characteristics and personality that enable them to be willing and able to perform most of these activities.

It is pertinent at this point to emphasize that clinical and research skills are not included on the preceding lists. While many of the underlying characteristics and skills noted are almost certainly essential to an individual becoming a successful clinician or researcher, clinical or research talents in themselves probably bear little direct relationship to administrative abilities. For example, Greenblatt (1972) writes: "The qualities that make a good manager are, to a large extent, separate and distinct from those which make a good doctor . . ." (p. 380). This is not to imply that clinical skills might not be useful in an administrative position. In their study of senior psychiatric administrators, Greenblatt and Rose (1977) found that although most believed "psychiatric training was not essential for psychiatric administration," it was perceived to be important for its "direct applicability to the tasks of administration and the use the administrator made of it on a personal and interpersonal level" (p. 627). My own view is that clinical or research talents and accomplishments can contribute to administrative success in two major ways. First, they can lead to increased self-confidence that gives a young psychiatrist the courage to assume an administrative position and to make difficult decisions. Second, they can provide a depth of understanding about specific issues that will have to be addressed in the process of administering any mental health organization.

Most authors agree that an individual's inherent capabilities can and should be improved by training. In other words, "born" administrators can indeed be "made better." For example, Greenblatt (1972) comments: "Training for administrative psychiatry rests on the assumption that although the basic mental and personality equipment necessary for the complex task of administration is probably inborn, there are precepts, experiences, concepts, and philosophies that may improve a person's skill and effectiveness in his role" (p. 380). Barton (1973) proposes that "the administrator should be trained in administration . . ." and points out that there is "an identifiable body of knowledge in administration that can be transmitted" (p. 18). Cozza and Hales (1992) write: "If leadership is development of character, then it is brought about by a complex process in which personal characteristics, experiences, and situational variables all play a part" (p. 43). The actual process of strengthening an administrator's innate talents falls under the purview of an educational curriculum in administration and will be addressed in the next section.

Pursuing a Sound Educational Curriculum: How Does a Capable Person Become an Effective Administrator?

Young psychiatrists who are at the point of contemplating the answer to the question guiding this section should have a least made a preliminary decision that they might want to become an administrator and a self-assessment that they do indeed possess those characteristics that would enable them to perform most of the skills required to be effective. What should be the next step along the path toward an administrative career? Returning to our educational framework can provide the answers to this question and considerable help with career development.

Given a willing and capable trainee, the essence of any educational curriculum consists of at least three elements: knowledge, skill, and attitude objectives; a combination of didactics, experiences, and supervision sufficient to attain the objectives; and a means of evaluation to assess progress toward achieving the objectives and to suggest other educational activities that might be needed. Adopting this approach now helps us to focus on those issues that must be addressed as part of a sound educational curriculum in psychiatric administration. Although it is to be expected that this type of educational methodology would be part of any modern program of formal training, I also believe this same process should guide the efforts of those who prefer to take the more common "learning by doing" approach to a career in psychiatric administration.

Educational Objectives in Administration
Educational objectives are the specific knowledge, skills, and attitudes a young psychiatrist should possess who has completed a period of formal

or informal training in administration. They form the basis for the design of the training components of the curriculum.

Knowledge objectives are the content areas of the information that administrators are expected to know. The Committee on Administrative Psychiatry of the American Psychiatric Association recommends that psychiatric administrators be knowledgeable about the following: broad categories of administrative principles and theory, psychiatric care administration, fiscal management, and law and ethics (American Psychiatric Association Committee on Administrative Psychiatry 1996). Greenblatt (1972) suggests that the "subject matter to be mastered" should include the "dynamics of institutional change, sociology of groups, systems of organization, program and budget planning, communications and public relations, labor relations, law and psychiatry, community organization, political science, public health and epidemiology, management science, and, finally, fund-raising" (p. 381).

Skill objectives are those tasks administrators are expected to perform. They would include most of the ones outlined in Table 28–2. Like the list provided by Cozza and Hales (1992) mentioned earlier, other authors have proposed similar skills they believe administrators must be able to perform. Among other abilities, Barton (1973) suggests investigation, planning, forecasting, organizing, coordination, control, inspections, and evaluation. Foley (1973) proposes the skills of planning, organizing, staffing, directing, coordinating, reporting, and budgeting.

Attitude objectives are the outlook and perspectives that form the basis for the manner in which administrators do their job. They would certainly include most of those characteristics listed in Table 28–1 that a young psychiatrist would bring to a training experience. A major goal of the curriculum should be to ensure that those innate talents are strengthened and any deficiencies identified and corrected to the extent possible. Making major changes in attitudes in the context of a voluntary training experience is easier said than done. It might well be impossible. At the least, it could require a level of supervision and control that might outstrip the resources available. This is the main reason I believe young psychiatrists who do not possess most of the characteristics in Table 28–1 would be well advised to pursue a career other than administration.

It is important to recognize that an educational curriculum is not static. Although the broad subcategories within the knowledge, skill, and attitude objectives will most likely remain similar to those I have listed, specific components of those categories will change over the years with advances in administrative theory and practice and the evolution of mental health systems. For example, knowledge, skill, and attitudes concerning such topics as total quality management and managed care would have been much less relevant in 1970 than they are today. Other issues unknown to us now will surely be dominant themes in 2010. Part of the challenge in the design of any sound educational curriculum is to constantly modify its objectives to ensure that they provide a solid foundation for relevant didactics, experiences, and supervision.

A Training Program in Administration

The training program consists of the combination of didactics, experiences, and supervision sufficient to enable a young psychiatrist to accomplish the desired educational objectives in administration. In a formal training program sponsored by an educational institution (e.g., MPA, MPH), these components will be required, and the trainee may appear to have little input into their design. In an informal learning-by-doing approach, however, "trainees" will be responsible for arranging their own program of education. Actually, I believe this will be true to a significant degree even for those individuals who complete formal training. Taking personal responsibility for aspects of one's formal education is also crucial to its success and establishes a pattern for effective continuing education and lifelong learning. Greenblatt and Rose (1977) discovered that most of the senior psychiatric administrators they studied "learned about administration by doing rather than studying. Some learned from other colleagues in administration or from knowledgeable individuals in related fields" (p. 629). On the other hand, Barton (1973) states: "It is too costly to use a trial-and-error approach. A time for learning and a mode for continuing education in administration are essential if we are to have efficient management . . ." (p. 23).

Barton may well be correct about the inefficiencies inherent in the "trial-and-error" approach to education, but it seems likely that this will continue to be the most common route to administrative expertise for the foreseeable future. While my remaining comments about didactics, experiences, and supervision in administration may be most pertinent to this informal method, I also believe they are relevant to the content and process of formal programs as well.

Didactics in administration should be designed to cover the topics included in the knowledge objectives of the curriculum. A number of excellent textbooks are available (Barton and Barton 1983; Feldman 1979; Talbott and Kaplan 1983; Talbott et al. 1992), and the Committee on Administrative Psychiatry has prepared a list of recommended references included in Appendix 28–A at the end of this chapter (American Psychiatric Association Committee on Administrative Psychiatry 1996). Several universities and other organizations also provide regular continuing education seminars on topics pertinent to administration. For example, the Department of Psychiatry at Tulane University School of Medicine sponsors an annual program titled "New Dimensions in Mental Health Administration" covering such issues as budgeting, managed care, marketing, organizational theory, human resources administration, regulatory and review mechanisms, ethics, and psychiatry and the law (Tulane University Center for Continuing Education 1996). Through a combination of self-directed study and enrollment in seminars, it is quite possible for any motivated young psychiatrist to obtain the required didactic information to meet the specific knowledge objectives.

Administrative experiences enable a young psychiatrist to become proficient in the skills necessary to be an effective administrator. An individual cannot learn to become an administrator by merely reading a book or going to seminars. Just as a physician must have graduated exposure to patient care in order to become an effective clinician, so must a young psychiatrist plan for progressive administrative experiences to learn the required skills. For as Barton (1973) notes: The best administrators usually are those who "move up the power structure to higher posts of leadership . . ." (p. 10).

From the beginning of residency training, many opportunities are available to begin the process of learning about psychiatric administration (Arnold et al. 1991). Each rotation in a psychiatric residency takes place in the context of a clinical service that must be administered. This is also true for the entire educational program itself. These rotations and educational programs can be used to begin to learn some of the important administrative skills listed in Table 28–2. Unfortunately, many of these opportunities are missed because residents and faculty are often preoccupied with learning and teaching clinical psychiatry. Specific administrative objectives are frequently not given high priority. The opportunities are usually available, however, for willing young psychiatrists who have identified specific skills they want to learn and who make their interest known to faculty who can assist them. As is true in most educational experiences, the amount learned about administration early in a residency usually depends on the initiative of the trainee. Later in the residency, more formal administrative electives and/or chief residency experiences are usually available to those who have demonstrated special interest and ability (Faulkner 1979). These more-structured administrative experiences provide excellent opportunities to select an area of activity in which to begin to study the process of administration in more detail. Many academic departments of psychiatry have created specific roles for senior residents in various clinical service, educational, or research programs. It is in those experiences that the resident should have time to focus on developing the specific administrative skills outlined in Table 28–2.

After residency, most entry-level positions in academic, public, and private mental health organizations carry at least some administrative responsibilities (Dressler 1978). As one moves up the career ladder, opportunities to learn more-sophisticated skills are readily available since they become more integral parts of the positions themselves (Reese 1972). Figure 28–1 presents examples of possible administrative career pathways in academic psychiatry. Similar pathways could be developed for administrative careers in the public sector, managed care, and so on. Although Figure 28–1 is obviously simplified, somewhat idealized, and certainly not relevant to every academic department of psychiatry, it does convey the important messages that there are multiple possible administrative career pathways and that an administrative career should probably proceed through stages of increasing responsibility and authority. This multilevel concept of administrative career pathways is consistent with Dressler's three-tiered "top management (executive), middle management (supervisor), and lower management (clinician)" scheme described earlier (Dressler 1978). For example, in Figure 28–1, the clinical psychiatrist "delivers clinical services to patients," the clinical service chief and director of clinical services are "responsible for the operation of a particular service element or elements," and the vice chair and chair generally "determine institutional policies and priorities."

It should be pointed out that although the entry into an academic administrative career does not have to be through a chief residency, it frequently is. The specific number of different levels in a career pathway will vary somewhat from academic department to department and usually is a reflection of the size and complexity of the academic system (e.g., some departments have assistant clinical service chiefs or assistant training directors; some departments have no vice-chair). Rather than the specific focus implied in Figure 28–1, the first level after the chief residency is frequently a generic junior faculty position with a mixture of clinical, teaching, and

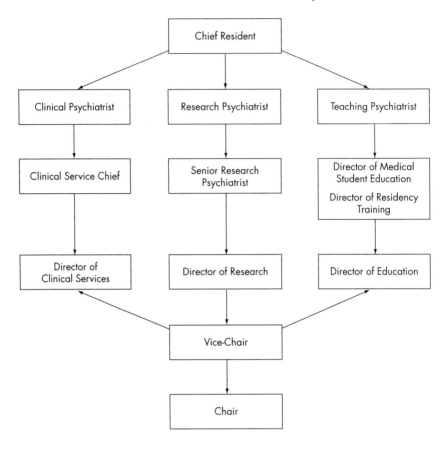

Figure 28–1. Possible administrative career pathways in administrative psychiatry.

research responsibilities. The specific nature of this position will usually be determined by the required duties for which a salary is paid. It is at this point in the career pathway that young psychiatrists usually determine which major aspect of their career to emphasize. Changes in career focus are fairly common at this level, as young psychiatrists learn more about the different aspects of their first academic position. It is also true, however, that career pathways are frequently determined by the opportunities that present themselves. A measure of good luck and timing can not only determine one's ultimate career pathway, but can also have an impact on the speed of ascent up the ladder. Of course, it is also true that one can take specific steps to prepare for the opportunities that will inevitably arise during a career. Taking part in an ongoing administrative educational program will enable the young psychiatrist to capitalize on those opportunities. After one moves up the career ladder, it becomes more difficult to change pathways since competitiveness for higher positions usually depends on positive experiences at lower levels. It should be emphasized, however, that academic administrators at all levels usually maintain some balance of clinical, research, and teaching activities, even though they may focus predominantly on one area. To become a chair of an academic department of psychiatry, for example, generally requires significant accomplishments in clinical work, research, teaching, and administration.

Supervision by competent psychiatric administrators must also be an integral part of any legitimate curriculum (Faulkner 1979). It is essential in order to master the required skills and to ensure the development of appropriate attitudes concerning administrative activities. In informal training experiences, young psychiatrists must seek out those competent administrators who can help to mentor trainees' development. Greenblatt and Rose (1977) found that many of the senior administrators they studied "acknowledged the influence of teachers or other prominent professionals on their career interests" (p. 627). Barton (1973) writes: "Classroom experiences cannot substitute for an ongoing, supervised experience with a preceptor who is an expert in administration" (p. 18). Most academic, public, and private mental health organizations have skilled administrators willing to assist an eager young psychiatrist who approaches them for help. As with the acquisition of skills, the limiting factor here will usually be the desire and initiative of the potential trainee.

It is relevant to note that "supervision" comes in many direct and indirect forms. Astute trainees will keep their eyes open for opportunities to learn from not only the successes of those around them but also from their mistakes. As one of the senior administrators in the Greenblatt and Rose (1977) study noted: "I learned from him what I didn't want to be" (p. 627).

Evaluation of Progress Toward Administrative Objectives

Evaluation mechanisms are those processes of assessing the progress a young psychiatrist has made toward meeting specific educational objectives in administration. In formal training programs, evaluation takes the form of regular feedback from faculty and perhaps even grades. Although this type of structure might not be possible in an informal approach to training in administration, some type of evaluation is still crucial to its success. Young psychiatrists should solicit constructive feedback about their performance from supervisors and mentors as well as suggestions for additional training experiences that might be helpful to their development. In doing so, the original educational objectives should always be used as the basis for a structured evaluation. This process should never be allowed to evolve into an informal "chat" between colleagues. Perhaps even more important than feedback from supervisors, all young psychiatrists involved in either formal or informal training should periodically do a self-assessment of their progress toward meeting the objectives of their educational program. This approach toward self-appraisal also establishes a constructive pattern that can become the basis for continuing education. Since educational objectives do change over time, regular self-assessment and efforts to upgrade one's talents must become a significant component of any effective administrator's career.

Avoiding Crucial Administrative Mistakes

At this point, it should be clear that I believe the keys to becoming an effective administrator lie in setting a specific goal to be one, having the required characteristics to assume the role, and completing a well-designed curriculum in administration. It also follows that I believe the inability to fulfill any of the three components of this educational framework will most likely result in serious administrative problems. There are many aspects of the three components in the educational framework I describe, and no psychiatrist can be expected to totally master each and every issue. Every psychiatric administrator will have strengths and weaknesses. I do believe, however, the ability to address the major issues I have outlined will increase the likelihood that a young psychiatrist will become an effective administrator.

Oftentimes it appears to be easier to learn from mistakes that are made than from successes. These are frequently painful lessons, because they usually are learned after the damage has been done. Perhaps it is the sharpness of the pain that "drives home" the message. After nearly 20 years in administrative roles at various levels in different organizations, I have either observed or experienced firsthand a number of these "educational opportunities," several of them on multiple occasions. I have come to believe that the 10 administrative mistakes listed in Table 28–3 and discussed next

Table 28–3. Ten administrative mistakes

1. Misunderstanding responsibility and authority
2. Unwillingness to fulfill a crucial component of an administrative position
3. Inadequate preparation
4. Failure to find a mentor
5. Inability to learn from mistakes
6. Failure to be a positive role model
7. Cultural insensitivity
8. Confusion about the source of power
9. Failure to protect a supervisor
10. Agreeing to work for an incompetent supervisor

should be avoided if one is to become an effective administrator. Limitations of space and my own knowledge prevent a complete listing or thorough discussion of all possible administrative errors. In fact, each specific aspect of the entire framework I discuss earlier could be seen as the basis for a potential administrative mistake. The 10 mistakes I will describe are merely those that seem very pertinent to me. They are not presented in any order of priority.

1. *Misunderstanding responsibility or authority.* To do any job, one must know what that job is and what resources may be brought to bear on its completion. Accepting an administrative position without clarifying these issues in advance can result in unexpected responsibilities or inadequate resources to be effective. Either situation might easily lead to an evaluation of performance that is less than optimal.
2. *Unwillingness to fulfill a crucial component of an administrative position.* As stated earlier, an effective psychiatric administrator must be willing and able to manage, administer, *and* lead an organization. The inability to recognize or accept the fact that all administrative positions require one to manage routine tasks, administer complex and often politically charged interactions between systems, and lead an organization's visionary and ceremonial activities may result in significant problems. Administrator's are unlikely to be successful unless they accept each facet of their position as a challenge worthy of their attention.
3. *Inadequate preparation.* The training program I outlined earlier may also serve as a measure of readiness to accept a specific administrative

role. Unfortunately, this assessment is frequently the responsibility of the potential candidate for a position, because those with the authority to appoint are not always the best judges of administrative capability. They often err by assuming medical training, clinical skills, or research success to be indicators of potential and readiness for an administrative position. Comparing the knowledge, skills, and attitudes that will actually be required with an individual's progress in a program of administrative education may help prevent the acceptance of a position for which one is obviously not prepared. The responsibility for bad administrative outcomes are rarely shouldered by those making inappropriate appointments. The blame is usually placed on the appointee, underscoring the importance of some caution in the acceptance of administrative positions. An early appointment to an important administrative role may certainly be ego-inflating, but a bad outcome due to inadequate preparation can have just the opposite effect. It may also permanently derail a promising administrative career.

4. *Failure to find a mentor.* A difficult path is always easier to follow with an experienced guide who encourages a traveler to challenge himself or herself but not to exceed the traveler's ability or readiness for the journey. Although the traveler might well arrive at the destination by himself or herself, it will most certainly take longer and there will undoubtedly be many detours along the way. So it is with an administrative career. A mentor might not be absolutely necessary, but one may certainly prevent many trial-and-error experiences. In a current era that emphasizes managerial efficiency, young administrators will not be afforded the luxury of making many significant mistakes before their supervisor comes to believe that they must be replaced.

5. *Inability to learn from mistakes.* Even in systems that are forgiving of error, most will clearly expect an administrator to identify whatever knowledge, skills, or attitudes were responsible for the problem and to demonstrate that they have been corrected. Repetitive, serious mistakes of the same type will almost always doom one's position. The educational framework I have described can help form the basis to identify where specific problems lie and to develop a program of continuing education. A mentor may be especially helpful to this process, since it must be implemented as quickly as possible.

6. *Failure to be a positive role model.* Like it or not, all administrators will find themselves in the "spotlight." This is especially true as they move

up the chain of command. Administrators must take care to ensure that they conducts themselves in a positive, professional manner that engenders respect from those around them. Dress and demeanor should always be appropriate and above reproach. Peers and supervisors will frequently base their judgment of an administrator's abilities on these factors. Younger members of an organization observe their leader's conduct closely, and many will try to model their own behavior after what they see. It is always easier to heed the advice and follow the lead of someone you respect. This is especially true during times of crises when difficult decisions must be made. No administrator will succeed for long without the respect of others.

7. *Cultural insensitivity.* Every organization has its own unique culture that forms the basis for acceptable behavior. These standards affect almost all facets of an organization, including interpersonal relationships between staff, administrative style, and so on. While administrators may recognize correctly that aspects of the prevailing cultural norms clearly need to change, they would be well advised to proceed cautiously. Too vigorous an assault on the traditions of an organization are threatening and may provoke tremendous resistance at all levels. Even worse, an administrator's supervisor might well be left with an impression that the administrator is not only ineffective but also insensitive.

8. *Confusion about the source of power.* Young administrators are frequently concerned with the location of their position on the organizational chart and how close it is to the top, where they believe real authority and power surely must reside. Although the support of those at higher levels in an organization is essential for administrative effectiveness, that support will not exist for long without the endorsement of peers and staff at lower levels. Disgruntled employees are only too willing to make their views known to top administrators, politicians, and even the press. A steady stream of complaints will cut short any administrative career. Care must be taken by administrators to communicate with and involve employees at all levels in the administrators' vision and plans for the organization.

9. *Failure to protect a supervisor.* The relationship between administrators and supervisors is obviously crucial to job security. It is important to keep one's supervisor satisfied and confident in one's ability and loyalty. This is accomplished by not only fulfilling administrative duties well, but also by protecting the supervisor from embarrassment and surprise.

Keeping a supervisor well informed and following the administrative chain of command are important components of this protection. Few things will undermine a relationship with a supervisor faster than for that supervisor to be "blind-sided" by major problems or to discover that someone has gone "above his head" without his approval. An administrative crisis will be the likely result, and its resolution might well be a "terminal event" for the young psychiatric administrator.

10. *Agreeing to work for an incompetent supervisor.* At first glance, this problem might well appear to have little to do with the administrator. In many situations, this is indeed the case, since the abilities of one's supervisor may not always be apparent initially. Quite often, however, good evidence is readily available for those willing to examine it. The educational framework I have described to guide the administrator's career may also be used to help assess the training and experience of a prospective supervisor. In addition, close questioning of others who have been supervised by this individual will frequently reveal strengths and weaknesses. Administrators who accept a position without this type of information should realize that they are embarking upon a risky venture. They should also be prepared to accept whatever consequences come their way.

Conclusion

In summary, the growing need for competent psychiatric administrators for our mental health system will most likely continue to be an issue for the foreseeable future. In fact, expanding administrative roles may well provide additional career opportunities for talented young psychiatrists. To be successful, a young psychiatrist should be willing and able to manage, administer, *and* lead an organization. I believe this requires specific innate and/or learned characteristics, the pursuit of a carefully designed educational curriculum in administration, and the ability to avoid crucial administrative mistakes along the way. While always a challenge, an administrative career can certainly be stimulating and rewarding for those with the right attitude and the willingness to devote themselves to the task.

References

American Psychiatric Association Committee on Administrative Psychiatry: Information Bulletin for Applicants. Washington, DC, American Psychiatric Association, 1996

Arnold WN, Rodenhauser P, Greenblatt M: Residency education in administrative psychiatry. Academic Psychiatry 15:188–194, 1991

Barton WE: Administration in Psychiatry. Springfield, IL, Charles C Thomas, 1962

Barton WE: Training in administration for psychiatrists. Psychiatric Annals 3:8–26, 1973

Barton WE, Barton GM: Mental Health Administration: Principles and Practice. New York, Human Sciences Press, 1983

Cozza SJ, Hales RE: Leadership, in Textbook of Administrative Psychiatry. Edited by Talbott JA, Hales RE, Keill SL. Washington, DC, American Psychiatric Press, 1992, pp 31–58

Dressler DM: Becoming an administrator: the vicissitudes of middle management in mental health organizations. Am J Psychiatry 125:357–360, 1978

Faulkner LR: Negotiating a chief residency: an educational opportunity in administration. Psychiatric Opinion 16:36–38, 1979

Feldman S (ed): The Administration of Mental Health Services, 2nd Edition. Springfield, IL, Charles C Thomas, 1979

Foley AR: Models for training in administration. Psychiatric Annals 3:54–81, 1973

Freedman AM: The medical administrator's life: here today and here tomorrow. Arch Gen Psychiatry 27:418–422, 1972

Greenblatt M: Administrative psychiatry. Am J Psychiatry 128:1249–1256, 1972

Greenblatt M, Rose SO: Illustrious psychiatric administrators. Am J Psychiatry 134:626–630, 1977

Levinson DJ, Klerman GL: The clinician-executive. Psychiatry 30:3–15, 1967

McConkey DD: Are you an administrator, a manager, or a leader? Business Horizons (September-October):15–21, 1989

Neufeldt V (ed): Webster's New World Dictionary. New York, Warner Books, 1990

Reese WG: An essay on administration. Am J Psychiatry 128:1249–1256, 1972

Talbott JA: Management, administration, leadership: what's in a name? Psychiatr Q 58:229–242, 1987

Talbott JA, Kaplan SR (eds): Psychiatric Administration: A Comprehensive Text for the Clinician Executive. New York, Grune & Stratton, 1983

Talbott JA, Hales RE, Keill SL: Textbook of Administrative Psychiatry. Washington, DC, American Psychiatric Association Press, 1992

Tulane University Center for Continuing Education: New Dimensions in Mental Health Administration, 15th Edition. New Orleans, LA, Tulane University, 1996

Selected References from the Suggested Resources of the American Psychiatric Association Committee on Administrative Psychiatry 1994

American Psychiatric Association: The Principles of Medical Ethics, With Annotations Especially Applicable to Psychiatry. Washington, DC, American Psychiatric Press, 1989

Appelbaum PS, Gutheil TG: Clinical Handbook of Psychiatry and the Law, 2nd Edition. Baltimore, MD, Williams & Williams, 1991

Barton WE, Barton GM: Mental Health Administration: Principles and Practice, Vols I, II. New York, Human Science Press, 1982

Berman HJ, Weeks LE, Kukla SF: The Financial Management of Hospitals, 8th Edition. Ann Arbor, MI, Health Administration Press, 1994

Cleverly WO: Essentials of Health Care Finance, 3rd Edition. Gaithersburg, MD, Aspen, 1992

Deming W: Out of the Crisis. Cambridge, MA, MIT Center for Advanced Engineering Study, 1986

Elpers JR: Community Psychiatry, in Comprehensive Textbook of Psychiatry, 6th Edition. Edited by Kaplan HI, Freeman AM, Sadock BJ. Baltimore, MD, Williams & Wilkins, 1995

Ewalt P: From Clinician to Manager in Middle Management and Mental Health: New Directions for Mental Health Services, Vol 8. San Francisco, CA, Jossey-Bass, 1980

Feldman S: The Administration of Mental Health Services. Springfield, IL, Charles C Thomas, 1980

Feldman S: The middle management muddle. Administration in Mental Health 8:3–11, 1980

Feldman JL, Fitzpatrick RJ: Managed Mental Health Care. Washington, DC, American Psychiatric Press, 1993

Greenblatt M: The Anatomy of Psychiatric Administration. New York, Plenum, 1992

Kennedy JA: Fundamentals of Psychiatric Treatment Planning. Washington, DC, American Psychiatric Press, 1992

Mattson MR: Manual of Psychiatric Quality Assurance. Washington, DC, American Psychiatric Press, 1992

Talbott JA, Hales RE, and Keill SL (eds): Textbook of Administrative Psychiatry. Washington, DC, American Psychiatric Press, 1992

Walton M: Deming Management at Work. New York, G. P. Putnam's Sons, 1990

29

Health Care Systems and Academic Psychiatry

Donald R. Ross, M.D., and Steven S. Sharfstein, M.D.

Managed health care is in the business of procuring cost-effective medical care for patients who are covered subscribers. It exists primarily to manage costs. Purchasers of health care insurance (employers, taxpayers) need to control and want to reduce the amount they are paying for health care. Managed care companies do that for them. The quality of care is a factor, but not the central factor. The key descriptor for the type of care purchased is "value"—quality divided by cost.

Academic psychiatry exists for three reasons: (1) to teach psychiatry to the next generation of physicians; (2) to advance knowledge about mental illness and treatment through scientific research;. and (3) to provide state-of-the-art care to difficult to treat patients. The key operative term for the type of care provided within academic psychiatry is "excellence"—cost is a secondary factor, kept in the background. Since academic medical centers are often located in large metropolitan areas, their patients usually include a high proportion of indigent patients who have no health insurance.

Managed health care and academic psychiatry speak different languages, move and breathe in different milieus. Managed care emphasizes the *business* aspects of medicine. Many of the principles of business are brought boldly into the arena of patient care—customer relations, productivity, critical pathways, continuous quality improvement. Academic psychiatry emphasizes the *clinical* aspects of medicine. It holds sacred the relationship of doctor and patient. The principles held forth include the healing relationship, confidentiality, scientific advancement, thoroughness, ethics, and the deep knowledge and traditions of medicine. This difference in emphasis, of intellectual and emotional milieus, breeds an easy antipathy and disrespect of one group for the other.

However, medicine has always been a business as well as a clinical calling. The force with which managed care has penetrated the clinical practice of psychiatry has made it clear that there are certain areas, previously ignored, that require the attention of academic psychiatry. These include broadening the focus to the care of populations of patients instead of only the care of individual patients. It includes evaluating expensive treatments with well-designed outcome studies. It includes making choices among treatments of uncertain effectiveness and different costs. It includes greater attention to patients' concerns about comfort, convenience, and availability of their doctors. Working from the other direction, managed care needs to recognize the key importance of the special bond patients form with their doctors. Otherwise, it will damage the product it is managing. Patients need caring doctors even within cost-effective systems of care. In addition, the advancement of knowledge through scientific research is essential for the development of more cost-effective treatments in the future. Finally, making sure future psychiatrists are well trained is in the long-term best interests of managed care's customers—both patients and their employers.

All this presents a series of challenges to both managed care organizations and departments of academic psychiatry that need urgent attention. Many of these challenges directly impinge upon the training of psychiatric residents. These challenges include the following:

1. What should be the *goals* of training residents in psychiatry?
2. How should academic psychiatry departments and residency training be *funded*?
3. As treatment approaches change rapidly in response to managed care, what *clinical rotations* should form the core of a training experience in psychiatry?
4. How should the *workload* of patient care within an academic setting be distributed among faculty and residents, and how should each be held *accountable*?
5. What should be the *didactic* content of residency education?
6. What should be the role of *research*?
7. Are there *new opportunities* for departments of psychiatry within academic medical centers?

Goals of Psychiatric Education

The goals of psychiatric education must be more clearly defined. Residents need to be trained for the jobs they will be filling, and, to a large extent, that means jobs in managed systems of care. But they also need to be trained in the scientific and humanistic fundamentals of psychiatry. Certainly there is a significant overlap between these two goals. But there are also areas of conflict and questions of where to place educational emphasis. One current area of conflict is whether to train residents in the intricacies of long-term psychodynamic psychotherapy. Such training is a basic building block of knowledge about mental illness and its treatment, at least as this has been defined up to this point. It teaches par excellence skills in empathy and the role of narrative in understanding patients. It is also clear that a psychiatrist working in a managed care environment will have little or no opportunity to practice this modality of treatment. Psychodynamic psychotherapy training takes considerable time and resources. What should its role be in residency education?

One can't answer this question without a broader discussion of the relative roles of job training versus a deeper education in psychiatric fundamentals. Unfortunately, this "discussion" easily can devolve into a polemic about the need to stay true to core values. But while academic psychiatrists wax eloquent on that soapbox, managed care companies will continue to change the mode of psychiatric practice out from under them. This is a real problem. Instead, a meaningful dialogue must begin between academic psychiatry and managed care. Without this, the question of goals for the education of future psychiatrists will remain conflicted and unclear. Until this is resolved, fewer and fewer high-quality medical students will choose to enter psychiatry.

Funding

The driving force pushing academic psychiatry into dialogue with managed health care is funding. More and more, managed care companies have control over the flow of patients and the patient care dollars that go with them. Having developed in a different era, academic medical centers have become complex systems of semiautonomous departments, many of which act as independent fiefdoms of power and ego. Distribution of funding within the medical center is often Byzantine and decentralized. Managed care, with its business orientation, demands a more streamlined partner. The managed care company is interested in negotiating with a representative for the academic medical center that can speak for all of its parts. If the academic medical center is to successfully compete for managed care contracts, it will need a streamlined internal administrative structure.

Funding for residency education is especially endangered. This funding has traditionally come from higher patient rates, direct and indirect payments from Medicare, support for resident stipends from the Veterans Administration, and state funding. Higher patient rates are increasingly untenable because managed care contracts will go to a lower bidder. Federal and state support for residency education are threatened as taxpayers demand a reduction in the tax burden from their legislators. A medical education superfund supported by an "all payers tax" has been proposed and was part of the ill-fated Clinton health plan. The argument for such a fund is that medical education and research are critical resources that support and advance the entire health care industry. However, no such superfund has been approved or financed.

In today's market, it is critical to stay abreast of the current formulae for funding residency positions. It is essential to ascertain when resident services can be reimbursed directly and when they cannot. Even when they cannot be reimbursed, when does resident service reduce the time and effort of the attending physician and thus represent a cost offset? Inpatient rotations and on-call duty are good examples of where residents can pay for their keep with "sweat equity" even when their services cannot be directly reimbursed. However, outpatient services are more problematic. Recently, Medicare has stated unambiguously that services billed under Part B in the name of the attending doctor require the continual attendance of the attending doctor. If a resident is seeing a Medicare patient one-on-one in psychotherapy or medication evaluation, either the institution cannot bill for that service or the attending needs to be right there. In such a situation, the service the resident provides becomes redundant or free. New models of funding and new models of delivery of outpatient care are needed.

The upshot of these changes in funding is that it is no longer so clear that residents are a financial asset to a psychiatry department. It is critical for academic psychiatry departments to "right-size" their residency programs. In most cases this means downsizing the program. Sharing residents with additional participating institutions and outright merger of residency training programs are strategies that also address this issue. There will be more pressure to use residents in service areas where they can earn their keep. This will require vigilance on the part of the training program to balance the need for reimbursable services with the need for quality educational opportunities. All training sites must have clear and convincing educational value.

The problem of funding faculty time for resident supervision and teaching must also be addressed. It is critical that adequate time be set aside for the training director and other key teachers to provide effective core teaching and leadership for the program. Other than these few designated and partially funded positions, many academic departments simply expect and require their faculty to teach gratis. However, as faculty are required to provide more direct clinical services, they will feel more and more pressure to cut corners somewhere. The potential for resentment over their uncompensated teaching time will grow if there is not some mechanism to ensure fairness in teaching assignments or direct compensation for teaching and supervision. The use of part-time clinical faculty to provide more of the teaching and supervision is feasible. As a rule, they volunteer their services, usually for 2 hours per week. However, they too are under significant pressure to see greater numbers of patients at lower fees. Many academic departments are experiencing difficulty in recruiting volunteer faculty for teaching. Furthermore, it is important to strike a balance between full-time faculty and part-time clinical faculty to assure the residents the benefit of top teachers and role models within the department. Residents need mentors with whom they can work side by side on the inpatient units and in the outpatient clinics.

Clinical Rotations

It is clear that under the cost-conscious eye of managed care, the clinical use of the inpatient unit is rapidly shifting to a short-term crisis stabilization site. Inpatient treatment is reserved for actively suicidal, homicidal, or disorganized psychotic patients. If the patient does not need 24-hour nursing care, he or she will not be authorized for continued inpatient treatment. The interventions emphasized on the inpatient service are crisis assessment and management, rapid start of medications to reduce symptoms, and mobilization of family, community, and outpatient resources. More active ongoing treatment (psychotherapy, medication adjustments, a more comprehensive evaluation) take place in alternative and less expensive settings. In addition, the extremely short lengths of stay (4–10 days) do not allow residents to see patients move from states of severe depression to euthymia or from psychotic states to compensated states. For these reasons, the use of clinical work on inpatient units as the backbone of training in PGY-1 and PGY-2 years of residency needs to be questioned.

Clinical teaching rotations need to be structured so that the resident can follow the patient from acute hospitalization to day hospital, and from there to the halfway house and outpatient status. These "continuum of care" rotations can provide residents with the continuity of care experience necessary for optimal learning about the treatment of patients with severe mental illnesses. This continuum of care model, with the same doctor following the patient throughout the continuum of sites and services, also provides better care for patients. In more traditional models of care, these patients have been vulnerable to fragmented care when they are passed from provider to provider.

However, there are certain problems with the continuum of care model for residency training. For example, the essential requirements for accreditation set forth by the Residency Review Committee (RRC) for Psychiatry insist that residents spend a minimum of 9 months full-time or its equivalent working on an inpatient unit. That requirement was established when the learning objectives for an inpatient rotation were quite different from what can be learned there today. This speaks to the need for flexibility within the RRC as academic psychiatry adjusts to the major changes in the practice of clinical psychiatry due to managed care. On the other hand, the RRC still needs to serve a stabilizing function so that the training of residents does not chase after every "innovation" in the delivery of psychiatric care.

Creativity in the use of outpatient settings for training residents is also vitally important. Here again, managed care has had a major impact on the mode of practice of psychiatry. The emphasis in on short-term, problem-focused interventions. Longer-term psychotherapy with the goal of more fundamental character change is "not a covered benefit" in most managed care systems. Also, most psychotherapy is provided by less-trained and less-expensive mental health professionals. Emphasis is placed on group therapy and psychoeducational sessions when these approaches are possible. Psychiatrist time is reserved for diagnostic evaluation, consultation, and medication management. Even here, the pressure is on efficiency and cost savings. In capitated systems of reimbursement, phone calls may be better than visits, home visits better than risking a hospitalization. These are some of the issues that need to be considered in designing and utilizing the kaleidoscopic array of outpatient services for teaching.

The issue of psychotherapy training comes front and center in outpatient settings. First, residents clearly need to become proficient in at least one or two forms of short-term, problem-focused psychotherapies. Interpersonal therapy and cognitive-behavioral therapy are perhaps the best studied and most easily taught. Brief psychodynamic psychotherapy is appealing, but it may be more complex and has been proven effective for a relatively narrow spectrum of patients. Solution-focused psychotherapy has become popular, but it lacks the theoretical and interpersonal depth felt necessary by most psychiatric educators. Whatever short-term approach is taught, supervisors who are expert in that school of therapy are necessary. Residents should have the opportunity to treat a number of patients using these brief, focused models.

Second, longer-term psychodynamic psychotherapy offers a more comprehensive foundation for understanding a wider variety of illnesses, personality styles, group behavior, and even organizational dysfunction. Despite the fact that residents may have very limited opportunity to practice this type of psychotherapy after training, the experience of learning it during residency gives them a much stronger foundation to master the subtleties of clinical practice that will confront them for a professional lifetime. As one important example of this, sophisticated supportive psychotherapy is built on the principles and experience of long-term psychodynamic psychotherapy. Provisions must be made for residents to have a significant experience in long-term psychodynamic psychotherapy, even though it will likely be a cost drain on the program.

Third, it is essential that the future psychiatrist develop the ability to skillfully serve as a medication manager. This is usually done in collaboration with a social worker who is providing psychotherapy for the patient. This experience should not be left to its own devices but should be supervised and given the same serious attention that the psychotherapy training is given during residency.

Clinical rotations in outpatient psychiatry may benefit from the use of novel settings. Using a community mental health center as the core of an outpatient psychiatry experience often works well. Community mental health centers (CMHCs) can offer a variety of outpatient roles for the psychiatrist-in-training and often can provide state funding for the resident's stipend. However, the changing "marketplace" is putting CHMCs under increasing pressure to accept managed care plans including managed Medicaid. This setting may soon face the same economic problems for trainees as other training sites. Placing residents in the offices of primary care physicians, HMOs, EAPs, and even prisons or jails may be useful. Under managed care, primary care doctors are becoming the major gate-keepers to psychiatric care. Future psychiatrists need to develop an easy rapport with primary care doctors if they are to succeed in future managed care settings. Some time spent working directly within primary care prac-tices could help psychiatric residents develop a greater sensitivity to the needs of primary care doctors and their patients and a better sense of how to be most helpful.

Faculty supervision of residents within outpatient settings is more problematic than on the inpatient services. The traditional model has the resident treating the patient behind a closed door, with the resident later reporting to the supervisor what happened from his or her perspective. More direct supervision using one-way vision rooms, videotapes, or the supervisor in attendance may be necessary, especially early in training. Every patient should be presented to a supervisor upon admission and the treatment plan reviewed. There should be a mechanism for regular review of each case under the care of a resident. Managed care companies frequently don't allow residents to treat outpatients. Those that do demand greater accountability from attending supervisors. Capitated contracts allow greater flexibility for integrating residents into the role of primary doctor. Some programs have gone to the model of a "firm" or group practice model of faculty and res-idents treating a panel of patients across the continuum of treatment set-tings from inpatient to outpatient. Additional innovative models need to be piloted and presented at forums such as the annual meeting of the American Association of Directors of Psychiatric Residency Training (AADPRT).

Finally, a PGY-4 rotation within a formal managed care setting can be very valuable. The resident works as an apprentice to a managed care psy-chiatrist. Such an experience should include some experience as a utilization reviewer (under supervision) in addition to providing primary patient care within the structure of the managed care provider. This is a powerful sen-sitizing experience that helps the future psychiatrist engage in more pro-ductive exchanges with managed care reviewers after graduation.

Accountability and Workload

With the restructuring of clinical rotations for residents, other problems arise. The first is the problem of accountability of residents; this includes the necessity to "credential" residents to provide progressively more independent services. Managed care companies have focused considerable energy on accountability. This includes defining the qualifications of the providers who are allowed to treat patients. This is both a quality assurance measure and a way to control costs. Residents enter their training with little in the way of specific knowledge or skill to treat psychiatric patients. They need careful supervision and specific didactic instruction that build on their developing competencies. Managed care companies usually deny residents access to patients, citing their lack of necessary credentials. Of course, this does not take into account that it is the "resident plus supervisor" who provides the care. But is this really the case? How closely attached to the resident is the supervisor? Does the supervisor supervise each patient encounter and each major treatment decision, or does the resident simply present a summary of the most pressing treatment problems for an hour a week? Is the level of supervision different for a PGY-1 resident compared with a PGY-2 resident and different again for a more-advanced resident? This is a critical area where residency programs need to develop guidelines and specific expectations. This could be done productively in collaboration and consultation with managed care.

Such an internal "credentialing" of residents requires that educational expectations and skill acquisition be formally articulated and assessed at each step of advancement. This, in turn, requires that careful attention be paid to the nature of each clinical rotation. The rotation must be designed so that residents will learn what they need to learn to move to the next level.

Direct faculty involvement, supervision, and teaching should be heavily concentrated in key areas such as intake assessment, triage of acute problems, emergency room visits, inpatient admissions, and initial treatment planning. Special focus must be given to suicidal and other high-risk patients. Residents can be given more room to operate independently as they demonstrate expertise in these key areas. Ongoing treatment should be assessed using other principles made familiar by managed care. For example, are treatment goals clearly delineated? Has the patient been an active partner in developing these goals? How is the treatment progressing toward the achievement of these goals? For difficult and long-term cases, has the treatment been periodically reevaluated? These principles of progressively credentialing residents and tailoring supervision to the needs of the resident and patient are sound educational principles that are fully in accordance with a managed care approach.

Another area that should become a routine aspect of residency education is regular feedback regarding productivity. How many "units of service" are residents expected to provide and how does this compare to what
they are actually providing? When residents are clear about what is expected of them, it is much easier for them to organize their time to meet
those expectations. This also allows the academic psychiatry department
to take a rational approach to financial budgeting and the design of systems
of care using residents.

Regular feedback about patient satisfaction is also very useful to residents. Again, managed care has led the way in reminding physicians that
the patient is also a "customer." If the patient isn't happy with something
about the doctor or the treatment, then that something is worth paying
attention to. Courtesy, timeliness of appointments, and availability by phone
outside regular working hours are areas that academic psychiatry has
tended to overlook but patients have found very important. Feedback from
other customers such as managed care reviewers, primary care doctors, and
other referring therapists is also very useful to residents in their education.
These have been neglected areas in many training programs until recently.

Under managed care rules, faculty members may need to provide more
direct clinical care to patients. In fact, in situations where funding for residency education is uncertain or the availability of high-quality resident
applicants is in doubt, it is prudent to design certain key services (such as
inpatient units) so that they are "resident proof." In other words, if residents
are not available, the faculty can provide the services without undue disruption to the department. To make this cost-effective, the service can make
intelligent use of physician assistants, nurse clinicians, and social workers
for various tasks. Residents become a "value-added" dimension to the service rather than the backbone of the direct work done. Paradoxically, this
can attract better resident applicants to the program. It improves resident
morale by making it clear that residents are valued by the health system
for something more than the amount of service they can provide.

When faculty are expected to provide more direct clinical service, their
role as teachers and supervisors need to be protected. It is a mistake to hold
faculty to certain productivity standards for direct patient services and not
give proportional credit for time spent teaching and supervising residents
or medical students. One solution to this is the establishment of a "relative
value unit" system where all services are given specific productivity value.
Teaching and supervision are included and are assigned and monitored with

the same care as direct patient services. This protects teaching time, reaffirms the academic identity of the faculty member, and assures the resident and student adequate supervision.

Didactics

The didactic curriculum taught to psychiatric residents needs to be modified in specific ways to effectively respond to managed care. Residents still need a strong basic knowledge in descriptive psychiatry, neuroscience, psychopharmacology, psychopathology, and psychodynamics. In addition, new course work needs to be offered in the economics of health care, business principles in health care delivery, and the ethics of population-based psychiatric care. Emphasis on crisis intervention, brief focused therapies, psychoeducation, and the assessment of risk should enhance more traditional areas of instruction. In an effort to ensure quality instruction and provide it in a cost-effective manner, there is serious discussion about a standardized didactic core curriculum that would be offered in every U.S. residency program in the PGY-1 and PGY-1 years. This could be delivered via videotape or interactive CD-ROM and augmented with faculty-led discussion groups.

In addition, specific didactic material and model curricula have been or will soon be developed in association with key clinical rotations. These include the diagnosis and treatment of chemical dependency, treatment of the chronically psychotic patient, and strategies of managing patients with treatment resistant depression. Increasingly, core competencies in both knowledge base and clinical skills will become standardized.

Research

As managed care comes to dominate the clinical practice of psychiatry, research takes on added significance and a different slant. Grant monies for psychiatric research have always been a significant revenue source for academic psychiatry departments. This source of revenue is managed care independent. Consequently, it serves as an important economic buffer, protecting the department from the full economic impact of managed care related changes. However, getting patients for research protocols is more difficult within managed care systems. Usually managed care requires the treating psychiatrist to follow strict guidelines that stress cost effectiveness.

Washout periods, double-blind drug trials, and other essentials of research design are not within these guidelines.

However, there are research opportunities, especially in the arena of clinical outcome studies. These should interest managed care. Treatment outcome studies are very important from both business and clinical perspectives. They are especially needed when new models of care are promulgated that promise to be cost-effective. Both managed care and academic psychiatry need to study the effectiveness of psychotherapies that are brief and focused. Both need to study the outcome of early intervention approaches that aim to prevent relapse or rehospitalization. Also, it would be well worth studying the clinical outcome and cost-effectiveness of using residents as primary therapists, especially for complex patients who need both psychotherapy and medication management.

New Opportunities

If this new era of managed care is a crisis for academic psychiatry, it also offers new and exciting opportunities. Just as one example, the interface of psychiatry and primary care offers a number of possibilities. This new era could create a niche for some psychiatrists to become primary care doctors for the chronically mentally ill. Pilot training programs should be funded that focus on the medical and psychiatric skills needed to treat chronic patients. Medical rotations could be integrated throughout all 4 years of the residency. Also, there is an increased need for psychiatrists to effectively teach residents in family medicine, pediatrics, and gynecology. These primary care doctors will need to recognize common psychiatric disorders and know how to treat and when to refer. The care of patients who are heavy users of medical and surgical care may benefit from innovative strategies that utilize the unique talents of psychiatrists.

In conclusion, major changes are upon us. They are powered by a new cost consciousness that currently is made operational by managed care. New financial incentives with an emphasis on less costly treatment settings, efficient care, and fewer highly trained specialists present a formidable challenge to American psychiatry. Whatever form this will take eventually, there will be no going back. Psychiatrists should lead and not follow these market-driven changes. Academic psychiatry must change in order to train the psychiatrists for the future who will lead and participate in these new health care systems. This chapter has tried to outline some of the changes to residency training and faculty development that will be necessary to facilitate that forward movement, avoiding the worst pitfalls and making the most of the opportunities that lie ahead.

For Further Reading

Inglehart JK: Rapid changes for academic medical centers (part 1). N Engl J Med 331:1391–1395, 1994

Inglehart JK: Rapid changes for academic medical centers (part 2). N Engl J Med 332:407–411, 1995

Lazarus A: An annotated bibliography in managed care for psychiatric residents and faculty. Academic Psychiatry 19:65–73, 1995

Meyer RE, Sotsky SM: Managed care and the role and training of psychiatrists. Health Affairs 14:65–77, 1995

Schreter RK, Sharfstein SS, Schreter CA (eds): Managing care, not dollars: the continuum of mental health services. Washington, DC, American Psychiatric Press, 1997.

30

Academic Psychiatry and the Public Sector

**Alberto B. Santos, M.D., John J. Spollen, M.D.,
George W. Arana, M.D., and James C. Ballenger, M.D.**

Schizophrenia and other chronic psychotic disorders are severely debilitating for patients as well as for their caregivers. Persons suffering from schizophrenia occupy 25% of all hospital beds in the United States. Their yearly economic cost is around $20 billion for direct treatment and $45 billion in indirect expenses.

Despite this reality, the internationally known author E. F. Torrey (1983) noted, "There are very few doctors in the U.S. who either know anything about, or have any interest in schizophrenia" (pp. 99–100). This opinion is unfortunately widely shared by advocacy groups and may be an accurate historical reflection of the level of interest of U.S. general psychiatrists in these and other publicly financed patients.

Close collaborations between psychiatry training programs and public mental health service agencies in the United States have been the exception rather than the rule. For many years, there has been serious concern regarding the poor quality of psychiatric care in state hospitals and their failure to recruit well-trained psychiatrists. Advocacy groups have argued strongly for an increased level of collaboration between academia and public mental health systems. Despite these concerns and public outcry, linkages between university and state programs have been highly inconsistent, contributing to large variations across the nation in standards of practice for these populations.

More recently, however, as streams of financial support for academic departments of psychiatry have become further constricted, the financial incentives associated with collaborations with public sector agencies has become more appealing to academic programs. In this chapter, we (1) provide a brief history of the relationship between universities and the public sector; (2) overview past collaborative activities highlighting differences in linkage arrangements; and (3) note national initiatives that provide career-enhancing opportunities for residents and faculty.

History

State, County, and City Programs

State hospitals opened rapidly across the United States in the mid- to late 1800s with little university involvement. They remained isolated from their state's academic institutions and rarely attracted highly qualified graduates of psychiatric training programs. In university townships with nearby state facilities there was little interest in developing public-academic collaborative activities expressed by either party. The major exceptions were townships with an abundance of psychiatrists (i.e., Menninger Clinic, Boston State Hospital, Harvard and the Massachusetts Mental Health Center, Columbia and the New York State Psychiatric Institute, UCSF and the Langley Porter Institute, UCLA and the Neuropsychiatric Institute). Minor exceptions involved an occasional educational or research agreement. State hospitals generally got by with a few of the best-trained psychiatrists, while academic departments (driven by the popularity of psychoanalysis) had little interest in state hospital patient populations.

The utilization of antipsychotic medications facilitated the passage of legislation that resulted in a national movement away from centralized institutional care and towards localized services, allowing patients to be deinstitutionalized. Federally funded mental health centers which were set up in part to rehabilitate deinstitutionalized patients provided little of the services necessary to support community integration. The mental health centers overemphasized mental health at the expense of those suffering from serious and chronic mental illnesses and were widely criticized for operating therapy clinics for appointment-compliant patients and discriminating against individuals with chronic psychoses. As a result, large numbers of discharged patients did not receive adequate follow-up care (even appointments) and stopped their medications. Few had proper medication regimens prescribed upon discharge and half of those that remained on pharmacotherapy relapsed within the first postdischarge year (Hogarty 1984; Hogarty and Anderson 1986; Torrey 1983). To worsen matters, acute care services were not developed locally in parallel to the deinstitutionalization effort, and discharged patients who required rehospitalization were routinely returned to centralized facilities, creating the "revolving door" phenomenon.

Gradually, academic departments of psychiatry began to respond to this situation, in part as a result of the public outrage organized by the National Alliance for the Mentally Ill and critics such as Dr. Fuller Torrey. Facilitated by a series of national incentives (described later in this chapter), academic departments of psychiatry began to explore collaborative activities with public sector agencies and reported their findings in the professional literature.

The resulting wave of public-academic collaborations was predominantly oriented toward inpatient care (Talbott and Robinowitz 1986) and unfortunately contributed to the disproportionate amount of resources available to inpatients compared with outpatients. The predominance of hospital-based service, research, and training programs has restrained our field's movement toward more cost-effective service systems.

As public mental health service systems began transitioning resources from institutional to community-based settings, and as private health agencies began to shift their support from hospital to outpatient and home health care, public-academic collaborations likewise began to shift in focus from hospital to community-based settings. The shift was eventually reflected in training programs. By the 1990s more than half of the U.S. residency programs had training affiliations with their state's mental health authorities' hospitals and/or community mental health centers. Contracts were awarded to universities for specialized community-based services such as emergency or acute inpatient care, and supervised assignments were made for residents to treat public sector outpatients. In some university townships with local state hospitals, a large department might provide all psychiatric services for the hospital such that residents viewed the state hospital as an integral part of their training.

Federal Programs

The Veterans Administration (VA) serves as a quasi-capitated system of care for veterans of the Armed Services through 175 facilities nationwide. The VA is the largest psychiatric service system in the United States, using around 16% of the VA budget for the care of individuals with mental illness and substance abuse through a network of both acute and chronic care facilities.

The affiliation of VA with medical schools began shortly after World War II, as a nationwide mechanism to provide high-quality care for the servicemen returning from the war. VA senior medical staff members are selected in collaboration with the appropriate department chairperson and a "Dean's Committee," a joint body responsible for overseeing the affiliations whose membership includes the VA hospital director, major academic department chairs, and VA service chiefs of services. The presence and expansion of education and research programs are now explicit goals of the VA.

The partnership of VA and academe is mutually beneficial in that training programs benefit from additional educational resources, whereas the VA has the benefit of currency of practice standards and enhanced recruitment of clinicians to VA facilities.

One-tenth of the VA funded house staff positions are earmarked for psychiatry residents. In academic 1996–1997 the VA funded 836 (15%) of all U.S. psychiatry house staff positions. Nearly two-thirds of psychiatry residency training programs have some form of affiliation with the VA.

As the VA enters the health reform environment, it will be mold modern health care system that are capitated, prevention and community oriented, cost-sensitive, and consumer-friendly. With its specific population of war trauma patients, older geriatric populations, and chronically psychotic and dually diagnosed patients, it will serve as an important training ground for future psychiatrists.

A Patchwork of State/University Initiatives

The nature of linkage arrangements continues to vary widely across the United States (Douglas et al. 1994). Most prevalent are strictly educational agreements involving undergraduate, graduate, and continuing education programs; there are clinical services arrangements in which university faculty and trainees provide direct patient care for a specified public sector service; there are large integrative relationships in which the majority of the medical staff at a CMHC or hospital are also on faculty at the university and/or the administration of both components overlap considerably; and there are various unique administrative, consultative, and/or research agreements.

Examples of initiatives developed specifically to provide specialized education for psychiatric residents in the community-based practice of public psychiatry are the state-university linkages in Oregon, Wisconsin, and South Carolina. In Oregon, since 1973, representatives of the state senate, the state mental health agency, the medical school, the department of psychiatry, and facility administrators have worked together through a board that plans, fund-raises, develops, and monitors programs to ensure that psychiatrists trained in Oregon are able to meet the evolving needs of public sector patients (Cutler et al. 1993). Consistent with the evolution of public mental health theory and practice, the orientation of the curriculum has shifted from primary prevention/mental health consultation and crisis intervention to tertiary prevention and the care of the most seriously disabled populations. This increased emphasis on education about the delivery of services to persons with serious long-term mental illnesses is also evident in the programs in Madison, Wisconsin, and Charleston, South Carolina (Factor et al. 1988; Santos et al. 1994). These programs feature experiences that highlight advantages to field-based outreach and teamwork with nonmedical mental health professionals. Topics in the Madison program's didactic series (see Table 30–1) illustrate the growing emphasis on social and economic issues.

The collaborations in Charleston, South Carolina, initially limited resident involvement. Public sector and university administrators/providers would first develop a given service to fill a specific gap in the system. Once the usual administrative obstacles were overcome, it was relatively easy to overlap and integrate training and research components. This approach resulted in an exponential increase in the number of graduates taking public sector jobs, and facilitated the acquisition and implementation of several National Institute of Mental Health (NIMH)–funded services research projects.

Another example of a successful recruitment-oriented strategic affiliation is that between the Maryland Mental Hygiene Administration and the University of Maryland's department of psychiatry. In 1976 these agencies joined forces to recruit university graduates into state service. The strate-

Table 30–1. Topics included in the didactic series at the University of Wisconsin's community psychiatry program

- The role of the psychiatrist in community health.
- The treatment of persons with long-term mental illness in the community, including the principles of psychosocial rehabilitation.
- Economic considerations in mental health treatment, including different funding systems and their consequences.
- The assessment of disability, and criteria for entitlements.
- Sociological and policy considerations in mental health treatment, including the sociology of organizations.
- Long-term mental illness as a lifestyle.
- Psychotherapy with persons with serious long-term mental illness (including a psychoeducational approach to family work).
- Issues of social control, including whose agent is the psychiatrist; confidentiality; and involuntary and coercive treatment, including interpersonal and ethical aspects.
- Dangerousness and its prediction.
- Criminal behavior among persons with long-term mental illness.
- Transcultural psychiatry.
- Alcohol and drug abuse along with other long-term mental illness.

gies used included abolishing autonomous state hospital residency training, placing the state's research center under university control, and sending faculty and trainees to community mental health centers and state hospital facilities. More than 200 graduates (85% U.S. medical graduates) have accepted state service positions, including more than 30 former chief residents since the implementation of this program, a marked increase (Weintraub et al. 1991).

Another well-known integrative agreement is that between the University of Virginia and the Western State Hospital in Virginia (Yank et al. 1991a). Between 1979 and 1985 their union progressed from two faculty members providing direct patient care at the state hospital to the majority of the state hospital's medical staff holding full faculty appointments. Beginning in 1985 the psychiatry department chair became the state hospital facility director, and there was creation of the Western State Hospital division in the academic department. The union provided funds for increased faculty recruitment, assignment of all residents to Western State rotations, and establishment of a research unit in the state hospital (under direction of the University Director of Research) and led to JCAHO accreditation of the state hospital for the first time. In 1990 a visiting scholar position was established in the State Department of Mental Health to strengthen the link between the department and the academic community (Yank et al. 1991b). These initiatives brought the program in 1991 the first Exemplary Collaboration Award from the State-University Collaboration Project.

Virginia's visiting scholar component (Yank et al. 1991b) has been described as a "linchpin model" and has also been used in Oregon and South Carolina (Bray and Bevilacqua 1993; Godard and Hargrove 1991). The notion is to establish a leadership position in which support for state-university collaborative activities is provided by a person who, by working simultaneously in both governmental and academic settings, creates linkages between state facilities and their administration and university departments as well as between community mental health agencies and these departments. Ideally this would be someone who could command respect from both areas, navigate the political and professional waters with a deft rudder, and foster collaborative relationships between previously distant camps.

Finally, collaborations sometimes take the form of continuing education programs that target previously trained mental health providers to facilitate collaboration between higher education and state mental health agencies. The Mental Health Program of the Western Interstate Commission for Higher Education (WICHE) has striven since the early 1980s to strengthen linkages between college and university mental health programs and mental health agencies in western states (Davis 1991). As one of its many activities, for example, they cosponsored with participating states a series of conferences for academic faculty and public mental health providers. The impetus for these conferences was derived from the belief that most academic faculty had little knowledge of or interest in treating public sector patients. These conferences provoked interest in collaboration between the heretofore isolated groups and provided an arena to find common ground and discuss possible obstacles to collaboration.

Collaborations sometimes evolve in response to needs and opportunities (e.g., grant announcements). These opportunities can be addressed through specific activity contracts and agreements. Negotiating individual contractual agreements may provide greater flexibility for making changes and/or modifications to specific programs as needed. This stepwise approach to linkages protects all parties in that each new collaborative agreement represents a relatively small change in the system, which is less threatening than an all-sweeping contract involving major financial commitments. Further, the university is better able to assess its abilities to participate effectively in new projects on a case-by-case basis. Finally, this approach avoids assumptions of shared overall clinical responsibility for the catchment area. With such a stepwise approach, the university can agree to a series of activities that it can fulfill, not an open-ended series of problems and responsibilities related to the community, an undertaking the university cannot and should not enter into.

Conflict is likely to result from differing priorities and practice preferences (e.g., established state priority to care for patients with serious mental illness and a university educational mission involving a broader-based population, or practice pattern biases toward field-based versus traditional office/facility-based loci of care). Such conflicts can often be managed through the use of contracts tailored to the needs of each agency for each specific collaborative opportunity.

University departments sometimes contribute through "in-kind" services including part-time faculty, resident workforce, expertise, and political influence. The "hard money" for many projects can be identified through use of funds from empty M.D. public sector slots, for services, or from anticipated savings to existing programs (e.g., reducing state hospital admissions).

Table 30–2 highlights specific examples of state/university collaborative activities and illustrates the highly complementary relationship of public-academic activities and their potential capacity to improve access to and quality of services, to increase the number of well-trained professionals in the public sector, and to generate extramural financial support.

National Initiatives

A number of national initiatives have paralleled state initiatives to bridge the gap between academic and public sector psychiatry.

The American Psychiatric Association (APA)
APA's State-University Interdisciplinary Collaboration Project
The APA's State-University Interdisciplinary Collaboration Project was established in 1989 to improve the care of the mentally ill in the public system by initiating and enhancing collaborative relationships between each state's mental health programs and the departments of psychiatry in that state's universities (Talbott et al. 1991). Although collaborative relationships between many state mental health programs and university departments of

Table 30–2. Examples of state mental health agency collaborations with academic departments of psychiatry

States	Universities	Sites	Principal focus
California	UC/San Diego	Gifford Mental Health Clinic	Resident and psychology interns training, clinical research
	UCLA	Cararillo State Hospital	Clinical research, consultation, training psychology interns
	San Jose State U	Family-founded housing agency	Training nursing and O.T. students
Colorado	U Colorado	Area public mental health agencies	Resident training (stipend incentive)
Florida	U Miami	State Hospital	Services to sex offenders; training child residents
Georgia	Mercer U	Central Georgia CMHC	Training, consultation, evaluation
Louisiana	Tulane U	Rural outreach	Training residents
Kansas	U Kansas	Statewide service system	Training nursing and social work students
Kentucky	U Kentucky	Eastern St Hospital; Bluegrass CMHC	Resident training, consultation
Maryland	U Maryland	State Hospitals, state CMHCs	Resident training, clinical and services research
Massachusetts	U Mass	State Hospitals and CMHCs	Staff recruitment, services, resident training
Mississippi	U Mississippi	State Hospital	Resident training (stipend incentive)
New Hampshire	Dartmouth U	State Hospital	Services, resident training, services research
New Mexico	U New Mexico	State Hospital; Indian Health Services	Training residents; public education
New York	Columbia U	Urban and rural outpatient clinics	Sub-specialty training in public psychiatry
	NYU	State Hospitals	Resident training
	Einstein-Montefiore	Bronx Children's Psychiatric Center	Research and clinical training
	Mount Sinai	Pilgrim Psychiatric Center	Faculty provides CME for State Hospital staff

(*continued*)

Table 30–2. Continued

States	Universities	Sites	Principal Focus
North Carolina	UNC-Chapel Hill	Dorthea Dix State Hospital	Training residents; clinical research
	Duke U	The John Umstead State Hospital	Training residents, clinical research
	East Carolina U	State Hospital, Goldsboro	Training residents (educational fund incentive)
Ohio	U Cincinnati; Xavier U	Several selected sites in area	Training residents, nurses, psychologists, social workers
	Wright State	Dayton CMHC	Training residents, nurses, psychologists, others
Oregon	Oregon Health Sciences U	State Hospital , community settings	Training residents, public mental health services research
Pennsylvania	Pennsylvania State U	Central Penn Psych Institute	Consultation, services, resident training
South Carolina	SC's 14 training programs	Statewide service system	Consortium coordinates missions with state
	MUSC	Charleston area CMHC	Training residents; services research
Virginia	U Virginia	Western State Hospital	Services, resident training, clinical research
	Medical College of Virginia	Central State Hospital	Staff recruitment, training, research
Washington	U Washington	Community Psychiatry Division	Public mental health services research, resident training

psychiatry had existed previously, there was a need for these programs to be expanded and strengthened, and for new programs to be started to improve services, training, and research.

The Project holds regional workshops and no-cost consultations for state departments of mental health and universities interested in developing joint interdisciplinary mental health projects.

The regional workshops explore ways in which collaborative efforts can be designed to meet individual state needs, to suggest initiatives for change, and to form collaborative information and support networks. The consultations provide technical assistance to organizers of an interdisciplinary state/university collaborative effort that involves consumers and families and is designed to establish or expand innovative activities in state priority areas. A consultation consists of up to two 2- to 3-day, on-site visits conducted by a team from the Project's multidisciplinary panel of experts. Telephone and written communication is ongoing between and after visits. To apply for this program the state commissioner of mental health, the chair or dean of university psychiatry, social work, psychology, and nursing programs, along with the director of a consumer and family alliance group must submit a jointly signed letter that describes:

- the nature of participation of the state department of mental health and the university;
- the reasons behind the choice of the particular problem area and how it was determined to be critical;
- the scope of the project;
- the expected outcomes;
- the role consumers and families play in the project;
- past state/university collaborations and interdisciplinary, educational, or service efforts; and
- a willingness to devote resources to support or match additional consultations and/or pilot studies.

Proposals should result in permanent academic and systems change and be responsive to issues of cultural diversity and their impact on service development. Applications should be no more than two single-spaced pages. Letters of support must accompany the application. Applications are accepted twice a year—on April 15 and October 15. Send applications to John

A. Talbott, M.D., c/o Alison Bondurant, Project Director at 1400 K Street, NW, Washington, DC 20005.

The Project also presents awards to states for their exemplary collaborative efforts, which are judged on their strength of service, research, education, and/or recruitment and retention efforts. In addition, it publishes journal articles and a quarterly newsletter to increase understanding and involvement in collaborative efforts and sponsors presentation at national meetings to foster the involvement and commitment of mental health professionals to improve services in public psychiatry. One of the desired outcomes of the Project is to enhance the recruitment and retention of psychiatrists interested in the care of adults with severe and persistent mental illnesses and youth with serious emotional disturbances. The Project is funded by a grant from the Center for Mental Health Services. For periodic updates on activities and information, you could request that your name be placed on the mailing list for the newsletter from this project. For further information, call Alison Bondurant (202) 682–6252 / Fax (202) 682–6348.

APA's Fellowship Program in Public Psychiatry.

The APA's Fellowship Program in Public Psychiatry was founded in 1980 to heighten resident's awareness of career opportunities in the public sector and to contribute to the professional development of residents interested in leadership roles within the public sector in future years. Residents are selected for their commitment to and accomplishments in public psychiatry. The program is supported by Mead Johnson Pharmaceuticals, a Bristol-Myers Squibb Company.

The fellowship program begins in the fall when the APA/Mead Johnson fellows attend the Institute on Psychiatric Services. They participate in sessions of their choosing and related activities designed to introduce them to timely issues in the field and to APA members who might serve as future mentors. During the fellowship year, the fellows are expected to plan presentations for the next Institute on Psychiatric Services. If the proposals are accepted, the fellows are guaranteed attendance and participation as faculty at the second Institute.

Each accredited psychiatric residency program is invited to nominate one resident entering the PGY-3 or PGY-4 year (if in a five-year program). The nomination should be in the form of a letter from the department chair or training director, providing details about the candidate and those accomplishments and activities that would justify the candidate's selection. Accompanying this letter should be the application form to be completed by the resident, which includes a personal statement indicating the candidate's reasons for wanting the fellowship and the ways in which it will contribute to the individual's career plans. Submission of a nomination represents an explicit commitment by the residency program to permit the candidate, if selected, time off to attend APA meetings in their entirety during the fellowship year, as well as the candidate's willingness to do so.

The NASMHPD Research Institute

The National Association of State Mental Health Program Directors (NASMHPD) Research Institute, Inc. was founded in 1987 as a nonprofit affiliate of the association of state mental health directors in the United States (also known as state commissioners of mental health). Its mission is to respond to current needs for objective research, analysis, and basic information to facilitate the management and delivery of mental health services. It is also committed to enhancing the capacity of university-based researchers to collaborate with public mental health agencies in addressing the system's needs. The Institute collaborates with independent researchers, academic and professional organizations, government agencies/private foundations, and other sectors of the general public. In keeping with this commitment, they support training and technical consultation to the field.

NASMHPD's Public-Academic Fellows Program in Mental Health Services Research

NASMHPD's training initiatives include sponsorship of the Public-Academic Research Fellows Program. This unique two-year program provides an opportunity for persons who have received an M.D. or Ph.D. (psychiatric residents as well as junior faculty are eligible) to pursue a career in mental health services research at various sites across the United States. The program's goals are to improve the fellow's knowledge and understanding of public mental health systems and services and to increase their theoretical, methodological, and analytic skills. Upon completion of the Program, fellows will be expected to pursue mental health services research careers in public agencies and/or academic institutions.

Approved training sites are listed in Table 30–3. Each site that has been approved as a host setting for a research fellow has the following characteristics:

Table 30–3. Approved NASMHPD services research training sites, 1996

New York Office of Mental Health/Center for Social Work Research, State University of New York at Albany (Albany)

Connecticut Department of Mental Health/Yale University, Connecticut Mental Health Center (Hartford)

Massachusetts Mental Health Center Department of Psychiatry, School of Medicine, Harvard University (Boston)

Philadelphia Office of Mental Health and Mental Retardation/Department of Psychiatry, School of Medicine, University of Pennsylvania (Philadelphia)

Pennsylvania Office of Mental Health (Harrisburg)/Department of Psychiatry, School of Medicine, University of Pennsylvania (Philadelphia)

Washington Division of Mental Health (Olympia)/School of Social Work University, University of Washington (Seattle)

Illinois Department of Mental Health/Department of Psychiatry, University of Chicago (Chicago)

Indiana Division of Mental Health/Department of Psychology, Indiana University-Purdue University of Indianapolis (Indianapolis)

South Carolina Department of Mental Health/Department of Psychiatry and Behavioral Sciences, Medical University of South Carolina (Charleston)

South Carolina Department of Mental Health/Department of Psychiatry and the School of Public Health, University of South Carolina (Columbia)

Massachusetts Department of Mental Health/John F. Kennedy School of Government, Harvard University (Boston)

Colorado Division of Mental Health/Department of Psychiatry, University of Colorado (Denver)

Illinois Department of Mental Health/Northwestern University Medical School (Chicago)

District of Columbia Commission on Mental Health Services (Washington, DC)/School of Hygiene and Public Health, The Johns Hopkins University (Baltimore, MD)

Maryland Mental Hygiene Administration/School of Hygiene and Public Health, The Johns Hopkins University (Baltimore)

Ohio Department of Mental Health/College of Social Work, The Ohio State University (Columbus)

Maine Department of Mental Health (Augusta)/Muskie Institute at the University of Southern Maine (Portland)

New York State Psychiatric Institute/School of Public Health, Columbia University (New York City)

Florida Mental Health Institute/University of South Florida (Tampa)

Western Interstate Commission on Higher Education/Colorado Department of Mental Health/and University of Colorado Department of Psychiatry (Denver)

(continued)

Table 30–3. Continued

San Francisco Department of Health (SF General Hospital)/University of
California at San Francisco

Virginia Department of Mental Health and the Department of Psychiatry, the
Southeastern Rural Mental Health Center, and the Department of Health
Administration at UVA (Charlottesville); and the Commonwealth Institute for
Child and Family Studies at Medical College of VA (Richmond)

New Hampshire Division of Mental Health/New Hampshire-Dartmouth
Psychiatric Research Center, Dartmouth Medical School (Hanover)

Cuyahoga County Community Mental Health Board/School of Applied Sciences,
Case Western Reserve University (Cleveland)

Missouri Institute of Mental Health, University of Missouri/St. Louis University
(St. Louis)

- A collaborative working relationship between the public agency and
  an academic institution
- An ongoing services research project being conducted under the aus-
  pices of the public agency in which the fellow will participate;
- Availability of academic education and training experiences in research methodology via courses, directed study, tutorial, or other
  university-sponsored activities;
- A research "mentor" (either at the agency or the university) who will
  be the fellow's primary resource person to assist in integrating the
  fellowship experiences
- Specific individuals at the agency and university who will serves as
  codirectors of the fellowship program at each site and who will participate actively in designing and monitoring a training experience
  for each fellow

To ensure a relevant and high-quality experience, the NASMHPD Research Institute will require that a formal learning contract be developed
that reflects the agency, academic center, and fellow's roles, responsibilities,
and contributions. The fellow's experience in the Program will be monitored
by the NASMHPD Research Institute through site visits and periodic reporting. It is required that the fellows spend at least half their work week
in the public mental health agency, with their remaining time pursuing
further education in research methods at the academic institution.

All stipends for fellowships are for two years of full-time (12 months) research training. The fellowship may not be held concurrently with another federally sponsored fellowship. Current annual full-time federally stipulated stipends range from $18,600 for fellows with no postdoctoral experience to $32,300 per year for postdoctoral trainees (including psychiatry residents) with seven or more years of relevant postdoctoral experience. Relevant postdoctoral experience includes activities beyond the doctoral degree such as internship, residency, teaching, or providing services. Research fellows who are recipients of stipends under this NIMH training grant must agree to engage in health-related research and/or teaching for a period equal to the length of support if the fellowship is terminated before month 12. During a typical 24-month fellowship, months 13 to 24 satisfy the payback requirement. Payback requirements are determined and monitored by the NIH. Supplementation of the stipend by the public mental health agency and/or the university from nonfederal funds is both permitted and encouraged.

The annual stipend is paid directly to each to each fellow on a monthly basis from the NASMHPD Research Institute. Up to $2,500 per fellowship year will also be available to the university-based course tuition expenses associated with the fellow's academic training.

Additional funds for travel, hotel, and meals are made available for fellows, and their assigned university faculty and mental health agency staff from their host agency site and academic institution. The seminar is held in conjunction with the NASMHPD Research Institute's Annual Conference on State Mental Health Agency Research conducted each October. Funding for the program is provided by the Services Research Branch, Division of Applied and Services Research, National Institute of Mental Health.

For further information, contact: Noel Mazade, Ph.D., NASMHPD Research Institute, Inc., 66 Canal Center Plaza, Suite 302, Alexandria, VA 22314, Phone (703) 739–9333/ Fax (703) 548–9517.

The National Alliance for the Mentally Ill

The National Alliance for the Mentally Ill (NAMI) is a unique grassroots organization to which training directors can be closely allied. NAMI began when a group of more than 200 persons met in Madison, Wisconsin, in 1979 to consider how to help themselves and their mentally ill relatives. NAMI families are often relatives of persons with these illnesses who have been frustrated by systems that accommodate slowly and poorly to advances in the field. The founders of NAMI were determined to make an organization governed for and by families and "consumers" (the term is used because as consumers of various health and support services, they want to be involved in the development and management of those services, and in guiding the underlying research). From the beginning, NAMI was focused on the unmet needs of people with schizophrenia and manic-depressive illness.

NAMI families found courage and hope in joining together to advocate for needed changes in public policy and attitudes (i.e., stigmatization from decades of blame for causing their relatives' mental disorder). By 1980 this grassroots family movement had achieved incorporation, received nonprofit tax-exempt status, and elected an initial board of directors. Early efforts centered on making connections with small family support groups across the nation. An annual conference was planned, and a newsletter was published. NAMI opened its first office in Washington, DC, in 1982 and began the work of influencing Congress, the administration, and key decision makers. NAMI advocates for greater attention to those afflicted with schizophrenia and affective disorders and greater government and business accountability.

In 1996 NAMI's lobbying efforts facilitated the passage of legislation that includes a landmark provision requiring insurance plans providing mental health benefits to set the same level of yearly and lifetime coverage for these benefits as for other medical conditions (despite strong lobbying against it by the business community).

More and more families, consumers, and providers join NAMI each year and embrace their mental illness agenda. Today there are more than 140,000 members and approximately 1,000 affiliates in all 50 states. Our department of psychiatry has paid for our residents' membership in NAMI for the past 10 years. We have found this to be an efficient means to introduce residents to advocacy and encourage their active participation. NAMI also sponsors a Curriculum and Training Network that disseminates educational information, and a yearly Excellence in Training Award. For more information, call (703) 524–7600 / Fax (703) 524–9094.

The Substance Abuse and Mental Health Service Administration

The Substance Abuse and Mental Health Service Administration (SAMHSA) is charged by its authorizing legislation with establishing and implementing a national program to improve treatment and prevention services to individuals with mental illness and substance abuse disorders, and to protect the legal rights of these individuals. The agency is authorized to carry out key functions through its three centers, the Center for Mental Health Services, the Center for Substance Abuse Prevention, and the Center for Substance Abuse Treatment.

At present, SAMHSA's primary mental health training initiative concerns managed care and addresses psychiatry workforce needs. The Health Care Delivery Systems program of the Center for Substance Abuse Prevention has established guidelines for substance abuse prevention related to internal management and service delivery for managed care organizations and hospitals. Developed by an expert panel, these guidelines serve as benchmarks for comprehensive substance abuse prevention services within managed care settings. The program offers a computerized organizational assessment tool and a one-day overview course to managed care organizations and hospitals. A comprehensive four-day course is also available. For further information, contact the CSAP Project Officer, Veronica M. Friel, Ph.D., at (301) 443–5276.

The Center for Mental Health Services (CMHS) recently convened a planning meeting for their primary mental health training initiative concerning managed care and will soon move toward implementation of the plan. For questions about the CMHS plan, call Dr. Paul Wohlford (301) 443–3503.

The Center for Mental Health Services (and its predecessor, the NIMH Psychiatry Education Branch) generously supported psychiatry residency programs through mental health clinical training grants to universities. These programs, however, have been terminated. SAMHSA currently supports a few training programs that are sponsored and administered by professional organizations (i.e., the APA's Minority Fellowship Program). SAMHSA's new director, Nelba Chavez, would welcome a dialogue on how training directors (through AADPRT or the APA) might join SAMHSA in ensuring that programs are served by a well-trained workforce (N. Chavez, personal communication).

One of SAMHSA's most important functions is the administration of the state block grant program. In 1995 SAMHSA had a budget of approximately $2.4 billion, of which about $1. 5 billion was channeled directly to states in the form of block grants. Each state uses monies from these block grants to (1) carry out the plan submitted by the state for the fiscal year involved as required by Public Law 99–660, (2) to evaluate the state's programs and services carried out under the plan, and (3) to support educational activities related to providing services under the plan. We strongly encourage you to contact the chair of your state's mental health planning council for specific information on how to get involved with this process (see Appendix 30–A). Other questions about state planning and the mental health services block grants should be directed to Carol T. Bush, Ph.D., R.N., at SAMHSA (301) 443–4257.

Discussion

Whatever their nature, initial collaborative activities should be strategically planned to maximize chances of success and future growth. The resolution of previous public-academic conflicts ("bury the hatchet") may be necessary to focus on the future benefits of a public-academic alliance. The parties should approach collaborations openly, recognizing that extensive efforts may be necessary to establish and maintain a reasonable level of trust among agency administrators, public sector providers, and academic faculty. Initial efforts may need to focus on the education of the two groups regarding the goals, values, styles, problems, limitations, and demands of the two very different systems. This will facilitate the identification of, and long-term commitment to, a set of shared goals and strategies that are important enough to allow both agencies to relinquish former attitudes and concentrate on the present and future of the proposed collaboration. The hurts, slights, and rejections of the past and the very real gulf that often develops between these systems can be gradually overcome, principally through a "new day" philosophy involving new people and new programs. The former animosity and distrust should eventually yield to a shared vision, complementary to both systems. Mutual benefits of such collaborations can be experienced quickly as the university acquires research opportunities, new sources of revenue, and training sites that allow residents to experience evolving methods of caring for public sector patients. The public agencies are able to meet their need for well-qualified professionals to fill empty slots, and obtain access to the specialized expertise and technologies available at the university. Over time, public sector personnel come to appreciate the stimulating, morale-supporting aspects of having academic medical center trainees and research activities on-site. The collaboration that evolves, then, is derived from two very different entities with a complementary overlap of interests, needs, values, and activities.

Planned relationships often fail because critical personnel do not embrace the stated goals of the collaboration sufficiently to exert the effort needed. They are often fraught with personnel who are divided because of agency allegiance, who are consumed by ill will, work at complete odds with each other, and unfortunately, all too frequently, fail to consider the consequences these actions have on the evolving collaboration and the benefits to patients served by the agencies. It is therefore imperative that leaders at all levels share a high degree of commitment to these linkages and to what they represent, that they practice a high level of patience and perseverance, and that they maintain a sense of humor about the inevitable conflicts that will emerge. This obviously applies to the departmental chair and key faculty, and the local and state public agency directors, all of whom need to know each other well, and eventually respect and trust each other. These leaders must be prepared to make most of the decisions in these collaborative efforts because consensus of everyone in their mutual organizations is almost certainly too complex to ever achieve. Of course, when agency leaders happen to be friends and colleagues and stable in their respective positions, a higher degree of success is likely to be enjoyed. Such relationships strengthen mutual trust and facilitate exchange of "favors." Clearly, this is an evolutionary process where longevity in the leadership will afford greater stability in such endeavors.

Stipends for residency training are often linked to hospital operating budgets; therefore, it is difficult to finance non-hospital-based clinical training experiences. However, as suggested by Steven Sharfstein, "The only way that our residents are going to understand episodes of care within the reality of current economic constraints is to be able to follow the patients regardless of their setting" (American Association of Directors of Psychiatry Residency Training 1991). Exposure to service delivery models other than hospital and office-based aftercare provides trainees a practical lesson in medical economics in that some of these programs demonstrate cost containment without jeopardizing the quality of care. Psychiatrists with this training will be better able to project the potential benefits and limitations of rehabilitation efforts, appreciate the fluid nature of psychiatric symptoms, discriminate baseline from relapse characteristics, and competently assess functional deficits. Thus, while reduced hospital revenues currently threaten to disrupt traditional methods of financing graduate medical education, the situation presents an important opportunity for restructuring training curricula through these types of collaboration (Diamond et al. 1993).

In conceptualizing and formulating initial service and training activities, plans should be developed that maximize chances of success and future growth. Therefore, preacknowledged and postevaluated outcomes should include what are desired as goals (e.g., favorable training experiences for residents, positive regard from public sector clinicians about the involvement of university personnel, and/or enhanced recruitment of qualified psychiatrists into public sector jobs).

To ensure success, PAL rotations should be administered and supervised by faculty with proven records of effective teaching and the ability to integrate and apply biological and psychosocial knowledge to the community-based care of patients. It is helpful if the identified core PAL faculty members also occupy leadership positions within the training program's administration. The training program may need to recruit new academic faculty from both inside and outside the department who share PAL concerns and who would be well received by both trainees and public sector clinicians (e.g., competent clinicians and teachers, eager to mentor residents and who are successful in public settings). These new faculty positions can be supported by the public sector from allocated funds for physicians' salaries. Potential faculty who are clinically, theoretically, or philosophically "out of date," or those unable to effectively work in complex systems should not be considered for appointment to these new teaching services. Faculty assignment will require careful consideration, and only those faculty willing to embrace and support the philosophy, spirit, and success of the collaboration should be utilized.

In keeping with principles of community-based services, faculty should agree to place a premium on the following:

- Continuity of care and avoidance of treatment dropout or "falling through the cracks"
- Reduction of system-dependent institutional care
- Development of consistent standards of care for public and private training environments

A popular teaching method is on-site and in vivo role modeling where faculty and residents travel and work together as a team. Through this approach the residents assume more and more responsibility over time as determined by the attending. In this way, faculty can readily monitor a resident's role satisfaction and the appropriateness of workloads; can respond in a timely manner to feedback; and can directly impart the necessary knowledge, skills, and attitudes to function effectively in community systems. This apprenticeship model appears to hold greater educational value than other approaches where residents do not have the opportunity to observe their attendings in direct service provision, or where residents are not observed routinely conducting clinical interviews.

Faculty should always provide residents with an optimistic long-range vision for both the future of their patients and the public system, thereby nurturing their sense of responsibility for these patients. Residents should be oriented to the many components of the system, but primary emphasis is best placed on the larger picture of administrative systems and processes that can provide good care for these publicly funded patients.

Faculty should not assume that a resident can work naturally in a service system without appropriate preparation and supervision; therefore, resident involvement in political or administrative conflicts should be discouraged. Arguably, the approach that is most likely to lead to desired outcomes is to develop the new collaborative services initially using only faculty psychiatrists (without residents). This will allow for time to establish an efficient system and to identify and overcome interagency administrative problems before adding training components.

Well-designed public psychiatry training experiences will be considered upbeat relative to other residency rotations as they convey a "can-do" attitude to difficult clinical and social problems. As a result, these experiences can often become one of the most popular aspects of a training program.

Poorly planned or implemented programs can result in negative experiences and perpetuate the dearth of qualified psychiatrists in the public sector. Dr. L. Faulkner's "prescription for disaster" outlined here provides directions to a certain failure in formulating a public training experience (Faulkner 1994):

- Be vague about what you want the educational program to accomplish. Do not identify any educational objectives (knowledge, skills, attitudes) for the training experience.
- Have unrealistic expectations about what your trainees should learn from their public training experience. Demand that they get experience unavailable in the public setting.
- Send only your very inexperienced trainees into public settings.

Make sure that the supervisory requirements outstrip available public resources.

- Do not allow your trainees to be exposed to any interesting or unique programs available in the public setting.
- Isolate your trainees from the best staff in the public setting. Assign them to work with the least competent clinicians.
- Do not allow your trainees any input about which public program they will be assigned to or what they will be expected to do.
- Provide your trainees with inadequate or incompetent supervision. Arrange for supervision to be done on a catch-as-catch-can basis by individuals who are overtly hostile to academics.
- Ensure that any seminars on public mental health have as little relevance as possible to the experimental component of the trainee rotation. It is preferable not to have a seminar at all, but if one must take place, be sure to prohibit trainees from discussing their current experiences.
- Do not evaluate the performance of your trainees, the training experience, or the faculty supervision. If you must evaluate your trainees, do not base the evaluations on any specific educational objectives. Never solicit or heed feedback from trainees about their experience or faculty supervision.
- Charge the public setting dearly for the privilege of working with your trainees. Be sure that your financial negotiations with the public setting emphasize the worth of the trainees' service and denigrate the value of their educational experience.

Conclusion

Sometimes by design and accompanied by luck, it is possible to achieve a shift in the perceived complementarity of the goals of the university and those of the public mental health system, and a systematic expansion of mental health care linkages can occur. This may be triggered by the demands of citizen groups, or by changes in agency leadership (e.g., state commissioner, department chair, local CMHC director) with corresponding changes in focus (e.g., emphasis on community-based care of adults with chronic psychoses and/or children with serious emotional disturbances).

Several factors are critical to the successful integration of public-academic experiences into training programs: (1) identification of *mutually* beneficial goals followed, at times, by extraordinary efforts to build and maintain good working interagency relationships; (2) striving for stability through effective long-term planning; (3) carefully selecting as training experiences the high-quality, efficient services implemented to fill service system gaps; (4) focusing on a broader span of experiences in the lives of patients (rather than only illness episodes); (5) choosing faculty with a history of dedication to, and effectiveness in, teaching; (6) providing trainees with an extremely well supervised environment; and (7) surmounting program administrative problems prior to introducing a training component. University faculty, public mental health specialists, and the consumers of mental health services stand to gain immeasurably as alliances between the academic community and the public mental health community are strengthened.

References

American Association of Directors of Psychiatry Residency Training: Managed care and residency training. American Association of Directors of Psychiatry Residency Training Newsletter 17:2–6, 1991

Bray JD, Bevilacqua JJ: A multidisciplinary public-academic liaison to improve public mental health services in South Carolina. Hosp Community Psychiatry 44:985–990, 1993

Cutler DL, Wilson WH, Godard SL, et al: Collaboration for training. Adm Policy Ment Health 20:449–458, 1993

Davis M: Public-academic linkages in Western states. Community Ment Health J 27:411–423, 1991

Diamond RJ, Factor RM, Stein LI: Response to "training residents for community psychiatric practice." Community Ment Health J 29:289–296, 1993

Douglas EJ, Faulkner LR, Talbott JA, et al: Administrative relationships between community mental health centers and academic departments. Am J Psychiatry 151:722–727, 1994

Factor RM, Stein LI, Diamond RJ: A model community psychiatry curriculum for psychiatry residents. Community Ment Health J 24:310–327, 1988

Faulkner L: Ten easy steps to failure of a public training experience. Hosp Community Psychiatry 45:101, 1994

Godard SL, Hargrove DS: Public-academic linkages: a "linchpin" model. Community Ment Health J 27:489–500, 1991

Hogarty GE: Depot neuroleptics: the relevance of psychosocial factors—a United States perspective. J Clin Psychiatry 45(5 Pt 2):36–42,1984

Hogarty GE, Anderson CM: Medication, family, psychoeducation, and social skills training: first year relapse results of a controlled study. Psychopharmacol Bull 22:860–862, 1986

Santos AB, Ballenger JC, Bevilacqua JJ, et al: A community-based public-academic liaison program. Am J Psychiatry 151:1181–1187, 1994

Talbott JA, Bray JD, Flaherty L, et al: State-university collaboration in psychiatry: the Pew Memorial Trust Program. Community Ment Health J 27:425–439, 1991

Torrey EF: Surviving Schizophrenia: A Family Manual. New York, Harper & Row, 1983

Weintraub W, Nyman G, Harbin H: The Maryland plan: the rest of the story. Hosp Community Psychiatry 42:52–55, 1991

Yank GR, Barber JW, Vieweg WVR, et al: Virginia's experience with state-university collaboration. Hosp Community Psychiatry 42:39–44, 1991a

Yank GR, Fox CJ, Davis KE: The Galt visiting scholar in public mental health: a review of a model of state-university collaboration. Community Ment Health J 27:455–471, 1991b

State Mental Health Planning Council Chairpersons (1995)

NOTE: The primary source of the information below is the letter from the Mental Health Planning Council and then the list of members of the MH Planning Council both located in the FY95 Mental Health Block Grant Application.

Alabama
Rogene Parris
Alabama Alliance
    for the Mentally Ill
2061 Fire Pink Court
Birmingham AL 35244
Tel: 205-987-8338
Fax: 205-987-8338

Alaska
Ed Krause
P.O. Box 51
Copper Center, Alaska 99573
Tel: 822-5241
Fax: 822-5247

Arizona
Dee Ann Barber
2122 E. Highland Ave.
Phoenix, AZ 85016
Tel: 602-622-7611
Fax: 602-624-7042

Arkansas
Sherry Brown
Texarcana School District
223 East Short 10th
Texarcana, AR 75502
Tel: 501-772-9815

California
Don Richardson
Department of Mental Health
1600 9th Street, Room 100
Sacramento, CA 95814
Tel: 916-654-2309

Colorado
Joseph N. deRaimes
Office of the City Attorney
PO Box 791
Boulder, CO 80306
Tel: 303-441-3020
Fax: 303-441-3859

Connecticut
Dr. Jean Adnopoz
Yale Child Study Center
South Frontage Road
Middletown, CT 06451
Tel: 203-785-4947
Phone: 203-347-9755

Philippa M. Coughlan, Ph.D.
Dir., Off. of Student MH
Weslyn University
New Haven, CT
Fax: 203-785-7402

Delaware
Jorge A. Pereira-Ogan, M.D.
Suite 22-B, Trolley Square
Wilmington, DE 19806
Tel: 302-571-9306, 302-654-6353
Fax: 302-654-1347

District of Columbia
Mattie Robinson
1307 Holbrook St., NE
Washington, DC 20002
Tel: 202-399-0558

Florida
Katie Vath
Government Relations Committee
Florida Alliance for the Mentally Ill
2069 Tocobaga Lane
Nokomis, FL 34275
Tel: 813-488-7780

Georgia
Cynthia Wainscott
Executive Dir.
MH Assoc of GA
620 Peachtree Street, NE
Suite 300 Atlanta, GA 30308
Tel: 404-875-7081
Fax: 404-607-8782

Hawaii
Robert Weads
State Council on Mental
Dept of Health
P.O. Box 3378
Honolulu, HI 96801
Tel: 808-244-9203
Fax: 808-877-8772

Idaho
Rose Marie Tiffany
HC 02, Box 237
St. Maries, ID 83861
Tel: 208-689-3603
Fax: 208-245-2544

Illinois
Boris Astrachan, M.D.
Dept. of Psychiatry
U of IL, College of Medicine
P.O. Box 6998 (MC 913)
Chicago, IL 60680
Tel: 312-996-6947
Fax: 312-413-1228

Indiana
Robert Levy, Ph.D.
2342 N. 7th Street
Terre Haute, IN 47804

Iowa
Peter Badami
407 North Fourth Street
Burlington, IA 52601
Tel: 319-754-4618
Fax: 319-754-4193

Kansas
David Seaton
Winfield Courier
201 E. 9th Street
Winfield, KS 67156
Tel: 316-221-1050
Fax: 316-221-1101

Kentucky
Robert Ray Hicks
631 Timothy Drive
Frankfort, KY 40601
Tel: 502-223-3034

Louisiana
William M. Coffey
Volunteers of America
3765 Government Street
Baton Rouge, LA 70806
Tel: 504-387-0061
Fax: 504-381-7963

Maine
Grace Leonard
University of Maine at Augusta
State House Station #40 or
46 University Drive
Augusta, ME 04333
Tel: 207-621-3257

Maryland
Livia Pazourek
Alliance for the Mentally Ill
in Anne Arundel County
578 Belmawr Place
Millersville, MD 21108
Tel: 410-768-2621
Fax: 410-760-6811

Massachusetts
Bernard Carey
130 Bowdoin Street, Suite 309
Boston, MA 02108
Tel: 617-742-7452
Fax: 617-742-1187

Judi Chamberlain
2 Dow Street
West Sommerville, MA 02144
Tel: 617-628-8438
Fax: 617-742-1187

Michigan
Sheila Faunce
916 Wick Court
Lansing, MI 48823
Tel: 517-373-1255
Fax: 517-335-6775

Minnesota
Cynthia Hart
951 Homestead Lane
Chanhassen, MN 55317
Tel: 612-496-3009
Fax: 612-949-3841

Mississippi
Steve Roark
Mental Health Center
P.O. Box 820691
Vicksbury, MS
Tel: 601-638-0031
Fax: 601-634-0234

Missouri
Paul Albert Emmons
Archway Communities
5652 Pershing Avenue
St. Louis, MO 63112
Tel: 314-751-4122
Fax: 314-361-7329

Montana
Liza Dyrdahl
PO Box 1784
Bozeman, MT 59771
Tel: 406-444-3964
Fax: 406-444-4920

Nebraska
Russell D. Pierce
2301 Deer Park Blvd. #7
Omaha, NE 68108
Tel: 402-733-2713

Nevada
Jerry Zadny
505 E. King Street, Rm. 603
Carson City, NV 89701

New Hampshire
Dorothy Walker, AMI
2 Dodier Ct.
Merrimack, NH 02054
Tel: 603-429-2044
Fax: 603-627-1166

New Jersey
Rose K. Ashin
Adult Council
Captial Center, CN 727
Trenton, NJ 08624-0727
Tel: 201-747-0624

Joan Mechlin
Children's Coordinating Council
Capital Center, CN 727
Trenton, NJ 08625-0727
Tel: 609-428-1300
Fax: 609-428-0350

New Mexico
Jose V. Torres
Division of Vocational Rehabilitation
435 St. Michael's Drive
Building D
Sante Fe, NM 87505
Tel: 505-827-3511
Fax: 505-827-3746

New York
Leila Salmon
44 Holland Avenue
Albany, NY 12229
Tel: 518-842-4852
Fax: 518-842-4852

North Carolina
M. W. Stancil
P.O. Box 188
Selma, NC 27807

North Dakota
Sister Paula Larson
Sacred Heart Priory
PO Box 364
Richardson, ND 58652
Tel: 701-974-2121
Fax: 702-224-2359

Ohio
Douglas DeVoe
Ohio Advocates for Mental Health
1068 Goodale Blvd.
Columbus, OH 43212-3831
Tel: 614-421-1121
Fax: 614-421-1108

Oklahoma
Dan O'Brien
RS #49
Support Emp. Unit
Dept. of Human Services
Tel: 405-556-5183
Fax: 405-528-4766

or
P.O. Box 53277
Oklahoma City, OK 73152
Tel: 405-271-8653

Oregon
Katherine Eaton
1631 E. 24th Ave.
Eugene, OR 97403
Tel: 503-344-2027

Pennsylvania
Donna N. McNelis, Dir. Conn MH Educ
Medical College of PA
P.O. Box 18589
Philadelphia, PA 19129
Tel: 215-842-4344
Fax: 215-735-2465

Glenda Fine Dir., Parents Inc-Network
Suite 902
311 South Juniper Street
Philadelphia, PA 19107
Tel: 215-735-2465
Fax: 215-843-9028

Rhode Island
Norman Orodenker, Esq.
600 New London Ave./Cottage 402
Cranston, RI 02920
Tel: 401-464-3291

Licht & Semonoff
One Park Road
Providence, RI 02903
Tel: 401-421-8030
Fax: 401-272-9408

South Carolina
Richard K. Harding
Two Richland Medical Park Suite 508
Columbia, SC 29203
Tel: 803-253-4698

South Dakota
Helen W. Dafoe
% Div of Mental Health
Hillsview Plaza
500 E. Captiol
Perre, SD
Tel: 605-773-5991

2201 W. 37 Street
Sioux Falls, SD 57105

Tennessee
William R. Busing
317 Louisiana Ave.
Oak Ridge, TN 37830
Tel: 615-531-TAMI

Texas
Reymyndo Rodriguez
Hogg Foundation for MH
PO Box 7998 Univ Station
Austin, TX 78713
Tel: 512-471-5011

Questions
Karen Hale
Acting Commissioner
Tel: 512-206-4588
or Deputy Comm. Steven Shon, MD
Tel: 512-206-4510

Utah
Delores Ottley
Dept. of Human Services
120 N. West
P.O. Box 45
Salt Lake City, UT 81145-0500
Tel: 801-538-4270
Fax: 801-524-6694

3085 Cindi Way
Ogden, UT 84403

Vermont
James L. Rivers
Board of Mental Health
c/o Dept of Mental Health
103 South Main Street
Waterbury, VT 05676
Tel: 802-241-2610

Virginia
Kia J. Bentley, Ph.D. Associatie
    Professor
VCU, School of Social Work
1001 W. Franklin Street
Richmond, VA 23284-2027
Tel: 804-367-1044
Fax: 804-828-0716

Washington
Arlene Engel
1301 S. 3rd Ave. # 3A
PO Box 250
Sequin, WA 98382-0250
Tel: 206-683-3496
Fax: 206-683-1846

West Virginia
Lynn Williams
c/o Office of Behavioral Health Service
RM B-717—Building C
Capitol Complex
Charleston, WV 25305
Tel: 304-558-0627
Fax: 304-623-9088

108 Summit Court
Clarksburg, WV 26301

Wisconsin
Larry Schomer
1 West Wilson Street
P.O. Box 7851
Madison, WI 53707

Wyoming
Rev. Roger Schmit
St. Paul's Newman Center Univ. Catholic
    Parish
1800 East Grand Ave.
Laramie, WY 82707-4316
Tel: 307-745-5461

Commonwealth of the Northern Mariana Islands
Juan L. Babauta (Vice-chairperson)
P.O. Box 1585
Saipan, MP 96950
Tel: 670-235-7706
Fax: 670-235-7778

Republic of Palau
Father John Paul Ililau
P.O. Box 6027
Koror, Palau PW 96940
Tel: 680-488-1002
Fax: 680-488-1211

Micronesia
Rosa H. Tacheliol
P.O. Box 127
Yap, FM 96943
Tel: 691-350-2146
Fax: 691-350-2341

Puerto Rico
Maria del Pilar Christian, MA, OTR
P.O. Box 191891
San Juan, PR 00919-1891
Tel: 809-791-5653

Virgin Islands
Thomas J. Dunn
Virgin Islands of the US

American Samoa
Rev. Ned Ripley
PO Box 1149
American Samoa, 96797
Tel: 684-633-2019
Fax: 684-633-1099

31

Canadian Solutions to Constricting Academic Resources

Paul E. Garfinkel, M.D.,
and Allan S. Kaplan, M.Sc., M.D., F.R.C.P.C.

The editors of this text have asked us to comment on scholarship in a Canadian university and faculty development in departments of psychiatry; we are pleased to do so. We have chosen to organize this discussion by briefly introducing the topic of scholarship in a clinical department and then describing some characteristics of Canadian settings that may differ from those in other countries and be either facilitative or problematic for scholarly work. However, it is important to note that scholarship in any country has more similarities than differences.

Scholarship

Scholarship has a variety of ingredients, but we wish to emphasize one central component—and that relates to attitude. Scholarship requires an attitude of critical enquiry, an attitude of self-scrutiny and an attitude of wanting to have one's work critiqued at a broad level. Burke et al. (1986) have described this aspect as the intellectual orientation of science; they commented that learning what questions to ask and how to pursue these with rigor is much more important than any technical skills that are mastered. Scholarship implies intellectual tolerance, but with clear standards, and the latter involve a relentless pursuit of scientific truth. It also implies a reflection on one's activities and making these more meaningful for future endeavors, both for oneself and for others.

Scholarship requires an acknowledgment that standards apply and that we all play by the same rules. And the rules involve review by our peers. It is true that such peer review has problems. For example, peer review can reflect an "old boys network," or a tendency to a conservative stance. Nevertheless, like democracy, peer review is the best system we've got (the British novelist E. M. Forster once wrote: "Two cheers for democracy: one because it admits variety, and two because it permits criticism." Forster thought two cheers "quite enough: there is no occasion to give three"). That corresponds to our view of peer review—it's not perfect, but it's the best we've got.

Clinical research is a new discipline; the first randomized controlled trials were reported in the late 1940s and early 1950s. Researchers then realized that when a large number of patients entered a clinical study, it allowed researchers to draw their conclusions more quickly and increased the chance that the study's findings would be valid. Furthermore, investigators soon appreciated the power of statistical analyses that permitted the evaluation of large groups to determine with some degree of certainty small differences between treatments.

In the 50 years since, many significant strides have been made, but with only modest progress in one key area—an increased ability to provide an array of effective treatments according to a particular person's specific needs. We need to be able to provide individualized care for each patient. It is simplistic, for example, to think that there is only one way to treat depression. This does not do justice to the complexities of us as human beings. Depression is not just the term to describe changes in brain chemistry, or a group of symptomatic affects or behaviors; it especially involves an experience of hopelessness and lost meaning. Depression will always require a variety of approaches, dependent on the particular person's unique needs. We are a long way from such tailored, flexible treatments at this time. And the only way to get there is through more scholarly work of a high quality.

Factors That Affect Scholarship in Canadian Psychiatry

A great deal more quality scholarship is required. What follows is a discussion of some factors that bear on this issue in Canada.

Atmosphere

Scholarship requires a particular atmosphere to flourish. This relates to what is valued and respected. An important aspect of this is the conceptual model created by the central department. Models are necessary to provide an anchor for all of us, and Canadian psychiatry has tended to a view of mental disorders that has breadth, that is multidimensional, with contributors from the social, cultural, interpersonal, intrapsychic, and physiologic domains. This can have the advantage of allowing an academic "home" for people with a variety of orientations. By contrast, psychiatry as a whole has often gone to extremes in attempting to explain mental illness. Examples include the extreme reliance on psychoanalytic interpretation in the 1950s or on community approaches in the 1960s and now on biological psychiatry and psychopharmacology. All have resulted in some gain, but often with an associated loss, as useful contributions from previous models have been abandoned with each new wave. The breadth to Canadian psychiatry may be a definite advantage in stimulating scholarship in areas currently not in vogue. And this has resulted in a considerable breadth to the psychiatric writing from this country (Rae-Grant and Fyfe 1996).

The atmosphere involves far more than the particular model of psychiatric illness. Also important are the types of scholarship that are valued. Boyer (1990) and Jacobs (1992) have suggested an expanded definition of scholarship in academic medicine. They proposed a fourfold definition of scholarship, which is overlapping and not exclusive. The components are (1) the scholarship of application, which includes building bridges between theory and practice and showing theory and practice in vital interaction; (2) the scholarship of teaching, which involves the transmission of knowledge in a way that is applicable and inspiring; (3) the scholarship of integration, which is described as a form of horizontal scholarship linking areas of study across disciplines and broadening the applications of research; and (4) the scholarship of discovery, which is defined as vertical scholarship through the generation of new knowledge. What is important is that all four forms of scholarship are of the highest standard—it is the quality that counts, rather than the particular area of study. It is advantageous to capitalize on the diversity of faculty utilizing the rich array of faculty talent to stimulate renewal of faculty, relating realistically both to contemporary clinical life and the promotion of scientific research.

Attitudes to Psychiatry Among the Public

Some difficulties with scholarship relate to public attitudes—perceptions of government, of our field, and of medicine have an impact. Stereotyping of psychiatry and of the mentally ill can be an impediment at many levels.

Attitudes to the mentally ill seem to have changed much more rapidly in the United States. In Canada, there remains a great deal of stigmatization. Commonly, the mental illnesses are still viewed as moral problems, so patients get blamed for their illnesses; or those closest to them—their families—are blamed; or people are so frightened by mental disorder that they want to keep the patients physically distant and not be reminded of these illnesses. These are all barriers to successful collaboration with the public and with government regarding improving care of the mentally ill. Fortunately, these attitudes are slowly beginning to change; there is a difference beginning to emerge here even in the last 5 years.

The results of this stigmatization are apparent in public funding of psychiatric research in Canada. The population of Canada is only one-tenth that of the United States; even when adjusted on a per capita basis, however, federal and provincial agencies provide far less support for psychiatric research than in the United States. The per capita funding for this research in the United States has been estimated to be approximately $3.50 (Lam and El-Guebaly 1994). The corresponding figure in Canada is about $1.00. Although this discrepancy relates partly to reduced levels of medical research funding in general, it is more marked in Canada for psychiatric research. For example, research funding for all mental illness and addictions in the United States accounts for 4.7% of all health research support (Pincus and Fine 1992). In Canada, the figure is 3.7%, 20% lower. The costs for these groups of illnesses to the two countries are not dissimilar on a percentage basis (psychiatric disorders account for 14% of Canada's health care costs; the corresponding figure in the United States is 12%). A recent study by Lam and El-Guebaly (1994) quantified aspects of this funding issue in Canada. On average, psychiatric disorders are investigated at about $4 per patient per year, a fraction of what is devoted to other medical conditions. In Ontario, Canada's most populous province, with more than 10 million people, the Ministry of Health spends $1.3 billion on the provision of mental health services. A fraction of 1% of this goes to research on mental illness.

This stigmatization also has a bearing on private philanthropy, which is not as well developed as it is in the United States. Furthermore, there is less private giving in Canada in general. With a tendency to rely on the government for provision of the social support network, there is also a tendency to expect that government will provide for research. And there are some differences in the tax laws regarding inheritance that make it less desirable to establish charitable foundations in Canada. As a result, there is less opportunity to fund research outside the traditional government agencies.

In Canada, there is a real need to sensitize our public to the issues of our patients. And in this regard many academic leaders in Canada could do better, both in sharing their knowledge as fully as possible and in forming partnerships with an eager group of families and patients. Mystery and evasiveness have no place in the research process. An important function in this regard is one of translation—translation of basic science to clinicians and students, and translation of new understanding to a broad public.

The Separation of Teaching and Research

Another impediment relates to the way in which teaching can be separated from research. The two, in fact, go together. Education must be closely intertwined with research and scholarship—it can never be just training. As Michaels (1994) recently commented, in education our task is having people know, to know how to learn and how to learn for the future. By contrast, training involves learning to do something—it is the apprenticeship component of skill acquisition. Clearly, a good postgraduate program must encompass the two. A residency program that ignores training issues will graduate residents who can't get jobs; a residency program that ignores scholarship issues will graduate clinicians who are unable to critically evaluate developments and maintain their competence.

We can improve our scholarship by seeing that our best mentors are more fully involved with students. This is a key part of the strategy in the University of Toronto Provostial White Paper on university objectives entitled "Planning for 2000" (1995). The plan here is to directly link teaching and research. The first objective in the strategy is to ensure that " the great majority of courses at all levels of the undergraduate curriculum as well as the graduate curriculum are taught by professors who are engaged in active programs of research and scholarship." Concern has been expressed that this could denigrate the role of clinician-teachers in a faculty of medicine. It is not meant to. It is recognized that many clinician-teachers are not directly involved in research, but they should be involved in scholarly activity. And these scholarly pursuits will vary widely. Many involve collaborations in research studies or in clinical trials, or in establishment of new clinical programs, or in development of continuing education or in related activities best described as creative professional endeavors. What is most important, clinician-teachers should be part of an academic unit with an active program of research and scholarship that they bring to bear in their teaching activities.

At the postgraduate level, training programs should be asked to link teaching and research. Thus, for the most part, postgraduate medical education should be delivered by teachers who are part of a community of scholars. This simply reaffirms the fact that postgraduate teaching includes more than an apprenticeship element (as valuable as this may be). We must expose our students to teachers who are intimately involved in academic scholarly pursuits. In this regard, residency programs in psychiatry in Canada, as in the United States, have made research training optional and the exception rather than the rule. However, this requires careful reconsideration, especially in view of the importance of critical evaluation to future practitioners.

Faculty Development

An important concern relates to the "quick fix." Here we are referring to the recruitment of faculty who have not been properly prepared for the academic world. We must learn to focus on the long-term perspective. This is particularly important in our approach to priority programs and their key underpinning, the recruitment and development of people. All too often, academic departments have relaxed their standards to take in faculty not adequately prepared for scholarship, then give them the responsibilities and duties, and then judge them harshly. It is partly out of respect for our students and partly out of respect for our faculty that we must insist on ensuring our faculty have the necessary skills for the academic life. This includes not only postgraduate training in other centers (to bring back unique skills), but also advanced studies in neurobiology, in clinical epidemiology, in education, in learning how to teach, and in other relevant fields. Any department that takes seriously its responsibility for the career development and promotion of its faculty must see that new staff are properly trained.

In this regard, the chair's hiring policy greatly affects the behavior of senior residents interested in pursuing the academic life (Garfinkel et al.

1989). If the chair discourages filling university geographic full-time positions with people fresh out of residency training, residents eager for academic careers will pursue the appropriate studies to prepare them for their later scholarly careers.

Mentors

A relative lack of mentors can be a significant hindrance to the development of a new generation of scholars. The critical role that mentors play has been described in business, sports, the arts, a variety of professions, and, to some extent, in medicine and psychiatry (Levinson 1978). Those who have been mentored are generally happier with their careers and derive more pleasure from their work than do nonmentored colleagues (Roche 1979). The mentor is more than just an experienced colleague helping in career development; the mentor is a trusted adviser with whom a close personal relationship develops. Identification, sponsoring, modeling, and counseling are components of the mentoring experience, besides the apprenticeship; these result in what Levinson (1978) called "realization of the dream" and both personal and professional growth (Colwill 1990).

Concerning the development of clinician-investigators, Cohen (1986) and Burke et al. (1986) have observed that young professionals must learn how to handle the frustrations and rejections of granting agencies, journal editors, and administrators; the feelings of rivalry and competitiveness of peers; and the multiple demands on their time that encroach on family life. Regular close contact with an experienced colleague who has also had to live with these same concerns provides an invaluable identification. A mentoring experience can be both particularly valuable and feasible during fellowship training, a critical period for the development of future clinician-investigators (Kirsling and Kochar 1990).

The problem here is a definite shortage of such senior colleagues well suited to the role of a scholarly mentor. This is especially so for women, who are strikingly underrepresented in senior academic positions (Levinson et al. 1989). And this can be a self-perpetuating problem. Kirsling and Kochar (1990) surveyed a variety of senior medical faculty and found that 90% had a mentor; among these, 81% who had a mentor indicated that they had served as a mentor to a younger medical colleague. By contrast, those not exposed to mentorship were themselves less likely to serve in this capacity later in their own academic careers. One of the most important issues regarding the mentor is our relative lack of understanding of the ingredients for this task. A capacity for nurturance and self-scrutiny, a sense of security with regard to one's professional identity, and the ability to derive satisfaction from one's students' performance have been described as essential personal qualities of a good mentor (Swensen et al. 1995).

In a previous part of this chapter, we commented on the need for students to be exposed to scientists and clinician-scholars regularly. But not all successful scientists or scholars become valued mentors; some, for example, can be quite competitive with their younger colleagues, and some are so invested in their own careers that they are not prepared to devote the time and energy to such relationships. To be a valued mentor requires not only successfully doing the work oneself, but it also requires a maturity characterized by reaching a phase of generativity in one's life (Levinson 1978). It also requires that mentors understand their younger colleague's interests and skills and have a broad perspective on what will be needed by our society. One problem some mentors have is a tendency to re-create themselves in their students, at times ignoring the student's unique strengths and the value of the area being pursued.

Very Large Geographic Distances and a Cooperative Spirit

Canada is a huge country, with a population of less than 30 million people. Academic centers are separated by great distances that can be an impediment to active, intellectual collaboration. Although this problem is significantly reduced in an age of vastly improved communication, there is still less of a concentration of scholars in the large cities, which in many American counterparts sustain two or more medical schools.

All 16 medical schools in Canada are government-financed public institutions, a very different situation than exists in the United States. Partly because of this, there is less of a competitive spirit among investigators in Canada. Although some competition is healthy in an academic environment, much of it can result in redundancy, wasted resources, and a loss of the ability to pool talented intellectual resources. Recently, there have been some impressive examples of cross-Canada linkage in scholarly work. Kennedy et al. (1995) have linked 16 groups across the country to form the Canadian Network for Mood and Anxiety Treatments (CANMAT)—to facilitate standardized approaches to quantitative research, diagnosis, and treatment. This collaboration also facilitates recruitment of participants for studies and a commitment to best practice models, professional and public education.

Government Regulations Regarding Physicians

Until recently, Canada encouraged physicians from other countries to train in our universities and, at times, to settle here. Since 1990 concern has increased about the possible oversupply of physicians; as a result, most provincial governments have passed laws that greatly restrict physician entry. This has a significant impact on who is recruited into Canadian residency programs and, regrettably, on recruitment for academic positions. Even though these restrictive new regulations are recent and have not yet had their real impact on the academic life, unless they are changed they will have a very significant negative effect on scholarship in Canadian medical schools. This is because quality of scholarship is heavily dependent on forming groupings linked much more to ideas and pursuit of knowledge than to country of birth.

Funding

Funding is a significant issue everywhere. How academic departments are funded, how research is funded, and how people are funded have an important bearing on the product of the academic enterprise. It is difficult to expect our faculty members to be scholarly when they are being bombarded by many conflicting pressures, including generating a significant component of their incomes; yet this is what we ask of many people.

For the past 25 years the Canadian people have had a system of national health insurance. The fundamental principles of this approach are universality, comprehensiveness, and public funding from taxation. This system is Canada's most successful and popular public program. We think of it not just as a mechanism of paying bills, but as an important symbol of helping one another, which is at the heart of the Canadian experience.

However, the government's fully tax-supported single-payer system is increasingly facing demands from its users that are outstripping resources available. This is leading primarily to more difficulty accessing the system, especially for elective procedures. The government is now encouraging movement away from the fee-for-service model of care to a mixed blended compensation package, with some physicians remunerated through salaries funded through a capitation-like system. In addition, to contain spiraling health care costs, specific ceilings on billings to the Ontario Health Insurance Plan (OHIP) have recently been introduced.

On balance, this health plan has positive implications for academic clinical groups, including flexibility regarding the financing of academic work. There is less pressure on the department to develop new ways to generate clinical earnings, or to be selective regarding who is being taken into treatment; also, at this time in most provinces, a variety of psychiatric treatments are available through the plan, based solely on clinical need, not on the patient's finances. Third-party involvement in decision making is therefore modest. In some provinces, some funding is available for indirect care—which can also be a balancing phenomenon for providing work with the multidisciplinary team. Also, since two-thirds of the funding for the academic group is generated from clinical earnings, academic groups have to spend a significant amount of time on patient care. Although this means that the academic staff members are very busy, it also keeps most members of a clinical department rooted in clinical concerns.

Remuneration for Canadian academic psychiatrists is made up of funds from a variety of sources—including fee-for-service clinical billings to OHIP, hard university support, and, for a few researchers, support from foundations (however, in Canada, research grants do not pay for investigators' time). The academic support for faculty has been somewhat protected by the formation of group practice plans that pool professional income and then redistribute the money according to the academic and clinical duties that individuals perform. Because these plans have a degree of flexibility (they are reviewed annually), there can be a distribution of funds according to the types of scholarship that the department wishes to emphasize; this can be a significant advantage in stimulating particular types of academic work. These plans are usually administered according to a predetermined set of principles by the chair and an advisory committee.

In addition to paying for the time of the academic faculty, the group practice plan serves as a business, which can at times use funds for adjunctive support. This can be very useful to the academic enterprise. For example, support for academic secretaries and computer and statistical assistance may all be provided from the academic practice plan. As a result, faculty who do not have external grant support may derive some assistance, especially in getting started. This can be particularly beneficial for people who are working in areas unlikely to be funded by granting agencies. In addition, some of these plans have developed "minisabbaticals" that provide staff with time for more intensive research and study.

Model of an Academic Group Practice Plan

Since funding has become such an important concern in academic medical departments in Canada and because clinical practice incomes have become so much a part of the earnings of Canadian academic psychiatrists (a typical figure would be that 70% of income is generated from clinical fees), it is probably useful to describe the function of one such partnership. The goal of these group practice plans is not to inhibit clinical practice, but rather to place a plan in the appropriate context for an academic group. The philosophical underpinnings of the plan involve the following:

1. A desire to support the academic goals of the hospital and the central university department
2. A need to promote a sense of collegiality and of fairness among participating faculty
3. A desire to support a level of funding capable of attracting and retaining the best faculty
4. A need to permit accountability back to the hospital chief and then to the university chair

Some specific ingredients to this plan are outlined in Table 31–1. Many of the ingredients (such as a hard base of support, a job description set annually, ceilings that increase with academic rank) are not different from those that exist in many U.S. university departments, but they did represent a marked change when they were introduced in 1990. What may be somewhat different is the presence of the Academic Trust Fund. This represents the pooled incomes of each partner above his or her ceiling (50% of all money earned above the ceiling is kept by the individual and 50% is retained by the Trust)—to 20% above the ceiling; at that point only 33% goes back to the individual. The Trust Fund is obligated to expend all its monies at the end of each year, to partners only and to stimulate the academic enterprise of the particular hospital site. Experience has shown that ceilings should be set so that approximately 5% of total partnership income is recaptured and redistributed so as to promote academic productivity but not risk producing resentment from the less productive members. In this plan, the maximum total award for any individual is $30,000. A copy of the Trust Fund criteria for distribution to partners of one hospital is provided in Table 31–2.

Table 31–1. Principles of agreement

1. There shall be ceilings on income. Each Associate's ceiling shall be set by the Chairman of the Department of Psychiatry on the advice of the Senior Advisory Committee and the Associates' Executive Committee amongst others.
2. Ideally, hard University funds or the equivalent from other sources shall be disbursed to all Associates with exceptions according to the Psychiatrist-in-Chief discretion. This shall be reviewed annually.
3. Each Associate shall have a performance review which shall be reviewed annually.
4. Ceilings on income shall increase with academic rank. These shall be reviewed annually.
5. Overage income above ceilings shall be directed to eligible individuals on a sliding scale with the remainder placed in the Academic Trust Fund.
6. The money in the Academic Trust Fund shall be used to stimulate academic activity for specific Associates and shall be distributed to individual Associates by certain priorities.
7. The Psychiatrist-in-Chief has access to the statements of gross income of each Associate.
8. The Associates' Executive Committee shall review, propose and advocate with respect to the implementation and outcomes of any of the principles 1 to 7 inclusive
9. There shall be a mechanism of appeal for all of the principles 1 to 7 inclusive. Its structure and process shall be established through consultation with the Psychiatrist-in-Chief.

When this practice plan was introduced in 1990, there was concern that this might reduce incomes of assistant professors too much or that it would put too much control in the hands of the hospital chiefs and university chair. Nevertheless, there was a recognition that change was necessary—for example, the final incomes for assistant professors were higher than those of professors in 1989; and a small number of the faculty were doing almost all the academic and administrative work of the department. Five years later, a formal and anonymous review of the plan was conducted. The results indicated widespread acceptance of the plan; for example, 84% felt the Trust Fund was overall a good thing; and over 90% felt the criteria were clear. Seventy percent thought that the categories were fair. But there was also a need expressed to communicate better how hard funds were allocated (by 45%); 48% thought the ceilings on income were too low. These results showed an approval of the partnership principles, but with a need

Table 31–2. Award categories for the Academic Trust Fund for 1996

Category	Description of category	Maximun for category
1	Principal investigator (PI) for research operating grant funded from peer-reviewed sources	$20,000
2	Coinvestigator for research operating grant funded from peer-reviewed sources	$10,000
3	Principal investigator for research operating grant funded from non-peer-reviewed sources	$10,000
4	Coinvestigator for research operating grant funded from non-peer-reviewed sources	$ 5,000
5	Teaching	$ 6,000
6	Supervising postdoctoral student, graduate student and fellow	$ 6,000
7	Creative professional development	$ 5,000
8	Awards	$ 4,000
9	Peer-reviewed publications and book chapters	$ 2,000
10	Scientific presentations	$ 2,000
11	Special circumstances	$10,000
Total maximum for any individual		$30,000

for some fine-tuning. At the same time, the income of partners clearly reflected academic rank and academic activities.

Conclusions

This is a particularly exciting time in academic psychiatry. We are witnessing significant progress in so many areas—in the reliability of diagnoses, in neurosciences, in molecular biology, in epidemiology, in the conduct of treatment trials, and in rehabilitation, as a few examples. At the same time, Canadian psychiatry has been able to attract outstanding people to the field to pursue the scholarly life. It is now the task of the senior group of academics to see that this new generation is both properly prepared for scholarly careers able to conduct work in a receptive environment. Although the latter involves many things, it especially involves a respect for the breadth to the field and for the nature of scholarship. This is not meant to imply that we should return to a view that anything goes; rather, properly pursued, this view is associated with an elevation in standards because it insists on rigorous review and validation both from within and externally. A broad public now demands this of us, and they are right to do so.

References

Boyer EL: Scholarship Reconsidered: Priorities of the Professoriate. The Carnegie Foundation for the Advancement of Education. Princeton, NJ, Princeton University Press, 1990

Burke JD Jr, Incus HA, Pardes H: The clinician-researcher in psychiatry. Am J Psychiatry 143:968–975, 1986

Cohen DJ: Research in child psychiatry: lines of personal, institutional and career development, in Clinical Research Careers in Psychiatry. Edited by Incus HA, Pardes H. Washington, DC, American Psychiatric Press, 1986, pp 57–78

Colwill JM: Reflections on mentoring. Fam Med 22:181, 1990

Garfinkel PE, Goldbloom DS, Kaplan AS, Kennedy S: The clinician-investigator interface in psychiatry: I. Values and problems. Can J Psychiatry 34:361–363, 1989.

Jacobs MB: Faculty status for clinician-educators: borderlines for evaluation and promotion. Acad Med 68:126–128, 1992

Kennedy S, Bradwejn J, Vaccarino S: CANMAT: Canadian Network for Mood and Anxiety Treatments. Toronto, Canada, Cameron McCheery Productions, 1995

Kirsling RA, Kochar MS: Mentors in graduate medical education at the Medical College of Wisconsin. Acad Med 65:272–274, 1990

Lam RW, El-Guebaly N: Research funding of psychiatric disorders in Canada: a snapshot, 1990–1991. Can J Psychiatry 39:141–146, 1994

Levinson DJ: The Seasons of a Man's Life. New York, Knopf, 1978

Levinson W, Tolle SW, Lewis C: Women in academic medicine. Combining career and family. N Engl J Med 321:1511–1517, 1989

Michaels R: New approaches to training needed now. Psychiatric News, June 17, 1994, p 14

Pincus HA, Fine T: The "anatomy" of research funding of mental illness and addictive disorders. Arch Gen Psychiatry 49:573–579, 1992

Rae-Grant Q, Fyfe I: Canada: images in psychiatry, in Images in Psychiatry. Edited by Rae-Grant Q. Washington, DC, American Psychiatric Press, 1996, pp 1–10

Roche G: Much ado about mentors. Harvard Business Review 57:14–28, 1979

Swensen JR, Boyle A, Last J, et al: Mentorship in medical education. Annals Royal College of Physicians and Surgeons of Canada 28:165–168, 1995

University of Toronto: Provostial White Paper: Planning for 2000. Toronto, Canada, University of Toronto, 1995

Index

*Page numbers printed in **boldface** type refer to tables or figures*